MERRITT'S
NEUROLOGY
HANDBOOK

SECOND EDITION

MERRITT'S NEUROLOGY HANDBOOK

SECOND EDITION

Pietro Mazzoni, MD, PhD

Assistant Professor of Neurology
Department of Neurology
Columbia University
Neurological Institute of New York
Columbia University Medical Center
New York, New York

Toni Shih Pearson, MBBS

Fellow in Pediatric Neurology
Department of Neurology
Columbia University
Neurological Institute of New York
Columbia University Medical Center
New York, New York

Lewis P. Rowland, MD

Professor of Neurology
Chairman Emeritus
Department of Neurology
Columbia University
Neurological Institute of New York
Columbia University Medical Center
New York, New York

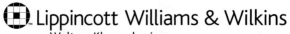
Lippincott Williams & Wilkins
a Wolters Kluwer business

Philadelphia • Baltimore • New York • London
Buenos Aires • Hong Kong • Sydney • Tokyo

Acquisitions Editor: Frances DeStefano
Developmental Editor: Louise Bierig
Managing Editor: Scott Scheidt
Project Manager: Bridgett Dougherty
Senior Manufacturing Manager: Benjamin Rivera
Marketing Manager: Kimberly Schonberger
Design Coordinator: Doug Smock
Production Service: TechBooks
Printer: R.R. Donnelley–Crawfordsville

Library of Congress Cataloging-in-Publication Data

Merritt's neurology handbook / [edited by] Pietro Mazzoni, Toni Pearson, Lewis P. Rowland, III.
  p. ; cm.
Concise version of: Meritt's neurology. 11th ed. 2005.
Includes bibliographical references and index.
ISBN-13: 9780781762700
ISBN-10: 0-7817-6270-7
  1. Nervous system–Diseases–Handbooks, manuals, etc. I. Mazzoni, Pietro. II. Pearson, Toni. III. Rowland, Lewis P. IV. Merrit, H. Houston (Hiram Houston), 1902–1979. V. Merrit's neurology. VI. Title: Neurology
  [DNLM: 1. Nervous System Diseases–Handbooks. WL 39 M572 2006]
RC343.4.M47 2006
616.8–dc22

2006016671

"A mamma e papà"

PM

"To Pepple"

TSP

"To Esther Rowland, my life support for 54 years, and my wondrous children: Andrew S. Rowland, Steven S. Rowland, and Joy Rosenthal"

LPR

The purpose of this handbook is to provide a concise, portable version of the essential information contained in the full 1200-page text of *Merritt's Neurology,* 11th edition. We have organized the material as an outline that can be accessed quickly, with chapter numbers and topics matching those of the original textbook. Many tables from the full textbook are included, along with new tables created specifically for the Handbook. To keep the volume to a manageable length, we omitted literature references, but they would be the same as those listed for each chapter in *Merritt's Neurology.*

We hope that the Handbook will be useful to diverse readers—medical students, residents in neurology and other specialties, nurses, neuropathologists, radiologists, other health professionals, journalists and general readers. It could be useful on the wards, in the office, or as a study guide for *Merritt's Neurology.*

We thank Scott Scheidt, Managing Editor at LWW, for pushing the project to completion with great perseverance; Frances DeStefano, Acquisitions Editor at LWW, for overseeing this endeavor; and Louise Bierig, Developmental Editor, for preparing the manuscript for production. We also wish to particularly acknowledge the contributions of 119 authors to the 11th edition of *Merritt's Neurology,* from which this handbook has been carved.

AChR	Acetylcholine receptor
AD	Alzheimer Disease
ADEM	Acute disseminated encephalomyelitis
AED	Anti-epileptic drug
AIDS	Acquired immunodeficiency syndrome
ALS	Amyotrophic lateral sclerosis
ATP	Adenosine triophosphate
AVM	Arteriovenous malformation
BAER	Brainstem auditory evoked response
CADASIL	Cerebral autosomal dominant arteriopathy with subcortical infarcts and leukoencephalopathy
cGy	centi-Gray units (a measure of radiation)
CIDP	Chronic inflammatory demyelinating polyneuropathy
CJD	Creutzfeldt-Jakob disease
CK	Creatine kinase
CMT	Charcot-Marie-Tooth disease
CMV	Cytomegalovirus
CNS	Central nervous system
CP	Cerebral palsy
CPS	Complex partial seizures
CSF	Cerebrospinal fluid
CT	Computed tomography
DNA	Deoxyribonucleic acid
DSM-IV	Diagnostic and statistical manual, version IV
DVT	Deep venous thrombosis
ECG	Electrocardiogram
EEG	Electroencephalogram
EMG	Electromyogram
FDG-PET	Fluorodeoxyglucose positron emission tomography
GBM	Glioblastoma multiforme
GBS	Guillain-Barré syndrome
GCS	Glasgow coma scale
HAART	Highly active anti-retroviral therapy
HD	Huntington disease
HIE	Hypoxic-ischemic encephalopathy
HIV	Human immunodeficiency virus
HMN	Hereditary motor neuropathy
HSAN	Hereditary sensory and autonomic neuropathy

HSV	Herpes simplex virus
HTLV	Human T-lymphotrophic virus
ICH	Intracerebral hemorrhage
ICP	Intracranial pressure
ICU	Intensive care unit
IVIG	Intravenous immunoglobulin
KSS	Kearns-Sayre syndrome
LHON	Leber hereditary optic neuropathy
LP	Lumbar puncture
M:F	Male:female ratio
MELAS	Mitochondrial encephalomyopathy with lactic acidosis and stroke
MERRF	Mitochondrial encephalomyopathy with ragged red fibers
MG	Myasthenia gravis
MLF	Medial longitudinal fasciculus
MRA	Magnetic resonance angiography
MRI	Magnetic resonance imaging
MS	Multiple sclerosis
mtDNA	Mitochondrial DNA
MuSK	Muscle-specific kinase
NARP	Neuropathy, ataxia, retinitis pigmentosa
NCS	Nerve conduction studies
NE	Norepinephrine
NF	Neurofibromatosis
NMJ	Neuromuscular junction
NPH	Normal pressure hydrocephalus
OH	Orthostatic hypotension
PCR	Polymerase chain reaction
PD	Parkinson disease
PEO	Progressive external ophthalmoplegia
PET	Positron emission tomography
PML	Progressive multifocal leukoencephalopathy
PNET	Primitive neuroectodermal tumor
PVL	Periventricular leukomalacia
RNA	Ribonucleic acid
RPR	Rapid plasma reagin
RT	Radiation therapy
SAH	Subarachnoid hemorrhage
SCA	Spinocerebellar ataxia
SDH	Subdural hematoma
SPECT	Single-photon emission computed tomography
SSEP	Somatosensory evoked potential
SSPE	Subacute sclerosing panencephalitis

SSRI	Selective serotonin reuptake inhibitor
TBI	Traumatic brain injury
TIA	Transient ischemic attack
TS	Tuberous sclerosis
VDRL	Venereal disease research laboratory test
VEP	Visual evoked potential

SECTION III ■ INFECTIONS OF THE NERVOUS SYSTEM

SECTION IV ■ CEREBROVASCULAR DISEASES

SECTION V ■ DISORDERS OF CEREBROSPINAL FLUIDS

SECTION VI ■ TUMORS

SECTION VII ■ TRAUMA

SECTION VIII ▪ BIRTH INJURIES AND DEVELOPMENTAL ABNORMALITIES

SECTION IX ▪ GENETIC DISEASES OF THE CENTRAL NERVOUS SYSTEM

SECTION X ▪ MITOCHONDRIAL DISORDERS

SECTION XXIV ■ ENVIRONMENTAL NEUROLOGY

SECTION XXV ■ REHABILITATION

SECTION XXVI ■ ETHICAL AND LEGAL GUIDELINES

MERRITT'S NEUROLOGY HANDBOOK

Section I
Symptoms of Neurologic Disorders

CHAPTER 1 ■ DELIRIUM AND DEMENTIA

DELIRIUM

DEFINITION

State of mental confusion; global mental dysfunction with prominent alteration, often fluctuating, of alertness or attention.

Common features: disorientation, fluctuating level of consciousness, inability to maintain attention, agitation. May progress for hours or days. Often worse at night. Usually reversible.

Variable features: drowsiness, restlessness, incoherence, irritability, emotional lability, perceptual misinterpretations (illusions), hallucinations.

ETIOLOGY

Primary Neurologic Disorders
Head injury, stroke, raised intracranial pressure, epilepsy, CNS infection.

Delirium tremens: follows alcohol withdrawal (24 to 48 hours); tremor, hallucinations, autonomic hyperactivity; potentially fatal.

Systemic Illness
Delirium present in 10–20% of patients in hospital.
  Systemic infection, dehydration (especially in older patients).
  Cardiovascular, endocrine, toxic-metabolic derangement.

Medications: atropine, barbiturates, benzodiazepines (chlordiazepoxide, diazepam, flurazepam), cimetidine, clonidine, cocaine, digitalis, dopamine agonists (pergolide, pramipexole, ropinirole), haloperidol and other neuroleptics, lithium, mephenytoin, meprobamate, opioids, phencyclidine hydrochloride (PCP), phenytoin, prednisone, propranolol, tricyclic antidepressants.

EVALUATION

History: trauma, alcohol use.
Examination: fever, jaundice, focal neurologic signs.
Laboratory data: serum electrolytes, complete blood count, liver and thyroid function tests, ESR, toxicology screen, syphilis serology, blood cultures, urine cultures, chest x-ray, ECG. Consider CT or MRI, CSF, EEG, HIV antibody titer, cardiac enzymes, blood gases, autoantibody screen.

MANAGEMENT

General supportive, symptomatic treatment: anxiolytic, antipsychotic medications. If known, treat underlying disease.

PROGNOSIS

Predictors of poor outcome: advanced age, multiple diseases.

DEMENTIA

DEFINITION

Cognition: includes memory, orientation, language, calculation, abstraction, insight, learning.
Dementia: progressive loss of cognition severe enough to interfere with daily social or occupational functions.
Chronic and progressive (months to years). In contrast to delirium: level of consciousness, alertness, awareness preserved until late in course. Rarely reversible.

ETIOLOGY

Alzheimer disease (AD): most frequent cause (>50%).
Vascular dementia (15–20%).

Neurodegenerative (other than AD): Parkinson disease, diffuse Lewy body disease, multiple system atrophy, corticobasal degeneration, frontotemporal dementia, Pick disease.

Infectious: subacute combined degeneration (HTLV-I), AIDS-dementia complex (HIV), prion diseases (e.g., Creutzfeldt-Jakob disease).

Potentially treatable: normal-pressure hydrocephalus (NPH), nutritional deficiencies (thiamine, cobalamin), metabolic abnormalities (hypothyroidism), inherited metabolic disorders (Wilson disease, metachromatic leukodystrophy, mitochondrial disorders, Kufs disease).

Mass lesions (subdural hematoma, brain tumor).

EVALUATION

History: trauma, alcohol use.

Routine: vitamin B_{12} level, serum RPR, thyroid function tests, head CT.

Consider: liver function tests, HIV tests, ceruloplasmin, neuropsychological tests, brain MRI, EEG, SPECT.

DIFFERENTIAL DIAGNOSIS

Age-associated memory impairment (mild cognitive impairment): mild memory loss in elderly not associated with other cognitive impairment.

Pseudodementia of depression: depression usually precedes memory problem. Neuropsychological tests may be atypical for dementia.

MENTAL STATUS EXAMINATION

Cognitive loss may not be evident in early delirium or dementia unless mental status is specifically tested. Most important and sensitive items: probably orientation to time, serial reversals, memorized words or phrases.

Information: Where were you born? What is your mother's name? Who is the President? When did World War II occur?

Orientation: Where are we? What place is this? What is the date? What time of day is it?

Concentration: spell "world" backwards; name months of year backwards.

Calculation: simple arithmetic, making change, counting backwards by 3s or 7s.

Reasoning, judgment, and memory: memorize 3 words and recall them 3 minutes later.

Higher intellectual dysfunction: aphasia (language); constructional apraxia (e.g., copying drawings); spatial disorientation; inability to carry out imagined acts (ideomotor apraxia; e.g., "Show me how you would light a match"); unilateral neglect.

Mini-mental state examination: (MMSE; available from Psychological Assessment Resources, Inc., Lutz, FL) quantitative test of cognitive function in few minutes at bedside. Maximum score 30 points. Score less than 24 consistent with dementia. However, pseudodementia of depression is also possible. Useful only as first step; does not replace history or detailed neuropsychological examination (see Chapter 20).

CHAPTER 2 ■ APHASIA, APRAXIA, AGNOSIA

APHASIA

DEFINITION

Disturbance of language.

Causes: stroke (most common cause); mass lesions (e.g., tumor); neurodegenerative diseases (e.g., primary progressive aphasia).

Left hemisphere dominant for language in 95% of right-handed people and most left-handed people.

MOTOR APHASIA

Lesion Location
Any gyrus of insula or upper bank of peri-Sylvian cortex from anterior inferior frontal region to anterior parietal.

Syndromes

Broca Aphasia (Major Motor Aphasia)
Speech intelligible but nonfluent. Small parts of speech (conjunctions, prepositions, etc.) reduced or absent (*telegraphic speech*).

Impaired: fluency, naming, repetition, writing.
Intact: verbal, written comprehension.

Usually late effect of stroke.

Speech Apraxia
Abnormal coordination of any part of motor apparatus of speech: breathing (dysphonia), articulation (dysarthria), emotional tone (aprosody).

Usually follows mutism.

Mutism
No speech output; comprehension intact; writing sometimes preserved.

Hemiparesis often present. Usually immediately after acute stroke.

SENSORY APHASIA

Lesion Location
Posterior temporal, posterior parietal, lateral occipital regions.

Syndromes

Wernicke Aphasia (Major Sensory Aphasia)
Nonsensical fluent speech (gibberish, "word salad").

Impaired: naming, repetition, verbal and written comprehension.
Intact: fluency.

Form of speech and writing (syntax) relatively preserved; content and meaning (semantics) impaired.

Paraphasic errors: literal (substitution of word part; e.g., "pinger" for "finger"); semantic (substitution of word meaning; e.g., "timer" for "watch").

Pure Word Deafness
Auditory comprehension impaired; speech, language, reading comprehension relatively spared.

    Good prognosis.

Alexia with Agraphia
Reading comprehension, writing impaired; spoken language and verbal comprehension less affected.

    Good prognosis.

CONDUCTION APHASIA

Lesion Location
Left temporal lobe or inferior parietal lobule (possibly in pathways connecting posterior language areas to anterior ones).

Syndrome
Impaired repetition; speech and comprehension otherwise relatively preserved. Rare.

GLOBAL APHASIA

Lesion Location
Large lesions involving many gyri; dominant hemisphere.

Syndrome
No speech output, no comprehension.

ANOMIC APHASIA

Lesion Location
Little localizing value. Seen in Alzheimer disease.

Syndrome
Difficulty naming objects, with literal or semantic paraphasias.

THALAMIC APHASIA

Lesion Location
Posterior thalamic nuclei with connections to language areas.

Syndrome
Fluctuations of speech with changes in level of consciousness.

APRAXIA

Impaired execution of learned movements, not explained by deficits of comprehension, strength, sensation, or coordination.

CLASSIFICATION SCHEMES

Periodically revised. Limited localizing value.

Selected types: limb-kinetic (poor dexterity); ideomotor (cannot make complex movement by imitation or on verbal command); ideational (cannot produce sequence of movements).

AGNOSIA

Inability to recognize previously familiar objects or object features despite normal vision, hearing, touch.
 Rule out aphasia, depressed consciousness.

Apperceptive: cannot name object in drawing; cannot copy it or match it to similar one.
Associative: cannot name object in drawing; can copy it and match it.
Examples: inability to discriminate or name colors (color agnosia), faces (prosopagnosia), sounds (auditory agnosia), words (pure word deafness).

CHAPTER 3 ■ SYNCOPE, SEIZURES, AND THEIR MIMICS

SYNCOPE

DEFINITION

Transient alteration of consciousness and loss of muscular tone due to acute, reversible global reduction in cerebral blood flow. Most common cause of loss of consciousness.

History: precipitating stimulus (heat, psychological stress), nature of fall (limp or swoon without injury); autonomic prodromal symptoms (light-headedness, sweating, palpitation, apprehension, feeling of impending faint).

Differences from most seizures: rhythmic movements, urinary incontinence rare; recovery within seconds of lying down; no post-ictal symptoms (headache, confusion, lethargy).

Few clonic jerks of arms and legs may occur (*convulsive syncope*).

Features: See Table 3.1.

NEUROCARDIOGENIC SYNCOPE

Mechanism: direct cardiac inhibition.
Features: adolescents, young adults. Usually seated or standing, not supine. Autonomic symptoms before spell. Bradycardia during spell.

Specific Etiologies

Vasovagal episode: provoking stimulus (e.g., pain, emotional shock) present. Predisposing background state usually present (e.g., fasting, hot and overcrowded room).
Carotid sinus syncope: unusual sensitivity of carotid sinus to normal mechanical pressure (e.g., head turning).
Micturition syncope: after emptying distended bladder.
Situational syncope: specific trigger (e.g., prolonged coughing, sneezing, micturition).

TABLE 3.1
SYNCOPE VS. SEIZURE: USEFUL DISTINGUISHING FEATURES

	Syncope	Seizure
Before Spell		
Trigger (position, emotion, Valsalva)	Common	Rare
Sweating & nausea	Common	Rare
Aura (e.g., déjà vu, smell) or unilateral symptoms	Rare	Common
During Spell (From Eyewitness)		
Pallor	Common	Rare
Cyanosis	Rare	Common
Duration of LOC	<20 secs	>60 secs
Movements	A few clonic or myoclonic jerks; brief tonic posturing (few secs); duration <15 secs; always begin after LOC	Prolonged tonic phase, then prolonged rhythmic clonic movements; duration >1 min; may begin at onset of LOC or before; unilateral jerking (partial seizure)

(*continued*)

TABLE 3.1

SYNCOPE VS. SEIZURE: USEFUL DISTINGUISHING FEATURES (Continued)

	Syncope	Seizure
Automatisms	Occasional	Common (in complex partial and secondarily generalized seizures)
Tongue biting, lateral	Rare	Occasional
Frothing/hypersalivation	Rare	Common
After Spell		
Confusion/disorientation	Rare; <30 secs	Common; several mins or longer
Diffuse myalgias	Rare, brief, usually shoulders/chest	Common, hours–days
CK elevation	Rare	Common (especially after 12 to 24 hours)
Features That are Not Helpful for Differentiating	Incontinence, prolactin level, dizziness, fear, injury other than lateral tongue biting, eye movements (rolling back), brief automatisms, vocalizations, visual or auditory hallucinations	Incontinence, prolactin level, dizziness, fear, injury other than lateral tongue biting, eye movements (rolling back), brief automatisms, vocalizations, visual or auditory hallucinations

CK, creatine kinase; LOC, loss of consciousness; min, minute; sec, second.

VASOMOTOR SYNCOPE

Mechanism: inability to maintain peripheral vascular tone (orthostatic hypotension).

Features: all ages affected. Invariably from upright posture. Tachycardia during spell.

Specific Etiologies

Primary autonomic failure: e.g., multiple system atrophy (Shy-Drager type).

Secondary autonomic failure: e.g., diabetes.

Drug-induced: variable individual susceptibility, increased by advanced age and debilitated state.

Drugs: antihypertensives, diuretics, beta-blockers, calcium channel blockers, arterial vasodilators, phenothiazines, levodopa, lithium.

Predisposing conditions: prolonged standing or bed rest, anemia, blood loss, malnutrition.

CARDIAC SYNCOPE

Mechanism: arrhythmia (brady- or tachyarrhythmia).

Features: all ages. Frequent spontaneous "pre-syncopal" symptoms. Inconstant relationship to posture. Arrhythmia frequently present during spell.

Specific Etiologies

Primary arrhythmias: sinus node dysfunction; atrioventricular conduction system disease; paroxysmal supraventricular, ventricular tachycardia.

Structural heart disease: outflow obstruction (syncope typically after exertion); failing myocardium (infarction, cardiomyopathy).

DIFFERENTIAL DIAGNOSIS

See Table 3.2.

SEIZURES

DEFINITION

Episodes of abnormal electrical activity in brain, manifesting as change in mental status, movement, or sensation.

TABLE 3.2
DIFFERENTIAL DIAGNOSIS OF SEIZURES AND SYNCOPE

Diagnosis	May be confused with: (seizure, syncope, or both)	Clinical features suggestive of diagnosis
Panic attack, hyperventilation	Seizure	Often with environmental trigger; severe fear; hyperventilation with perioral cyanosis, bilateral hand paresthesias, carpopedal spasm; no complete LOC; dyspnea; palpitations; >5 mins in duration (seizures are shorter); associated depression and phobias (95%), esp. agoraphobia; onset in young adulthood.
Cataplexy	Both	No LOC; other features of narcolepsy present (daytime somnolence, hypnagogic hallucinations, sleep paralysis); triggered by emotion, esp. laughter.
TIA, vertebrobasilar	Syncope	If transient loss of consciousness, virtually always accompanied by focal neurologic features (e.g., dysarthria, dysphagia, vertigo, diplopia, ataxia, unilateral weakness or numbness).
TIA, limb-shaking	Seizure	Non-rhythmic, coarse, 3 Hz to 12 Hz shaking of arm and/or leg contralateral to severe carotid stenosis. Can mimic focal seizures; due to borderline perfusion; may occur upon standing.

TIA with aphasia and other negative symptoms	Seizure	Recurrent isolated aphasia can be due to seizure; if recurrent with no infarct on imaging, consider focal seizures. Similarly with other recurrent, stereotyped negative symptoms initially diagnosed as TIA, including unilateral weakness or numbness.
Subclavian steal	Syncope	Vertebrobasilar ischemia triggered by arm exercise; focal neurologic symptoms, especially vertigo and other brainstem symptoms, with or without LOC.
Psychogenic (conversion disorder)	Both	Psychiatric history, esp. somatization; history of physical or sexual abuse; eyes closed and normal vital signs during spell; recurrent spells not responding to treatment; precipitation by hyperventilation or other suggestive techniques.
Fugue attacks	Seizure	Can be difficult to distinguish from nonconvulsive status epilepticus without EEG
Migraine (esp. basilar)	Both	Slow march of neurologic symptoms over > 5 mins and prolonged duration (usually 20–60 mins); posterior circulation symptoms; scintillating scotomata; subsequent headache (may be absent).
Hypoglycemia	Both	Long prodrome; no rapid recovery unless treated.
Transient global amnesia	Seizure	Prolonged spell (hours) with normal behavior except for amnesia; personal identity always intact (if not, suspect psychogenic etiology).

(continued)

TABLE 3.2

DIFFERENTIAL DIAGNOSIS OF SEIZURES AND SYNCOPE (*Continued*)

Diagnosis	May be confused with: (seizure, syncope, or both)	Clinical features suggestive of diagnosis
Sleep disorders (somnambulism, night terrors, confusional arousals, enuresis, REM behavior disorder, hypnagogic hallucinations, periodic limb movements, paroxysmal nocturnal dystonia)	Seizure	Sometimes difficult to distinguish from seizures without video/EEG monitoring, polysomnography, or both, esp. if no reliable witness. Paroxysmal nocturnal dystonia is probably epilepsy in many or most cases. Slow wave sleep parasomnias are usually in first third of night.
Staring/behavioral spells in patients with static encephalopathy or dementia	Seizure	Sometimes difficult to distinguish from seizures without video/EEG monitoring.
"Drop attacks"	Both	Can be due to cataplexy, cervical spine disease, basilar ischemia, vertigo attack (Meniere), seizures (myoclonic, tonic, atonic; rarely complex partial), or syncope (esp. cardiac).

Esp., especially; LOC, loss of consciousness; REM, rapid eye movement; TIA, transient ischemic attack.

FEATURES

Never consistently related to head or body posture. Movements stereotyped (automatisms, clonic jerks). Pre-ictal light-headedness, diaphoresis uncommon. Urinary incontinence, post-ictal confusion common.

See Table 3.1.

ETIOLOGY

See Chapter 141.

DIFFERENTIAL DIAGNOSIS

See Table 3.2.

CHAPTER 4 ■ COMA

DEFINITIONS

Consciousness: awareness of self and environment; requires both arousal and mental content; requires integrity of reticular activating system and cerebral cortex.

Lethargy, obtundation, stupor, coma: states of progressively reduced responsiveness to external stimuli.

Coma: deep, sustained unconsciousness. No volitional movement; no or little involuntary response to verbal stimuli, shouting, shaking, or pain.

Confusion, delirium: acute state of inattentiveness, altered mental content, and either agitation or decreased response to external stimuli.

EXAMINATION AND MAJOR DIAGNOSTIC PROCEDURES

INITIAL APPROACH

Detect and treat any life-threatening condition, e.g., protect airway, ensure adequate ventilation, stop hemorrhage, support circulation, monitor for arrhythmia.

If diagnosis unknown, draw blood for *glucose* determination; then give intravenous *thiamine* (50 mg) and 50% *dextrose* (1–2 ampules D50 solution). If opiate overdose possible, give intravenous *naloxone* (0.4 mg). If trauma suspected, assume damage to internal organs and cervical fracture until *radiographs* assure otherwise.

Obtain *history* from accompanying person, including ambulance team, police.

GENERAL EXAMINATION

Temperature
Fever: consider infection, heat stroke.
Hypothermia: cold exposure (especially with alcoholism), hypothyroidism, hypoglycemia, sepsis, or, infrequently, primary brain lesion.

Pulses
Asymmetry: dissecting aneurysm.

Head
Inspect and palpate scalp for signs of *trauma*. Blood in external ear canal (Battle sign) or around eyes (raccoon sign) suggests skull fracture. Inspect ears and nose for blood, CSF.

Neck
Stiff neck (on passive flexion, not lateral rotation or tilting): meningitis, subarachnoid hemorrhage, foramen magnum herniation.

Resistance in all directions: bone or joint disease, including fractures (exclude cervical fracture before checking for stiff neck).

Other Areas
Skin, nails, mucous membranes: pallor, cherry-redness, cyanosis, jaundice, sweating, uremic frost, myxedema, hypo- or

hyperpigmentation, petechiae, dehydration, decubitus ulcers, signs of trauma.

Breath: acetone, alcohol, fetor hepaticus.

Fundi: papilledema, hypertensive or diabetic retinopathy, retinal ischemia, Roth spots, granulomas, subhyaloid hemorrhages.

Urinary or fecal incontinence: unwitnessed seizure, especially if patient awakens spontaneously.

RESPIRATION

Cheyne-Stokes respiration (CSR): periods of hyperventilation and apnea alternating in crescendo-decrescendo fashion. Bilateral cerebral disease, including impending transtentorial herniation, upper brainstem lesions, metabolic encephalopathy. Patient usually not in imminent danger. "Short-cycle CSR" (*cluster breathing*), with less smooth waxing and waning: often posterior fossa lesion or dangerously elevated intracranial pressure.

Sustained hyperventilation: usually metabolic acidosis, pulmonary congestion, hepatic encephalopathy, or analgesic drugs; rarely, lesion in rostral brainstem.

Apneustic breathing: inspiratory pauses; pontine lesions (especially infarct); infrequently, metabolic coma or transtentorial herniation.

Ataxic breathing (Biot breathing): variably irregular rate and amplitude; medullary damage. Can progress to apnea (abruptly with posterior fossa lesions).

Ondine curse: loss of automatic respiration; preserved voluntary breathing; must be alert to breathe. Medullary lesion; as patient falls asleep, apnea can be fatal.

Stertorous breathing (i.e., inspiratory noise): airway obstruction.

Other ominous respiratory signs: end-expiratory pushing (like coughing); "fish-mouthing" (lower-jaw depression with inspiration).

PUPILS

Anisocoria: pupil inequality. If <0.5 mm in awake, otherwise normal person, likely physiologic. Always assumed to be pathologic in coma.

Parasympathetic lesions: e.g., oculomotor nerve compression in uncal herniation or after rupture of internal carotid artery aneurysm; pupil enlarges; ultimately, full dilation, no reaction to light.

Sympathetic lesions: intraparenchymal (e.g., hypothalamic injury or lateral medullary infarct) or extraparenchymal (e.g., invasion of superior cervical ganglion by lung cancer); Horner syndrome (miosis, ptosis, anhydrosis).

Combined sympathetic and parasympathetic lesions: e.g., midbrain destruction; one or both pupils in mid-position, unreactive.

Pinpoint but reactive pupils: pontine hemorrhage, opiate intoxication.

Fixed, dilated pupils: confirm with bright light. Consider (a) anticholinergic drugs (atropine, glutethimide, amitriptyline, antiparkinsonian agents); (b) hypothermia; (c) severe barbiturate intoxication (b and c can cause reversible picture simulating brain death); (d) ongoing or recent seizure (pupil abnormality may be unilateral); (e) anoxic-ischemic event (fixed pupils imply poor prognosis).

Some pupillary abnormalities due to local trauma, surgical scars.

EYELIDS AND EYE MOVEMENTS

Closed eyelids in comatose patient: lower pons intact.

Blinking: sign of reticular activity.

Conjugate eye deviation: (a) away from hemiparetic limbs: destructive cerebral lesion (on side of eye deviation); (b) toward paretic limbs: pontine lesion, seizure, or "wrong-way" gaze paresis of thalamic hemorrhage.

Eyes dysconjugate at rest: paresis of individual muscles, internuclear ophthalmoplegia, or preexisting tropia or phoria.

Roving eye movements: side-to-side, slow, smooth velocity movements: brainstem is intact. Fast, jerky movements suggest relative wakefulness.

Periodic alternating (ping-pong) gaze: repetitive smooth excursions to both sides; 2- to 3-second pauses in each direction; may follow bilateral cerebral infarct or cerebellar hemorrhage with an intact brainstem.

Oculocephalic reflex ("doll's-eyes" maneuver): be sure cervical injury excluded. Passively turn head from side to side. With intact reflex arc (vestibular-brainstem-eye muscles), eyes move conjugately in opposite direction.

Caloric tests: stimulate, more vigorously, same reflex arc as oculocephalic reflex. With head at 90 degrees, irrigate one ear with 30 to 100 mL ice water. *Normal, awake* person: nystagmus follows, with fast component in direction opposite irrigated ear. *Comatose* patient with intact reflex arc: slow deviation of eyes toward irrigated ear, usually for several minutes. *Simultaneous bilateral irrigation*: vertical deviation, upward after warm water and downward after cold water.

Oculocephalic or caloric testing may reveal intact eye movements, gaze palsy, individual muscle paresis, internuclear ophthalmoplegia, or no response. Cerebral hemisphere gaze paresis (*supranuclear ophthalmoplegia*) often overcome by these maneuvers; brainstem gaze palsies (*infranuclear ophthalmoplegia*) usually fixed.

Complete ophthalmoplegia: extensive brainstem damage or metabolic coma (especially barbiturate or phenytoin poisoning).

Unexplained dysconjugate eyes: brainstem or cranial nerve lesion (including abducens palsy due to increased intracranial pressure).

Downward eye deviation: thalamus or midbrain lesion; may be accompanied by unreactive pupils with inability to look up (*Parinaud syndrome*).

Skew deviation: one eye up, other eye down; cerebellum or brainstem (especially pontine tegmentum).

Retractatory convergence nystagmus: eyes retract and relax in orbit in oscillating fashion, converging during retraction phase. Due to midbrain lesions.

Ocular bobbing: involuntary conjugate brisk downward movements, slower upward movement. Destructive lesions of pontine tegmentum (lateral eye movements lost); also with cerebellar hemorrhage, metabolic encephalopathy, transtentorial herniation, lesion at cervical-medullary junction. Unilateral bobbing (nystagmoid jerking): pontine disease.

MOTOR EXAMINATION

Muscle tone: if asymmetric, consider structural lesion. *Paratonia (Gegenhalten)*: resistance to passive movement, increasing with movement velocity, continuing through full range of movement. Attributed to diffuse forebrain dysfunction, often accompanied by grasp reflex.

Motor responses: to stimuli may be appropriate, inappropriate, or absent. If absent, be sure absent also to noxious stimuli (e.g., pressure on sternum or supraorbital bone ridge; pinching neck or limbs; or squeezing muscle, tendon, or nail beds).

Posturing responses to noxious stimuli: most often, but not uniquely, hemisphere disease (including metabolic encephalopathy). (a) Decorticate rigidity: arms flexed, adducted, internally rotated; legs extended; (b) decerebrate rigidity: arms, legs extended; prognosis worse. Anatomic significance debated.

Lack of motor response to any stimulus: consider cervical trauma, Guillain-Barré neuropathy, locked-in state.

TESTS

CT OR MRI

Perform promptly if coma unexplained; before lumbar puncture if examination suggests focal lesion.

LP

Perform promptly if coma not explained by imaging. If imaging not readily available *and mass lesion not suspected on examination*, perform spinal tap cautiously, using 20- or 22-gauge needle. If imaging reveals frank transtentorial or foramen magnum herniation, decide about LP on individual basis.

EMERGENCY LABORATORY STUDIES

Blood levels of glucose, sodium, calcium, blood urea nitrogen, creatinine; arterial pH, PCO_2, PO_2; other electrolytes and liver function tests; blood and CSF cultures; blood or urine toxicology screening. Coagulation studies, other metabolic tests, depending on suspicion.

EEG

Can distinguish coma from psychic unresponsiveness and locked-in state. Always abnormal in true coma. May also reveal asymmetry or clinically unsuspected seizure activity.

Distinguishing status epilepticus from myoclonus (common after anoxic-ischemic brain damage) may be difficult.

LESION LOCALIZATION

Based on: response to stimuli (includes motor examination); pattern of respiration; pupils; eye movements.

COMA FROM SUPRATENTORIAL STRUCTURAL LESIONS

Lateral brain displacements depress consciousness. Downward brain displacement leads to coma from rostro-caudal brainstem dysfunction.

Uncal transtentorial herniation (e.g., due to subdural hematoma): early compression of oculomotor nerve by inferomedial temporal lobe causes ipsilateral pupillary enlargement first, then lethargy; unilateral, then bilateral fixed pupils; oculomotor palsy; CSR, hyperventilation, or ataxic breathing; flexor, then extensor posturing; progressive unresponsiveness. Hemiparesis may be ipsilateral to cerebral lesion (compression of contralateral midbrain peduncle against tentorial edge).

Central transtentorial herniation (e.g., thalamic hemorrhage): consciousness rapidly impaired; pupils normal or small, reactive to light; eye movements normal. CSR, paratonia, and flexor or extensor postures also seen. Then pupils fixed in mid-position, followed by unresponsiveness, ophthalmoplegia, and respiratory and postural abnormalities as seen in uncal herniation.

Causes of transtentorial herniation: hemorrhage (epidural, subdural, or intraparenchymal), infarct, infection (abscess or granuloma), and neoplasm.

COMA FROM INFRATENTORIAL STRUCTURAL LESIONS

May compress or directly destroy brainstem. Suggested by bilateral limb weakness or sensory loss, crossed cranial nerve and long tract signs, miosis, loss of lateral gaze with preserved vertical eye movements, dysconjugate gaze, ophthalmoplegia, short-cycle CSR, and abnormal breathing.

Clinical picture of *pontine hemorrhage* is characteristic: sudden coma, pinpoint but reactive pupils, no eye movements.

Upward brain herniation (transtentorial): signs not well defined. Include decerebrate posturing; initially small reactive pupils, then anisocoria.

Downward herniation (through foramen magnum): distortion of medulla by cerebellar tonsils; apnea, circulatory collapse.

Other (rare) brainstem causes of coma: MS, central pontine myelinolysis.

COMA FROM METABOLIC, DIFFUSE, OR MULTIFOCAL BRAIN DISEASE

Mental, respiratory abnormalities (early); tremor, asterixis, or multifocal myoclonus; paratonia, frontal release signs (snout, suck, grasp), flexor or extensor posturing. Pupils reactive (except with anticholinergic intoxication). Eyes may deviate downward. Lateralizing signs may occur with hypoglycemia, hyperglycemia, seizures. Etiologies in Table 4.1.

CONVERSION, CATATONIA

CONVERSION DISORDER UNRESPONSIVENESS

Usually with closed eyes, normal or rapid respirations, normal pupils. Eyelids may resist passive opening. Nystagmus with caloric testing. EEG pattern: normal wakefulness.

CATATONIA

Cataleptic posturing (limbs have "waxy" rigidity and, if placed in new position by examiner, remain there as if frozen), abnormal mental status (stupor, mutism, negativism, excitement), akinetic mutism (severe psychomotor retardation). Respirations normal or rapid; pupils large but reactive; eye movements normal. EEG usually normal. Most frequently seen in schizophrenia, depression, toxic psychosis.

TABLE 4.1

DIFFUSE BRAIN DISEASES OR METABOLIC DISORDERS THAT CAUSE COMA

Deprivation of oxygen, substrate, or metabolic cofactor
  Hypoxia
  Diffuse ischemia (cardiac disease, decreased peripheral circulatory resistance, increased cerebrovascular resistance, widespread small-vessel occlusion)
  Hypoglycemia
  Thiamine deficiency (Wernicke-Korsakoff syndrome)

Disease of organs other than brain
  Liver (hepatic coma, sedative hypersensitivity)
  Kidney (uremia)
  Lung (CO_2 narcosis)
  Pancreas (diabetes, hypoglycemia, exocrine pancreatic encephalopathy)
  Pituitary (apoplexy, sedative hypersensitivity)
  Thyroid (myxedema, thyrotoxicosis)
  Parathyroid (hypo- and hyperparathyroidism)
  Adrenal (Addison or Cushing disease, pheochromocytoma)
  Other systemic disease (cancer, porphyria, sepsis)

Exogenous poisons
  Sedatives and narcotics
  Psychotropic drugs
  Acid poisons (e.g., methyl alcohol, ethylene glycol)
  Others (e.g., anticonvulsants, heavy metals, cyanide)

Abnormalities of ionic or acid-base environment of CNS
  Water and sodium (hypo- and hypernatremia)
  Acidosis
  Alkalosis
  Magnesium (hyper- and hypomagnesemia)
  Calcium (hyper- and hypocalcemia)
  Phosphorus (hypophosphatemia)

Disordered temperature regulation
  Hypothermia
  Heat stroke

CNS inflammation or infiltration
  Leptomeningitis
  Encephalitis
  Acute toxic encephalopathy (e.g., Reye syndrome)
  Parainfectious encephalomyelitis
  Cerebral vasculitis
  Subarachnoid hemorrhage
  Carcinomatous meningitis

(continued)

TABLE 4.1

DIFFUSE BRAIN DISEASES OR METABOLIC DISORDERS THAT CAUSE COMA (*Continued*)

Primary neuronal or glial disorders
  CJD
  Marchiafava-Bignami disease
  Adrenoleukodystrophy
  Gliomatosis cerebri
  PML

Seizure and postictal states

Modified from Plum F, Posner JB. *The diagnosis of stupor and coma*, 3rd ed. Philadelphia; FA Davis, 1980.

TABLE 4.2

CRITERIA FOR DETERMINATION OF BRAIN DEATH

1. Coma, unresponsive to stimuli above foramen magnum.

2. Apnea off ventilator (with oxygenation) for a duration sufficient to produce hypercarbic respiratory drive (usually 10–20 min to achieve P_{CO_2} of 50–60 mm Hg).

3. Absence of cephalic reflexes, including pupillary, oculocephalic, oculovestibular (caloric), corneal, gag, sucking, swallowing, and extensor posturing. Purely spinal reflexes may be present, including tendon reflexes, plantar responses, and limb flexion to noxious stimuli.

4. Body temperature above 34°C.

5. Systemic circulation may be intact.

6. Diagnosis known to be structural disease or irreversible metabolic disturbance; absence of drug intoxication, including ethanol, sedatives, potentially anesthetizing agents, or paralyzing drugs.

7. In adults with known structural cause and without involvement of drugs or ethanol, at least 6 h absent brain function; for others, including those with anoxic-ischemic brain damage, at least 24 h observation plus negative drug screen.

8. Diagnosis of brain death inappropriate in infants younger than 7 d. Observation of at least 48 h for infants aged 7 d to 2 mo, at least 24 h for those aged 2 mo to 1 yr, and at least 12 h for those aged 1–5 yr (24 h if anoxic-ischemic brain damage). For older children, adult criteria apply.

9. Optional confirmatory studies include:
     EEG isoelectric for 30 minutes at maximal gain
     Absent brainstem evoked responses
     Absent cerebral circulation demonstrated by cerebral angiogram, radioisotope study, or MRA.

LOCKED-IN SYNDROME

Total paralysis of lower cranial nerve and limb muscles with preserved alertness and respiration. Patient does not speak or move, but can respond by blinking or slight eye movements.

Usually destruction of basis pontis (ventral pons) by infarct or central pontine myelinolysis. Rarely also seen in GBS, ALS.

VEGETATIVE STATE

Isolated diencephalic (thalamus and hypothalamus) and brainstem function after massive cerebral damage. Preserved sleep-wake cycles, cardiorespiratory function, primitive responses to stimuli; no evidence of awareness or meaningful speech.

Persistent vegetative state: survival for at least 1 month; improvement then unlikely.

BRAIN DEATH

Neither cerebrum nor brainstem functions. Only spontaneous activity is cardiovascular; apnea persists despite hypercarbia sufficient for respiratory drive; only spinal cord–mediated reflexes persist (Table 4.2).

Rarely lasts more than a few days; always followed by circulatory collapse. In the United States, brain death equated with legal death. Legislation concerning withdrawal of life support differs from state to state.

CHAPTER 5 ■ DIAGNOSIS OF PAIN AND PARESTHESIAS

DEFINITIONS

Neuropathic pain: lesion of the peripheral or central nervous system.

Somatic pain: stimulation of peripheral nerve endings by lesions in a ligament, joint capsule, muscle or bone.

Paresthesias: spontaneous abnormal sensations ("pins-and-needles") or lack of sensation (numbness). Abnormality anywhere along sensory pathway from peripheral nerves to sensory cortex. Persistent paresthesias imply likely neurologic abnormality.

Dysesthesias: disagreeably abnormal sensations evoked when area of abnormal sensation is touched; may be present with paresthesia.

NECK PAIN

Hints that neck pain is neurologic: (a) pain limited to neck but with abnormal neurologic signs; (b) radiation down ulnar or radial aspect of arm (radicular distribution), sometimes to fingers; (c) weakness and wasting of hand muscles innervated by affected root; (d) abnormal gait, bladder symptoms, loss of tendon reflexes in arms and overactive reflexes in legs (cervical spinal cord compression); (e) pain affected by movement of head and neck, exaggerated by Valsalva maneuvers (sneezing, coughing, straining during bowel movements).

ETIOLOGY

Isolated neck pain: bony abnormalities (e.g., cervical osteoarthritis) or local trauma.

Neck pain with neurologic symptoms or signs: cervical spondylosis most common. Before age 40: tumors, spinal arteriovenous malformations, congenital anomalies of the cervical-occipital region more common.

DIAGNOSIS

MRI or myelography.

LOW BACK PAIN

Most common cause: herniated nucleus pulposus.

Usually abrupt onset: often brought on by heavy lifting, twisting, or Valsalva maneuvers.

Other features: vigorous paraspinal muscle contractions ("splinting"), complete relief on lying down, radiation to buttocks or down posterior aspect of leg to thigh, knee, or foot.

Chronic low back pain: imaging indicated if neurologic abnormalities present on examination. Otherwise, diagnosis and treatment may be major challenge.

ARM PAIN

Non-neurologic causes: musculoskeletal disease (e.g., bursitis or arthritis).

BRACHIAL PLEXUS PATHOLOGY

Tumor: invasion of brachial plexus by lung or breast tumors, or metastases.

Brachial plexus neuritis: pain often poorly localized.

Thoracic outlet syndrome: pain evoked by particular arm positions. Examination may be normal.

Neuralgic amyotrophy: pain, weakness, and wasting of muscle; sensory loss. May be restricted to axillary nerve distribution (deltoid muscle).

ENTRAPMENT NEUROPATHIES

Pain in hands from entrapment of median nerve at wrist (carpal tunnel syndrome), or ulnar nerve at wrist, elbow. Paresthesias in distribution of affected nerve.

CAUSALGIA

See also Chapter 71.

Constant burning pain accompanied by trophic changes (red glossy skin, sweating in affected area, abnormalities of hair and nails).

Follows high-velocity missile wound (bullets or shrapnel) or crush injury. Emotional factors in chronic syndrome. May be relieved by sympathectomy.

Reflex sympathetic dystrophy (Complex Regional Pain Syndrome): local tissue swelling and bony changes accompanying causalgia. Similar changes after minor trauma.

LEG PAIN AND PARESTHESIA

Multiple symmetric peripheral neuropathy: major cause of bilateral foot pain and paresthesias. Usually glove-and-stocking distribution, worse at night. Pain characteristic of neuropathy with diabetes, alcohol, amyloid, cancer, HIV.

Occlusive vascular disease: increasing incidence with age; often with diabetes.

Diabetic mononeuritis multiplex: pain more restricted, onset usually abrupt. Both pain and motor findings improve in months to years.

Nutritional neuropathy: important cause of limb pain in areas of poverty. Also in patients on hemodialysis.

Tumor invasion of lumbosacral plexus: other signs of tumor usually evident.

TREATMENT OF CHRONIC LIMB PAIN

Relieve cause if possible.

Symptomatic therapy with analgesics, tricyclic drugs, monoamine oxidase inhibitors, transcutaneous nerve stimulation, dorsal column stimulation, cordotomy, acupuncture, and others. The long list of remedies attests to limitations of all.

CHAPTER 6 ■ DIZZINESS AND HEARING LOSS

TINNITUS

DEFINITION

Any abnormal sound arising within head, perceived in one or both ears, or inside head. Continuous, intermittent, or pulsatile.

OBJECTIVE TINNITUS

Heard by examiner as well as patient. Uncommon, but associated with serious conditions that mandate prompt diagnosis.

Etiology

Intravascular turbulence: aortic or carotid stenosis, arteriovenous malformations of head and neck, vascular tumors (e.g., glomus jugulare); aneurysms of abdomen, chest, head, neck; enlargement of sigmoid sinus and jugular vein; high blood pressure (typically pulsatile tinnitus); temporal arteritis.
Other causes: temporomandibular joint syndrome; palatal myoclonus.

Evaluation
Auscultation of ear, head, and neck indicated in all patients with tinnitus. Blood pressure, fundoscopic examination especially for pulsatile tinnitus.

SUBJECTIVE TINNITUS

Abnormality somewhere in auditory system from external ear to central auditory connections.

Etiology
Chronic exposure to loud noise; acoustic neuroma (often years before hearing loss or ataxia); compression or inflammation of vestibulocochlear nerve; otosclerosis; otitis; cerumen.

Evaluation

Otologic consultation, hearing tests for persistent tinnitus. Also consider auditory evoked potentials, MRI.

HEARING LOSS

CONDUCTIVE HEARING LOSS

Due to decreased mechanical transmission of sound waves in external or middle ear.

Etiology

Trauma, congenital cranial abnormalities, otosclerosis, ossicular discontinuity (trauma or erosion from chronic otitis media).

Evaluation

Patients speak with soft or normal voice because own voice sounds louder than background sounds in environment. In tuning fork test, sound conveyed by bone conduction is as loud as or louder than by air conduction (abnormal *Rinné test*). Sound of tuning fork in midline of forehead (*Weber test*) heard as though it originated on side of hearing loss. Audiometry, middle ear impedance test confirm diagnosis.

Treatment

Hearing aids, reconstructive microsurgery.

SENSORINEURAL HEARING LOSS

Due to decreased transmission of signals in auditory nerve or central auditory pathways. Most often with lesion in cochlea or cochlear nerve. Rarely from central auditory dysfunction.

Etiology

Excessive exposure to noise, ototoxic drugs, age-related cochlear degeneration, congenital cochlear defects, viral or bacterial infections.

Evaluation

Patients speak with loud voice. Air conduction greater than bone conduction (normal Rinné). Tuning fork louder in better ear on Weber test. Difficulty hearing words suggests central lesion. Audiometry, auditory evoked potentials for lesion localization. MRI of the brain and internal auditory canals with and without gadolinium for any asymmetric sensorineural hearing loss (possible cerebellopontine angle tumor).

Treatment
Hearing aid sufficient for most patients; cochlear implants.

DIZZINESS, DYSEQUILIBRIUM, VERTIGO

PURE DIZZINESS

Sensation of altered spatial orientation; light-headedness, "wooziness," sensation of swimming or floating. No spinning or dysequilibrium. No localizing value.

Circulatory, metabolic, endocrine, degenerative, or psychologic factors all potentially contributory. In advanced age, may be due to combination of normal decrease in vision, proprioception, and vestibular sensation.

VERTIGO

Any abnormal sensation of motion of patient or environment; sensation of spinning, swaying back and forth, or falling.

Peripheral origin: usually episodic or short-lasting; precipitating factor often present; may be accompanied by sweating, pallor, nausea, vomiting, nausea and vomiting; aggravated by head and body movement. Sometimes with hearing loss, tinnitus.

Central origin: constant; nystagmus in any direction including vertical. May be isolated or with other brainstem signs (diplopia, dysarthria, ataxia). Hearing loss unusual.

DYSEQUILIBRIUM

Feeling of unsteadiness, imbalance on walking; absent when sitting or recumbent. Suggests central lesion.

Diagnosis

History: previous episodes; family history; alcohol, drugs; depression (for psychogenic dizziness). Clues to **peripheral** origin: hearing loss, tinnitus or fullness. Clues to **central** origin: disorientation, depressed consciousness.

Examination: external ear (cholesteatoma, infection, middle ear tumor); nystagmus; gait; maneuvers to induce vertigo.

Studies: audiometry; electronystagmography; brain MRI with and without gadolinium.

Treatment

Primary goal is treatment of cause of vertigo, with symptomatic treatment if needed.

Vestibular suppressants: glycopyrrolate; scopolamine patch; meclizine; benzodiazepines. For acute severe vertigo: intramuscular promethazine, intravenous droperidol. Chronic dysequilibrium: vestibular rehabilitation.

COMMON CAUSES OF DIZZINESS AND HEARING LOSS

BENIGN PAROXYSMAL POSITIONAL VERTIGO

Recurrent vertigo brought on by changing head position; onset few seconds after position change, usually lasts less than a minute.

Etiology, Pathogenesis

Head trauma, labyrinthitis, aging. Probably due to dislodgement of calcium carbonate crystals (otoconia) from utricle and saccule into posterior semicircular canal.

Evaluation

Symptoms reproduced by positional tests. Patient asked to lie down quickly from sitting, with head extended and turned all the way to one side. Horizontal, torsional nystagmus (beating toward the floor if patient is lying down with head turned toward offending ear) with latency, fatigability.

Treatment Options

1) spontaneous resolution within weeks or months; 2) otolith repositioning maneuvers aimed at moving otoconia back into utricle (e.g., Epley maneuver); 3) vestibular suppressants (see above); 4) refractory cases: surgical section of posterior ampullary nerve, obliteration of posterior semicircular canal.

VESTIBULAR NEURITIS

Sudden, severe vertigo with nausea, vomiting, nystagmus; lasts several days.

Etiology, Pathogenesis
Unknown. Often follows viral illness. Symptoms result from sudden loss of function of one vestibular system.

Clinical Findings
Hearing not usually affected. Unsteadiness may persist for weeks.

Treatment
If necessary, short course of vestibular suppressants.

MÉNIÈRE DISEASE

See Chapter 144.

PERILYMPHATIC FISTULA

Sudden hearing loss, vertigo, following sudden change of pressure in middle ear or CSF.

Etiology
Weight-lifting, barotrauma of scuba diving or flying, or even nose blowing.

Treatment
Surgery to patch fistula may be necessary.

CEREBELLOPONTINE ANGLE TUMORS

Acoustic neuroma (schwannoma) most common.

Clinical Findings

Early: tinnitus, asymmetric hearing loss, persistent sense of unsteadiness or light-headedness (rather than true vertigo).
Late: loss of corneal reflex, cerebellar signs, nystagmus, unilateral facial weakness.

Evaluation

Audiometry: If sensorineural hearing loss found, consider electronystagmography, BAER, MRI with gadolinium.

DRUG TOXICITY

Aminoglycosides, intravenous loop diuretics, intravenous erythromycin, intravenous vancomycin, intravenous *cis*-platinum, anticonvulsants, alcohol, sedatives (benzodiazepines, phenobarbital), antihistamines, mood elevators, antidepressants. Ataxia, hearing loss may be permanent with aminoglycosides, intravenous loop diuretics, intravenous erythromycin, intravenous vancomycin, intravenous *cis*-platinum.

CARDIAC ARRHYTHMIA

Arrhythmias sufficient to lower cardiac output can cause dizziness; 24- to 48-hour continuous ECG monitoring may be helpful in diagnosis.

PRESBYCUSIS, PRESBYASTASIA

Age-related loss of hearing (presbycusis), balance (presbyastasia). Due to degradation of primary sensory signals (hearing, vision, proprioception) and their integration.

Treatment
Hearing aids (presbycusis); vestibular rehabilitation (presbyastasia).

HYPERVENTILATION

Acute anxiety attacks or panic attacks can cause vertigo, lightheadedness or dreamy state.

CHAPTER 7 ■ IMPAIRED VISION

OCULAR LESIONS

Causes: refractive error, opacity of ocular media, or retinal abnormality (e.g., retinal detachment, inflammation, hemorrhage, vascular occlusion). Sometimes with pain or soft-tissue swelling.

OPTIC NERVE LESIONS

Hallmarks: blurring, dimming, darkening of vision; decreased pupillary reaction to light; usually monocular.

Relative afferent pupillary defect: sign of optic nerve lesion; due to decreased transmission of visual signals through affected optic nerve. Elicited by shining light in one eye and then alternating to other eye (swinging flashlight test): affected pupil constricts with light on normal eye, dilates with light on affected eye, which constricts less rapidly, less completely and less persistently than normal eye.

Scotoma (limited area of absent vision, a "pathological" blind spot) may be present; usually central (surrounded by areas of normal vision), centrocecal (elongated shape of deficit covering fovea, extends to normal blind spot), or altitudinal (covers upper or lower half of visual field). May be symptomatic (recognized by patient) or found on visual field examination.

Bilateral optic nerve lesion: suggests hereditary, toxic, nutritional, demyelinating disorder.
Unilateral optic nerve lesion: ischemia, inflammation, compression.

OPTIC NERVE INFARCT (ANTERIOR ISCHEMIC OPTIC NEUROPATHY)

Patient usually older than 50.
Visual defect usually altitudinal, occasionally centrocecal, sudden onset, stable.

Etiology

Idiopathic (most common), temporal arteritis, carotid occlusive disease (rare).

OPTIC NEURITIS

Usually young adult.

Central or centrocecal scotoma; subacute progression, followed by gradual (partial or complete) resolution. Disc swollen (optic neuritis) or normal (retrobulbar neuritis). Local tenderness or pain on eye movement.

COMPRESSIVE OPTIC NEUROPATHY

Steady progression of visual loss. Disc may appear normal until optic atrophy ensues.

LESIONS OF OPTIC CHIASM

Characteristic visual defect: bitemporal hemianopia (due to compression of crossing fibers). Variants: (a) bitemporal superior quadrantanopia; (b) blind in one eye, superior temporal quadrantanopia in other eye.

Etiology

Compression of chiasm by pituitary tumor, craniopharyngioma, meningioma, aneurysm.

RETROCHIASMAL LESIONS

Homonymous hemianopia: loss of vision in right or left half of visual field in both eyes. Patient often not aware of defect; trouble reading may be only symptom. Visual acuity usually intact.

Lesion anterior to lateral geniculate nucleus: optic atrophy.

Retrogeniculate lesions: optokinetic nystagmus abnormal, especially with movement of test strip toward the lesion. Damage to optic radiation: homonymous quadrantanopia (superior for temporal radiations, inferior for parietal).

TRANSIENT VISUAL EVENTS

Formed visual hallucinations: temporal lobe lesions.

Unformed visual hallucinations: occipital; includes *scintillating homonymous scotoma* of migraine.

Phosphenes (light flashes): optic nerve lesions, eye movement.

Amaurosis fugax: transient visual obscuration, usually in one eye; ophthalmic-carotid hypoperfusion or embolization, cardiogenic emboli, vasospasm of migraine.

IMPAIRED OCULAR MOTILITY

See also Chapter 69.

NORMAL EYE MOVEMENTS

Saccades: rapid conjugate eye movements controlled by contralateral frontal lobe; rapidly redirect gaze to a new target.

Smooth pursuit movements: slow conjugate movements requiring intact ipsilateral occipital lobe; fixation maintained on slowly moving target.

Oculovestibular reflex: slow conjugate movement mediated by reflex arc in midbrain and neck proprioceptive pathways; stability of the retinal image maintained if head moves in relation to body or environment.

Vergence movements: slow disconjugate horizontal movements; alignment of visual axes maintained on looking at nearby objects.

Opticokinetic nystagmus (OKN): normal response of alternating pursuit movements and refixation saccades made when looking at objects moving across visual field (e.g., from a moving train), or a moving tape decorated with lines at regular intervals. Differentiates psychogenic blindness (OKN present) from bilateral occipital lesions (cerebral blindness or cortical blindness, OKN absent).

EYE MOVEMENT PATHWAYS

Cerebral cortex: contralateral frontal for saccades, ipsilateral occipitoparietal for pursuit. Project to ipsilateral *mid-*

brain and pontine eye movement centers. Horizontal movements: pontine paramedian reticular formation; vertical movements: rostral interstitial nucleus of the medial longitudinal fasciculus (MLF; midbrain). Project to *oculomotor nuclei.*

Horizontal conjugate movements: cranial nerve VI nucleus activates ipsilateral lateral rectus to abduct ipsilateral eye, contralateral third cranial nerve nucleus via MLF. Latter drives medial rectus muscle to adduct contralateral eye. Result: conjugate horizontal movement toward the side of the sixth cranial nerve nucleus, paresis of gaze to side of lesion.

Eye movements impaired in contralateral direction if lesion is in hemisphere (supranuclear paresis of gaze contralateral to lesion); paresis of gaze to side of lesion in pons (infranuclear). Vestibulo-ocular reflex preserved with supranuclear lesions.

DIPLOPIA (DOUBLE VISION)

Phoria: misalignment of visual axes when one eye is fixating.

Tropia: persistent misalignment, even when both eyes are fixating.

Diplopia: double vision. Results from tropia. Exception: if strabismus (squint) present from early childhood, useful vision in one eye is suppressed (*amblyopia*); no double vision.

Concomitant (comitant) tropia: constant in all directions of gaze; usually due to disruption of mechanisms responsible for combining binocular images into one. Rarely, psychogenic: convergence spasm; eyes forcefully maintained in convergence.

Incomitant (nonconcomitant) tropia: amount of misalignment varies with eye position. Limitation of action of one or more muscles (lesion in brainstem, cranial nerve, neuromuscular junction, or muscle); mechanical limitation of eye movement in orbit (orbital fractures).

Monocular diplopia: present even with other eye closed; disturbance of refractive media in the eye, psychogenic disease.

Mechanical Limitation of Ocular Motility

Orbital lesions, such as thyroid ophthalmopathy, orbital fracture, tumor. Velocity of saccades preserved.

Myasthenia Gravis

Eye movement abnormality usually involves muscles innervated by more than one nerve; may be unilateral or bilateral, often with ptosis. Diurnal fluctuation; ptosis increases after upgaze for 1 minute.

Third Nerve Palsy

Ptosis; paresis of medial, inferior, superior recti, inferior oblique; impaired adduction, vertical movements, and external rotation. May show large pupil, defective constriction, defective accommodation.

Additional involvement of second, fourth, and sixth cranial nerves suggests lesion in cavernous sinus, superior orbital fissure, or orbital apex. There may also be fifth cranial nerve (ophthalmic division) involvement and oculosympathetic defect (Horner syndrome: miosis, mild ptosis, incomplete and delayed pupil dilatation).

SUPRANUCLEAR AND INTERNUCLEAR OCULAR MOTILITY DEFECTS

Internuclear Ophthalmoplegia

Impaired adduction in horizontal conjugate gaze due to lesion in MLF. On attempting to look away from side of lesion, ipsilateral eye cannot adduct; contralateral eye abducts normally (often with nystagmus). Convergence may be intact.

Unilateral: ischemic lesion likely.
Bilateral: MS likely.

"One and a Half" Syndrome

Combination of ipsilateral gaze palsy and internuclear ophthalmoplegia; neither eye moves to side of lesion; eye ipsilateral to lesion cannot adduct; sole remaining horizontal movement is abduction of eye contralateral to lesion.

Unilateral pontine lesion involving both the MLF and prepontine reticular formation.

Sylvian Aqueduct Syndrome

(a) Impaired upgaze; can be evoked by downward moving OKN, where upward saccades impeded. (b) Convergence-retraction nystagmus (eyes converge and move rhythmically backward into orbits) on attempted upward gaze. (c) Sluggish pupillary response to light. (d) Lid retraction (Collier sign). Attributed to lesion of periaqueductal gray with inhibition of third cranial nerve neurons.

NYSTAGMUS

Involuntary rhythmic oscillation of eyes, generally conjugate and of equal amplitude; usually caused by lesions of cerebellar or vestibular connections.

Physiologic end-gaze nystagmus: fine regular horizontal conjugate jerking at extremes of lateral gaze. No pathologic significance.

Jerk nystagmus (not only at extreme lateral gaze): horizontal or rotary; central or peripheral vestibular disorder.

Vertical nystagmus: posterior fossa disease; sedative or anticonvulsant drugs.

Downbeating nystagmus in primary position: lesion at cervicomedullary junction. Contrast with *ocular bobbing*: total horizontal pontine gaze palsy; not rhythmic, coarser than nystagmus.

Upbeating nystagmus in primary position: lesion in pons, cerebellar vermis, or medulla.

Seesaw nystagmus: vertically dysconjugate with rotary element; lesion usually around optic chiasm.

Periodic alternating nystagmus: horizontal nystagmus with periodically alternating direction; lesion in lower brainstem.

Rebound nystagmus: horizontal jerk nystagmus in primary position transiently after sustained gaze to opposite side; lesion in cerebellar pathways.

Oscillopsia: the symptom of nystagmus; sensation of oscillatory movement of visual environment; rarely present.

OTHER OCULAR OSCILLATIONS

Ocular dysmetria: overshoot or terminal oscillation of saccades. Lesion in cerebellar system.

Ocular flutter: bursts of "back-to-back" saccades.

Opsoclonus: chaotic multidirectional conjugate saccades.

Square-wave jerks: small saccades interfering with fixation in forward gaze; characteristic of progressive supranuclear palsy.

Ocular myoclonus: rhythmic ocular oscillation, often vertical; may be seen with synchronous palatal myoclonus.

CHAPTER 8 ■ APPROACH TO HEADACHE AND FACIAL PAIN

HEADACHE

Usually benign; occasionally manifestation of serious illness.

Prevalence: occasional headaches, nearly 100% of population; severe headaches at least once a year, 40%.

GENERAL PRINCIPLES

Quality
Most headaches dull, deeply located, aching.

Sharp, jabbing (ice-pick like): usually benign headache.

Throbbing, "tight": nonspecific; reflect general head pain mechanisms.

Intensity
Little diagnostic value. Response to placebo (30%) not helpful in diagnosis. Headache due to brain tumor usually not severe.

"Worst headache of my life": characteristic of subarachnoid hemorrhage, but most frequently due to migraine.

Location
Occasionally informative. Temporal arteritis: local scalp tenderness, after age 60, malaise, high ESR. Posterior fossa lesion: occipito-nuchal headache. Supratentorial lesions: frontotemporal pain. Multifocal head pain: usually benign.

Time-Intensity Relationship

Ruptured aneurysm: pain peaks in an instant (thunderclap).

Cluster headache: 3- to 5-minute peak, 45-minute plateau, then tapers off. Migraine: build-up over hours, maintained for several hours. Brain tumor: sleep disruption.

Associated Factors

Cluster headache: relieved by oxygen inhalation.

Migraine: scintillating scotoma in aura; nausea, photophobia; provoked by red wine, sustained exertion, pungent odors, hunger, lack of sleep, weather change, menses. Relief by sleep. Positive family history.

Pituitary adenoma: visual field changes, amenorrhea, galactorrhea.

Brain metastases, carcinomatous meningitis: suspect if known cancer elsewhere or as cause of low CSF sugar with pleocytosis.

Meningitis: pain worse with eye or neck movement.

Posterior fossa mass or Arnold-Chiari malformation: abrupt onset with coughing.

Subdural hematoma, benign intracranial hypertension: worse in recumbent position.

Post-lumbar puncture headache: pain relieved by lying supine, brought on by sitting or standing.

Sinusitis: dark-green, purulent exudate.

Ophthalmic disease: red eye.

APPROACH TO THE PATIENT WITH HEADACHE

Acute, severe headache with stiff neck and fever: suspect meningitis (perform LP); without fever, subarachnoid hemorrhage.

Conditions characteristically associated with headache: infectious mononucleosis, systemic lupus erythematosus, chronic pulmonary failure with hypercapnia (early morning headache), Hashimoto thyroiditis, corticosteroid withdrawal, oral contraceptive and ovulation-promoting medications, inflammatory bowel disease, HIV–associated illnesses, acute blood pressure elevations (pheochromocytoma, malignant hypertension).

Subacute, chronic hypertension rarely causes headache. Recurrent headache more likely benign.

FACIAL PAIN

NEURALGIA

Paroxysmal, fleeting, often electric shock–like episodes of pain in cranial nerve distribution. Nerve demyelination activates pain-generating mechanism in brainstem. Most common: trigeminal, glossopharyngeal.

Trigger
Maneuvers provoke pain in neuralgia syndromes. Chewing: trigeminal neuralgia; also temporomandibular joint

dysfunction, giant cell arteritis (*jaw claudication*). Swallowing, taste: glossopharyngeal neuralgia; also *carotidynia* (facial migraine; due to carotid artery inflammation).

Most common origin of facial pain: dental; provocation by hot, cold, or sweet foods. Cold stimulus repeatedly induces dental pain. Neuralgia: pain cannot be induced repeatedly (refractory period).

Approach
History of trigger points, refractory period. Avoid reproducing pain on examination.

ATYPICAL FACIAL PAIN

Variable syndrome; pain vague, poorly localized, not elicited by trigger maneuvers. Usually psychogenic (depression); follow-up rarely reveals somatic cause (e.g., nasopharyngeal carcinoma).

OPHTHALMIC HERPES ZOSTER (SHINGLES)

Vesicular skin lesions in distribution of ophthalmic division of trigeminal nerve; pain may precede skin lesions; improves with antiviral treatment; often followed by shooting pain in same distribution (postherpetic neuralgia) or by paresthesias.

CHAPTER 9 ■ INVOLUNTARY MOVEMENTS AND RELATED SYNDROMES

INVOLUNTARY MOVEMENTS

ATHETOSIS

Continuous, slow, writhing movements of the limbs (distal and proximal), trunk, head, face, or tongue.

When brief, these merge with chorea (*choreoathetosis*). When sustained, they merge with dystonia (*athetotic dystonia*).

AKATHISIA

Restlessness. Inner component: bothersome urge to move. Motor component: movements made to relieve inner sensation.

Examples: crossing and uncrossing legs, caressing scalp or face, pacing floor, squirming in chair, picking at bedclothes.

Clinical setting: neuroleptic drug therapy, encephalopathy with confusional states, some dementias, Parkinson disease, levodopa toxicity.

BALLISMUS

Large-amplitude jerks, with flinging movements of limbs. Often unilateral (hemiballismus). Lesion usually in subthalamic nucleus.

CHOREA

Brief, irregular contractions; rapid, but not lightning-like.

Often affect individual muscles as seemingly random events, neither repetitive nor rhythmic (e.g., HD, Sydenham chorea).

Presumably disorders of caudate nucleus (see Chapters 109, 110).

DYSKINESIAS

Abnormal involuntary movements of one or multiple body regions. Most common appearance is of athetosis (see above). May be slow or fast. Most frequently continuous (see Chapter 117); sometimes intermittent (see "Paroxysmal Movement Disorders" below).

Usually evident at rest, increased by action, disappear during sleep (with exceptions).

Identified by appearance; EMG occasionally helps. Complex dyskinesias: choreoathetosis.

DYSTONIA

Sustained muscle contraction with twisting, repetitive movement, or abnormal postures.

Variably characterized by (a) sustained contraction of agonists and antagonists; (b) increase of involuntary contraction on attempted voluntary movement ("overflow"); (c) rhythmic interruption (*dystonic tremor*) of contraction when patient attempts to oppose them; (d) inappropriate or opposing contraction during specific voluntary motor *actions (action dystonia)*; and (e) *torsion spasm*, which may be as rapid as chorea, but differs because it is continuous and includes twisting (see also Chapter 113).

MYOCLONUS

Fast, lightning-like movements due to brief muscle contractions (Chapter 111). May be physiologic (e.g., hypnic jerks while falling asleep; hiccups), focal/diffuse, idiopathic/symptomatic, intermittent/rhythmic.

Asterixis: sudden loss of limb tone from brief pause in sustained muscle contraction. "Negative" myoclonus.

PERSISTENT MUSCLE STIFFNESS

Due to continuous muscle firing; idiopathic.

Syndromes: neuromyotonia, encephalomyelitis with rigidity (spinal interneuronitis), stiff-limb syndrome, stiff-person syndrome.

RESTLESS LEGS SYNDROME

Vague discomfort in legs, often described as *formication* (sensation of ants crawling under skin).

Typically in evening when person is relaxed and sitting, or lying down and attempting to fall asleep. Disappears when walking. Often familial.

Treatment: dopamine agonists, levodopa, opioids.

STEREOTYPED MOVEMENTS (STEREOTYPIES)

Simple or complex movements that repeat relatively regularly in almost identical fashion. May resemble tics, but usually in people with mental retardation, autism, schizophrenia; sometimes due to neuroleptic medication. Hands involved more often than cranial muscles (vs. tics).

Bursts of stereotypic shaking seen in otherwise normal children; usually resolve spontaneously.

Buccal-lingual dyskinesia (*Meige syndrome*): constant chewing movements, writhing and protrusion of tongue, puckering of lips.

TICS

Patterned sequences of coordinated movements appearing suddenly and intermittently. Occasionally simple, resembling myoclonic jerks; usually more complex. Typically rapid and brief; occasionally sustained (i.e., dystonic).

Examples: blinking, sniffing, head shaking, shrugging, complex facial distortions, arm-waving, touching body parts, jumping movements, making obscene gestures (*copropraxia*). Vocalization may be barking, throat clearing, squealing, uttering of obscenities (*coprolalia*), repeating one's own sounds (*palilalia*) or sounds of others (*echolalia*).

Features: feel compelling need to execute tic; release of "internal tension" on execution; suppressible for brief intervals or sometimes in public; variable severity; may be temporary or persist throughout life (Chapter 112).

Face, neck, shoulders more often affected than limbs.

TREMOR

Rhythmic oscillatory movement; alternating contractions of opposing muscles.

May be most evident when affected body part is (a) at rest (e.g., *parkinsonian* tremor); (b) with action (e.g., when writing or pouring water from a cup, as in *essential* tremor); (c) with maintained posture (e.g., with arms outstretched in front of body; severe parkinsonian or essential tremor); (d) with intention (e.g., when approaching target in reaching movement; *cerebellar* tremor).

Frequency may be low (3 to 5 Hz; parkinsonian tremor), high (10 to 15 Hz; essential tremor), variable (cerebellar tremor; *dystonic* tremor).

PAROXYSMAL MOVEMENT DISORDERS

Abnormal involuntary movements appear briefly on background of normal movements.

Likely due to abnormalities of membrane ion channels ("channelopathies").

PAROXYSMAL DYSKINESIAS

Bouts of any combination of dystonia, chorea, athetosis, ballismus. Unilateral or bilateral. May be severe enough to cause falls. Speech often affected, with inability to speak due to dystonia. No alteration of consciousness.

Usually inherited (autosomal dominant pattern).

Syndromes: See Table 9.1.

PAROXYSMAL HYPNOGENIC DYSKINESIAS

Short attacks: seconds to minutes. Sometimes due to supplementary sensorimotor seizures. Occur in sleep; respond to anticonvulsants.

Prolonged attacks: 2–50 minutes. Poor response to treatment.

EPISODIC ATAXIAS

See Table 9.2 and Chapter 108.

HYPEREKPLEXIA

Startle syndrome; complex motor responses to sudden tactile or verbal stimuli.

Motor response variable across cultures. May be hereditary or sporadic.

TABLE 9.1

CLINICAL FEATURES OF PAROXYSMAL KINESIGENIC (PKD), NONKINESIGENIC (PNKD), AND EXERTIONAL DYSKINESIA (PED)

Feature	PKD	PNKD	PED
Attack duration	<5 min	2 m–4 h	5 m–2 hr
Attack frequency	100/d–1/mo	3/d–2/y	1/d–2/mo
Trigger	Sudden movement, startle, hyperventilation	Nil	Prolonged exercise; muscle vibration; nerve stimulation; TMS of motor Cx.
Precipitant	Stress	EtOH, stress, caffeine, fatigue	Stress
Treatment	Anticonvulsants	Clonazepam, benzodiazepines, acetazolamide, antimuscarinics	Acetazolamide, antimuscarinics, benzodiazepines

Adapted from *Merritt's Textbook of Neurology, 11th Ed.*

DYSKINESIAS ATTRIBUTED TO PERIPHERAL DISORDERS

HEMIFACIAL SPASM

Intermittent brief or sustained contractions of facial muscles, due to bursts of spontaneous activity in facial nerve.

OTHERS

"Painful legs, moving toes"; "jumpy stumps"; "belly dancer's" dyskinesia; sustained muscle contractions of reflex sympathetic dystrophy.

TABLE 9.2
CLINICAL AND GENETIC FEATURES OF EPISODIC ATAXIAS

Type	Age at onset	Clinical	Acetazolamide response	Precipitant	Frequency/duration	Interictal
Myokymia, neuro-myotonia (EA-1)	2–15	Aura of weightlessness or weakness, then ataxia, dysarthria, tremor, facial twitching	In some kindreds; anticonvulsants may help	Startle, movement, exercise, excitement, fatigue	Up to 15 per day; usually one or less per day; seconds to minutes, usually 2–10 min	Myokymia, shortened Achilles tendon; PKD
Vestibular (EA-2)	0–40, usually 5–15	Ataxia, vertigo, nystagmus, dysarthria, HA, ptosis, ocular palsy, vermis atrophy	Very effective	stress, alcohol, fatigue, exercise, caffeine	daily to q 2 mos; usually hours; 5 min to weeks	Nystagmus, mild ataxia, less common: dysarthria, and progr. cerebellar
Ocular (EA-3)	20–50	Ataxia, diplopia, vertigo, nausea	No response	Sudden change in head position	Daily to year; minutes to hours	Symptoms gradually become constant
Tinnitus (EA-4)	1–41	Ataxia, tinnitus, falling, headache, blurred vision, vertigo, nausea	Effective	None	Daily; 10–30 minutes	Myokymia; some with ataxia

Adapted from *Merritt's Textbook of Neurology*, 11th ed.

PSYCHOGENIC MOVEMENT DISORDERS

Usually mixture of different types of movement, particularly shaking, paroxysmal disorders, fixed postures, or bizarre gaits.

Clues: inconsistency and incongruity of symptoms and signs, weakness due to reduced effort, variable sensory changes, sudden onset, marked slowness of voluntary movements without reduction of spontaneous movements, appearance of marked fatigue and exhaustion from involuntary movements.

Distractibility: disappearance of abnormal movement when attention is diverted to another task (e.g. listing months backwards, identifying object by touch).

Diagnosis suggested by incongruity of symptoms and signs, distractibility. Confirmed by relief of signs and symptoms using psychotherapy, suggestion, physiotherapy.

OTHER INVOLUNTARY MOVEMENTS

Convulsions, fasciculations, myokymia are described elsewhere.

CHAPTER 10 ■ SYNDROMES CAUSED BY WEAK MUSCLES

DEFINITIONS

Weakness: cannot exert normal force.
Paralysis, plegia: total loss of ability to contract muscle.
Paresis: partial loss, but often used interchangeably with plegia.
Hemiplegia: weakness of arm and leg on same side.
Monoplegia: weakness of one limb.
Paraplegia: weakness of both legs.

RECOGNITION OF WEAKNESS AND PSEUDOWEAKNESS

COMMON WEAKNESS SYMPTOMS

Cranial: ptosis of eyelids, diplopia, dysarthria, dysphagia; change in facial appearance.
Proximal limbs: difficulty lifting packages, combing hair, reaching overhead, climbing stairs, rising from chairs.
Distal limbs: difficulty turning keys or door knobs, difficulty using coins or buttons, footdrop.

CONDITIONS MIMICKING WEAKNESS

Subjective weakness without objective muscle weakness.

Chronic fatigue syndrome: easy fatigability, inability to do housework, need for prolonged rest after slight exertion. Often with myalgia, depression. No focal weakness on examination.
Fatigue of systemic illness: anemia, hypoventilation, congestive heart failure, cancer, systemic infection. Usually with other evidence of underlying disease.
Psychogenic weakness: somatoform disorder, depression, factitious disorder, malingering. Inconsistencies in history,

examination. Clues: misdirection of effort (give-way weakness, or intermittent instead of sustained effort in manual muscle tests; improvement of findings with distraction; histrionic behavior; exaggerated gait difficulty (patient staggers dramatically but does not fall).

Other: parkinsonism, severe sensory loss, joint inflammation. Examination clarifies.

PATTERNS OF WEAKNESS

Motor neuron disorder: overactive tendon reflexes with clonus, Hoffmann sign, Babinski sign; if chronic, may show no weakness on manual muscle tests but alternating movements slow and clumsy.

Lower motor neuron disorder: muscle weakness, wasting, fasciculations, loss of tendon reflexes. See Chapter 125.

Hemiparesis: weakness of arm and leg on same side with upper motor neuron signs: lesion in brain or cervical spinal cord. Stroke, mass lesion.

Paraparesis: weakness of both legs with upper motor neuron signs: lesion may affect corticospinal tracts bilaterally (brain, spinal cord) or lower motor neurons (e.g., Guillain-Barré syndrome). See Chapters 118–120.

Monomelic paresis: weakness of one leg or one arm with solely lower motor neuron signs. Herniated nucleus pulposus, brachial plexus neuritis (neuralgic amyotrophy), peripheral nerve entrapment syndromes, mononeuritis multiplex, ALS.

Neck weakness: floppy head or dropped head syndrome, diseases of motor unit. MG, ALS most common, or 'axial myopathy' of neck extensors. Often accompanied by involvement of lower cranial nerves (dysarthria, dysphagia) and upper cervical segments (difficulty raising arms).

Weakness of cranial muscles: see Chapters 7, 69.

CHAPTER 11 ■ GAIT DISORDERS

EXAMINING STANCE AND GAIT

Observe patient from the front, back, and sides. Ask patient to rise quickly from chair, walk at slow pace, then fast pace, then turn around; walking successively on toes, on heels, and tandem.

Note body and head posture (normal = erect), shoulders (no scoliosis or kyphosis), arm swing (present and equal), foot base (narrow), stride (full, symmetric, without shuffling), cadence (regular), speed, steadiness, turning (in one step).

GAIT IN HEMIPARESIS

Combined effects of spasticity, incoordination, weakness. Affected arm flexed at elbow and leg extended. Paretic leg swings outward at the hip (*circumduction*). Paretic arm moves little, remaining flexed and adducted; arm swing.

GAIT IN SPASTIC PARAPARESIS

Combined effects of spasticity, incoordination, weakness of both legs. Slow, stiff movements at knees and hips, with evident effort. Legs usually maintained extended or slightly flexed at hips and knees, often adducted at hips. Short steps, side-to-side trunk movements, circumduction of legs. Each leg may cross in front of the other (*"scissors gait"*).

GAIT IN PARKINSONISM

Combined effects of akinesia (difficulty initiating movement), dystonia (fixed abnormal posture), rigidity, and tremor.

Difficulty rising from chair. Flexed posture with few automatic limb movements. Reduced arm swing. Short steps, sometimes becoming successively shorter and more rapid (*festination*).

Several steps for turning. Poor recovery of balance when pulled from behind; normals restore balance with 1–2 steps. Motor *"freezing"* (sudden brief inability to move legs). Rest tremor often emerges during walking.

GAIT IN CEREBELLAR DISEASE

Wide-based stance, unsteady balance, cautious steps of variable length and cadence; lurching from side to side (*"ataxic gait"*).

Narrow-based stance difficult to attain with eyes open or closed. In mild disease, problem may appear only on tandem-walking.

Cerebellar vermis lesions: gait may be affected alone, without limb ataxia.

Unilateral lesions: gait predominantly affected on side ipsilateral to lesion; falling toward that side. Movement of limbs ipsilateral to lesion also affected (inaccurate reaching, intention tremor, decreased tone, scoliosis toward side of lesion).

Bilateral cerebellar hemisphere lesions: gait and limb movements affected on both sides.

GAIT IN SENSORY ATAXIA

Loss of proprioceptive sensation due to lesions of peripheral or central sensory fibers.

Wide-based stance, cautious steps of variable length, constantly watching the ground. Feet lifted higher than normal and flung abruptly to ground ("stomping gait").

Romberg sign: can stand with feet together, eyes open, but not with eyes closed.

PSYCHOGENIC GAIT DISORDERS

Bizarre gait, unlike any other disorder of gait evoked by neurologic disease. Objective signs of neurologic disease missing. Inconsistencies in examination sometimes present (e.g., positions demonstrating excellent balance briefly achieved in spite of difficulty walking just before or afterwards); usually do not fall or sustain injury despite dramatic staggering.

GAIT IN CEREBRAL PALSY

Cerebral palsy: diverse motor abnormalities caused by nonprogressive cerebral lesions present from birth or early infancy.

Mild injury: exaggerated tendon reflexes and extensor plantar responses with slight degree of inward turning of knees (*spastic diplegia*).

Slow, stiff walk; "scissoring" (crossing of feet at each step due to spasticity of hip adductors).

Extensive lesions: legs adducted and internally rotated at the hips, extended or slightly flexed at the knees, with plantar flexion at the ankles; arms adducted at the shoulders and flexed at the elbows and wrists (*spastic quadraplegia*).

Athetotic cerebral palsy: slow, writhing movements of arms and neck, with facial grimacing. Movements brought on by walking.

GAIT IN CHOREA

Brief movements randomly involving face, trunk, or limbs and occurring at random times. Result in sudden changes in trunk posture, walking speed, path.

GAIT IN DYSTONIA MUSCULORUM DEFORMANS

Inversion of one foot at ankle (often first symptom). Then other postural abnormalities, often exacerbated by walking.

GAIT IN MUSCULAR DYSTROPHY

Exaggerated lumbar lordosis and protuberant abdomen because of weak abdominal and paravertebral muscles. Legs spread apart; waddling motion of pelvis. Rising from floor or chair: forward trunk flexion, placement of hands on knees, followed by marching of hands up the thighs to push the trunk up (*Gower sign*).

GAIT DISORDERS ASSOCIATED WITH AGING

Not all indicative of disease.

CAUTIOUS GAIT

Often seen in healthy elderly people. Slightly wide base, short stride, slow speed, turning in several steps. No hesitancy in initiation of gait; no shuffling or freezing. Normal rhythm. Mild dysequilibrium in response to a push; difficulty balancing on one foot.

SUBCORTICAL DYSEQUILIBRIUM

Typical of progressive supranuclear palsy.

Difficulty maintaining upright posture; hyperextension of trunk and neck; parkinsonian signs.

Poor postural adjustments in response to jostling. Combination of postural instability and preserved speed of walking and turning characteristically results in falls on turning.

FRONTAL DYSEQUILIBRIUM

Difficulty walking, standing, or even sitting without support.

Balance problem: cannot bring legs under the center of gravity; falls back on rising from chair.

Wide base, shuffling steps, dysequilibrium. Hesitation in starting to walk or turn.

Usually with dementia, signs of frontal release (suck, snout, and grasp reflexes), motor perseveration, urinary incontinence, pseudobulbar palsy, exaggerated muscle stretch reflexes, and extensor plantar responses.

ISOLATED GAIT IGNITION FAILURE

Difficulty starting and continuing to walk without dementia, apraxia, parkinsonism, or poor balance.

Steps short and shallow (shuffling) initially, then normal.

"Freezing" of gait may occur with distraction.

"Magnetic gait" or "apraxia of gait": terms used for this disorder as well as for frontal dysequilibrium.

FRONTAL GAIT DISORDER

Often used to describe gait associated with normal pressure hydrocephalus (NPH). Wide base, short steps with shuffling, difficulty in gait initiation and turning, poor recovery with jostling. May be accompanied by urinary incontinence, dementia, frontal release signs (e.g., suck, snout, grasp reflexes). If accompanied by hydrocephalus on imaging, gait disorder may improve with ventriculoperitoneal shunting.

GAIT IN LOWER MOTOR NEURON DISORDERS

Distal weakness: footdrop, high step ("steppage gait"). Unilateral or bilateral, depending on nature of disorder (compression of one peroneal nerve vs. CMT, motor neuron disease.)

Proximal weakness: hip and pelvis muscles used to lift legs (*"waddling gait"*).

CHAPTER 12 ■ SIGNS AND SYMPTOMS IN NEUROLOGIC DIAGNOSIS

DIAGNOSTIC FACTORS

Ninety percent of neurologic diagnosis suggested by history. Objective evaluation (exam, laboratory tests, imaging studies) usually directed at confirming or excluding diagnoses raised by history.

Two questions addressed in parallel: (a) *Where is the lesion?* Cerebrum, basal ganglia, brainstem, cerebellum, spinal cord, peripheral nerves, neuromuscular junction, muscle? (b) *What is the nature of the disease?*

Answers derive from analysis of symptoms (Chapters 1–11) and additional considerations below.

AGE OF PATIENT

Examples: progressive paraparesis (spinal cord compression in child, MS in adult). Focal seizures (structural lesion more likely in adult than in child). Myopathic leg weakness (muscular dystrophy in child, polymyositis in adult).

SEX

X-linked diseases (almost always in boys), autoimmune diseases (women more often affected), pregnancy-related complications (women), head injury (more common in men).

ETHNICITY

Prevalence of particular diseases higher in some ethnic groups.

SOCIOECONOMIC FACTORS

Poverty associated with increased mortality: alcoholism, drug addiction, trauma, malnutrition, infections all play a role.

Inequities of access to medical care disadvantage the poor and geographically isolated globally. The 45 million US citizens without health insurance also have limited access.

TEMPO OF DISEASE

Abrupt onset: syncope, seizure, TIA, stroke. Variable recovery: syncope (seconds), seizure (minutes), TIA (minutes to hours), stroke (days to weeks).

Gradual progression: over hours (intoxication, infection, or subdural hematoma), days (GBS), weeks to months (most CNS tumors), years (heritable and degenerative diseases).

Remissions and exacerbations: MG (weeks), MS (days to weeks), some forms of peripheral neuropathy (weeks to months).

Episodic (usually hours): periodic paralysis, migraine headache, cluster headache, narcolepsy.

Long-standing (headache more likely tension or vascular; seizures more likely idiopathic) vs. recent-onset (headache more likely due to structural lesions; seizures more likely structural lesion or metabolic abnormality).

MEDICAL HISTORY

Common disorders (e.g., diabetes mellitus, hypertension, tumor metastases) cause characteristic neurologic symptoms.

Many medications for systemic diseases have neurologic adverse effects.

Cutaneous signs may point to neurologic disorder (e.g., neurofibromatosis type 1, tuberous sclerosis) or to systemic disorder with neurologic complications (e.g., lupus erythematosus).

IDENTIFYING SITE OF DISORDER

Cerebral hemispheres: seizures, delirium, dementia, or focal signs that can be attributed to a particular brain area (e.g., hemiplegia, aphasia, hemianopia).

Brain stem: cranial nerve palsies, cerebellar signs of ataxia, tremor, or dysarthria; ocular signs especially helpful in localizing brainstem lesions.

Basal ganglia: involuntary movements.

Spinal cord: spastic gait disorder, bilateral corticospinal signs, bladder symptoms. With neck or back pain: suspect compressive lesion. No pain: MS likely.

Peripheral nerves: usually both motor and sensory symptoms. Manifestations usually more severe distally ("glove-and-stocking" distribution).

Neuromuscular junction, muscle: limb or cranial muscle weakness without sensory symptoms (paresthesias).

Section II
How to Select Diagnostic Tests

Section II

How to Select
Diagnostic Tests

CHAPTER 13 ■ CT AND MRI

COMPUTED TOMOGRAPHY (CT)

DESCRIPTION

Based on x-rays; visual "slices" through body part showing tissue density. Gray scale of display from black (low density, e.g., fluid) to white (high density, e.g., bone).

Intravenous iodinated contrast agents enhance differences in tissue density, show vascular structures, reveal areas of blood-brain barrier breakdown. Contraindications to using contrast in CT studies include renal disease, allergy to iodine, shellfish.

CT faster and less expensive than MRI. CT preferred for imaging bone, calcium, acute hemorrhage. Major limitation: posterior fossa poorly visualized.

MRI now gold standard for identifying intracranial or spinal lesions.

CT ANGIOGRAM

Spiral technique used to obtain serial scans following injection of intravenous contrast bolus; then 3D reconstruction performed. Used to image vascular anatomy, pathology (e.g., aneurysms, stenosis).

CT PERFUSION

Repeated imaging of same brain region during rapid intravenous bolus contrast injection to assess brain perfusion. Can be quick screening test for acute ischemia in major vascular territories.

Acute Hematoma
Bright (hyperdense; hours to days); then same density as brain (weeks); then dark (hypodense; several weeks to months).

Nonhemorrhagic Infarction
Typically dark (low density). Earliest abnormality: loss of distinction between gray and white matter; sometimes visible

3 hours after infarct. Hypodensity usually visible within 24 hours, but may take weeks to appear.

MAGNETIC RESONANCE IMAGING (MRI)

DESCRIPTION

Superior to CT for most purposes. Images based on behavior of protons in various tissues when exposed to a strong magnetic field; brightness or darkness depends on tissue fat and water content.

Image weighting: MRI sequences designed to detect diverse abnormalities. See Table 13.1.

Gadolinium (contrast agent): bright on T1 (Table 13.1). Reveals vessels, areas of breakdown of blood-brain barrier (e.g., inflammation), neoplasms. Few adverse reactions (vs. iodinated contrast agents of CT).

Contraindications to MRI: some metallic implants (e.g., cardiac pacemakers, certain aneurysm clips). Pregnancy (especially first trimester) a relative contraindication, primarily because safety data are incomplete.

MAGNETIC RESONANCE ANGIOGRAPHY (MRA)

Provides map of blood vessels constructed from blood-flow signals. Sensitivity adjusted for arteries ("MR arteriogram") or veins ("MR venogram"). Unlike CT angiogram, does not require contrast injection.

Indications for brain MRA: possible venous sinus thrombosis, arteriovenous malformation, vascular tumors, TIA, stroke.

Detects aneurysms as small as 3 mm. Conventional angiography still the most sensitive examination for evaluation of intracranial aneurysms, arteriovenous malformations, occlusion of small arteries (e.g., vasculitis).

FUNCTIONAL MRI TECHNIQUES

MRI methods used to image physiologic processes.

Cerebral perfusion: Special techniques to identify underperfused regions distal to arterial stenosis or occlusion ("first pass" or "bolus tracking," "arterial spin labeling").

TABLE 13.1

IMAGE WEIGHTING SEQUENCES IN MRI

	T1	T2	T2-FLAIR	T2-GRE
Bright (hyperintense; high signal)	Fat Gadolinium Subacute hemorrhage (met-hemoglobin)	All fluids (including CSF, edema) Most lesions Subacute hemorrhage	Edema Most lesions	Flow-related enhancement (MR angiography)
Dark (hypointense; low signal)	CSF	Acute hemorrhage (deoxyhemoglobin) Old hemorrhage (hemosiderin)	CSF	Old hemorrhage (hemosiderin)
		Rapidly flowing blood, dense calcification, cortical bone, air		

FLAIR, fluid attenuated inversion recovery; GRE, gradient echo.

Diffusion: restricted water diffusion appears as high signal (bright) within minutes of infarction ("diffusion weighted imaging [DWI]").

MR spectroscopy: spectra of common tissue metabolites, including *N*-acetylaspartate, creatine, choline, lactate. Changes in amplitude of peaks may indicate pathologic processes (e.g., neuronal death).

Cerebral activation: electrical signaling among neurons correlates with local changes in cerebral blood oxygenation. Can reconstruct map of cerebral activation ("functional MRI").

ACUTE INFARCTION

MRI more sensitive and more specific than CT. Ischemia, infarction dark on T1, bright on T2, FLAIR after 6 to 12 hours. DWI technique shows ischemia (bright) within minutes of injury. MRA often used to assess patency of intracranial and neck vessels.

CHAPTER 14 ■ EEG AND EVOKED POTENTIALS

DEFINITIONS

Electroencephalography (EEG): recording spontaneous brain electrical activity.

Evoked potentials: electrical responses to specific sensory stimuli.

ELECTROENCEPHALOGRAPHY

NORMAL ADULT EEG

Awake Resting State

Alpha rhythm: 8–12 cycles per second (Hz), over parieto-occipital regions.

Beta rhythm, 13–25 Hz, over frontal regions.

Sleep Stages

Stage 1: alpha replaced by slower rhythm; vertex waves (high-voltage sharp waves at top of head) present.

Stage 2: sleep spindles (symmetric 12 to 14 Hz sinusoidal waves).

Stages 3, 4: high-voltage, widely distributed, slow wave activity.

Rapid eye movement (REM) stage: low-voltage mixed frequency activity together with rapid eye movements and generalized atonia; begins about 90 minutes after sleep onset.

REM in daytime EEG suggests sleep deprivation, withdrawal from REM-suppressant drugs, alcohol withdrawal, narcolepsy (see Chapter 145).

COMMON EEG ABNORMALITIES

Diffuse background slowing: the most common EEG abnormality. Nonspecific. Associated with diffuse encephalopathies of diverse causes, multiple structural abnormalities.

Focal slowing: localized parenchymal dysfunction; lesion seen on CT, MRI in 70% of cases.

Triphasic waves: generalized synchronous waves in brief runs; toxic metabolic encephalopathies (hepatic encephalopathy in 50%).

Epileptiform discharges: brief discharges of characteristic shape (spike, sharp, slow wave, or combinations of these); occur intermittently; strongly associated with seizure disorders; type of discharge may suggest specific epileptic syndrome.

Periodic lateralizing epileptiform discharges (PLEDs): seen with acute destructive cerebral lesion; focal epileptiform discharges recurring at 1–2 Hz over focally slow or low-voltage background. Acute cerebral infarct (35%); other mass lesions (26%); cerebral infection, anoxia, other causes (39%).

Generalized periodic sharp waves: recur at 0.5–1 Hz on attenuated background. Most common after cerebral anoxia; also seen in CJD.

CLINICAL UTILITY OF EEG

Epilepsy

EEG essential in diagnosis and classification of epilepsy (Table 14.1; see also Chapter 141).

Epileptiform discharges strongly suggest epilepsy. Recorded in 30% to 50% of patients with epilepsy on first routine EEG and in 60% to 90% by third routine EEG. Seen in 2.7% of adults without seizures and 1.5% to 3.5% of healthy normal children.

Specific epileptic syndrome often defined by type of interictal epileptiform discharge together with clinical features.

Dementia and Diffuse Encephalopathies

Toxic metabolic encephalopathy: triphasic waves.
Sedative-hypnotic medications: high-voltage beta activity.
HD: generalized voltage attenuation.
CJD: generalized periodic sharp waves (90% of patients within 12 weeks of symptom onset).
Alzheimer disease (advanced): diffuse slowing.

Focal Brain Lesions

EEG assesses epileptogenic potential of mass lesions.

TABLE 14.1

EPILEPTIFORM ABNORMALITIES IN THE COMMON EPILEPSY SYNDROMES

West syndrome
  No organized background rhythms (hypsarrhythmia)
  Random high-voltage, chaotic slow activity
  Multifocal epileptiform discharges
  Abrupt voltage attenuation (during spasm)

Lennox-Gastaut syndrome
  Slow generalized spike and wave (<2 Hz)
  Moderate-to-severe slowing of background rhythms

Childhood absence epilepsy
  Generalized 3–4 Hz spike-wave activity
  Usually precipitated by hyperventilation
  Normal background rhythms

Benign rolandic epilepsy
  Focal central-midtemporal sharp waves
  Normal background rhythms

Juvenile myoclonic epilepsy
  Generalized 4–8 Hz spikes and polyspike-wave discharges
  May be precipitated by photic stimulation
  Normal background rhythms

Localization-related epilepsy (e.g., temporal lobe seizures)
  Focal epileptiform discharges
  Occasional focal slowing
  Occasional mild slowing of background rhythms

Hemispheric TIAs: focal EEG abnormalities in half.
Hemisphere infarct: focal slowing, improves with time.
Neoplasm: focal slowing, worsens with time.

Cerebral Infections

Herpes encephalitis: focal EEG changes in more than 80%; PLEDs in more than 70% (2 to 30 days after symptom onset).
Subacute sclerosing panencephalitis: stereotyped bursts of high-voltage delta waves at regular intervals of 4 to 20 seconds. Virtually diagnostic of this disease.
HIV infection: nonspecific; usually diffuse slowing (especially AIDS-related dementia). Focal slowing with superimposed cerebral lesions, such as lymphoma, toxoplasmosis.

LONG-TERM EEG MONITORING

Computer-based systems for prolonged continuous EEG recording.

Applications

Epilepsy monitoring unit: EEG with simultaneous video recording. Improves diagnostic accuracy: 1) characterization of possible seizures; 2) determination of seizure type; 3) identification of seizure focus for surgical resection.

Intensive care unit: 1) management of status epilepticus; 2) detection of non-convulsive seizures; 3) management of drug-induced coma for increased ICP.

EVOKED POTENTIALS (EP)

PRINCIPLES OF EP RECORDING

EP: small electrical signal recorded at the scalp; produced by neural structures along visual, auditory, or somatosensory pathways in response to sensory stimulus.

Delayed responses arise from conduction delay along sensory pathways. Attenuation or loss of component waveforms results from conduction block or dysfunction along sensory pathways; affected component waveform reflects the site of dysfunction.

VISUAL EP (VEP)

Stimulus: checkerboard pattern. Delay of occipital positive signal (P100) to stimulation of one eye: dysfunction in visual pathways anterior to optic chiasm on side of that eye.

Delay of P100 to stimulation of either eye: dysfunction in visual pathways bilaterally (anterior or posterior to chiasm). Unilateral hemisphere lesion: no delay of P100.

Acute optic neuritis: delay and loss or severe attenuation of VEP; delay is permanent. VEPs abnormal in about 70% of patients with MS who have no history of optic neuritis.

Other causes of abnormal VEP: ocular disease (major refractive error, media opacities, glaucoma, retinopathies); compressive lesions of optic nerve (extrinsic tumors, optic nerve tumors); noncompressive optic nerve lesions (ischemic optic neuritis; nutritional or toxic amblyopia); diffuse CNS disease (adrenoleukodystrophy, Pelizaeus-Merzbacher disease, spinocerebellar degenerations, Parkinson disease).

Normal in psychogenic blindness.

BRAINSTEM AUDITORY EVOKED POTENTIALS (BAEP)

Stimulus: repetitive "click" sound.

Wave I: from peripheral portion of auditory nerve. Wave III: tegmentum in caudal pons. Wave V: inferior colliculus.

BAEPs often abnormal with structural brainstem lesions; almost always abnormal with brainstem glioma. Attenuated or delayed waves III, V.

Abnormal in >90% of patients with acoustic neuroma. Earliest abnormality: prolongation of I to III interpeak interval. Abnormal in 33% of patients with MS. Also used to assess hearing in infants.

SOMATOSENSORY EVOKED POTENTIALS (SSEP)

Stimulus: electrical stimulation of median and posterior tibial nerves; reflect sequential activation of structures along dorsal column–lemniscal system.

Components of median nerve SSEP: (a) Erb point potential (reflects brachial plexus integrity); (b) N13 (central gray matter of cervical cord); (c) P14 (lower brain stem); (d) N18 (rostral brain stem); (e) N20 (primary cortical somatosensory receiving area).

Posterior tibial SSEP: includes components generated in gray matter of lumbar spinal cord, brainstem, primary somatosensory cortex.

Altered by focal lesions (strokes, tumors, cervical spondylosis, syringomyelia), diffuse diseases (hereditary system degenerations, subacute combined degeneration, and vitamin E deficiency), and diseases specifically affecting myelin (MS, adrenoleukodystrophy, adrenomyeloneuropathy, metachromatic leukodystrophy, Pelizaeus-Merzbacher disease).

Abnormal in 50% to 60% of patients with MS, even without clinical signs or symptoms.

Abnormally large amplitude SSEPs (increased cortical excitability): progressive myoclonus epilepsy, photosensitive epilepsy, late infantile ceroid lipofuscinosis.

MOTOR EVOKED POTENTIALS

Stimulus: electric or magnetic pulse through scalp over the motor cortex. Response: limb movement.

Used to assess descending motor pathways (e.g., intraoperative monitoring, with SSEP, during surgery with risk of spinal cord injury).

CHAPTER 15 ■ NERVE CONDUCTION STUDIES, ELECTROMYOGRAPHY, AND MAGNETIC STIMULATION

NERVE CONDUCTION STUDIES

Measure speed and strength of electrical impulse conducted along motor or sensory peripheral nerve.

SNAP: *sensory nerve action potential*. Electrical signal traveling along sensory nerve. Recorded on skin surface overlying nerve; measured in microvolts.

Sensory nerve conduction: stimulate nerve (usually a pure sensory branch) distally, record SNAP proximally.

CMAP: *compound motor action potential*. Electrical signal from contracting muscle. Recorded on skin surface overlying muscle; measured in millivolts.

Motor nerve conduction: stimulate nerve proximally, record CMAP from muscle distally.

Amplitude of waveform: indicates strength of electrical impulse. Reduced with axonal loss.

Latency: time between stimulation and action potential (SNAP or CMAP).

Nerve conduction velocity: latency of action potential/distance between stimulation and recording sites. Slowing usually reflects demyelinating injury.

Conduction block: severe, focal demyelinating lesion prevents action potentials from being transmitted downstream, causing loss of waveform amplitude on one segment of the nerve.

F response: stimulate motor nerve antidromically (toward nerve root) with supramaximal intensity. Action potential reaches anterior horn cells via ventral root, then travels back down motor nerve orthodromically (in direction of normal flow); time for round trip = *F wave latency*. Measures integrity of proximal motor pathways (root, anterior horn cell); no synapse involved.

H reflex: electrical equivalent of ankle jerk reflex; stimulate sensory afferents of tibial nerve at knee, activating monosynaptic stretch reflex pathway to record soleus muscle contraction. Measures integrity of segmental reflex pathway, including sensory nerve and root, spinal segment (dorsal column, synapse, anterior horn), motor root and nerve. Mainly used to assess L5-S1 nerve root compression.

F and H responses (*late responses*) assess proximal segments; useful when distal nerve conduction studies are normal. Examples: late responses delayed or absent in proximal radiculopathy (e.g., GBS), motor neuron disease, MS, dorsal root damage. Absence of H and normal F: suggests dorsal root pathology.

ELECTROMYOGRAPHY (EMG)

Needle electrode inserted directly into a selected muscle records action potentials generated by muscle fibers at rest ("spontaneous activity") or during voluntary movement.

INSERTIONAL AND SPONTANEOUS ACTIVITY

Any spontaneous discharge in resting muscle following insertional activity is abnormal and may reflect neurogenic or myopathic disease.

Insertional activity: brief burst of electrical activity recorded when EMG needle is first moved into muscle. Normal when duration is few hundred milliseconds. Prolonged in denervating disorders (e.g., ALS), muscle inflammation (e.g., polymyositis).

Fibrillation potentials: discharges of single muscle fibers (denervating axonal injury, some myopathies—especially polymyositis).

Positive sharp waves: different shape but same implications as fibrillation potentials.

Complex repetitive discharges: spontaneous discharges of constant shape and frequency with abrupt onset and abrupt cessation (denervation, inflammatory myopathy).

Fasciculations: discharges of entire motor unit, usually resulting in contractions visible with naked eye (unlike fibrillations). Neurogenic origin (motor neuron disease, radiculopathy). Can be seen in otherwise normal people (benign fasciculations).

Myotonia: high frequency muscle fiber discharge of waxing and waning amplitude (myotonic dystrophy, congenital myotonia).

Myokymia: bursts of muscle activity as doublets or multiplets, often with cramps and visible continuous twitching (Guillain-Barré Syndrome, multiple sclerosis).

Electrical neuromyotonia: EMG pattern of continuous motor unit activity with high frequency, involuntary trains of single motor unit discharges.

Clinical neuromyotonia (Isaacs syndrome, Morvan syndrome): see Chapter 130.

MOTOR UNIT CONFIGURATION

Motor unit: all muscle fibers innervated by single axon.

Motor-unit action potential (MUAP): electrical wave-form, measured from muscle, generated by motor-unit activation; assess waveform duration, amplitude and morphology.

Neurogenic disease: abnormally large MUAPs with long duration, high amplitude, increased complexity. Reflect *collateral reinnervation*: motor units increase in size as surviving axons sprout to innervate adjacent muscle fibers to compensate for damaged axons.

Myopathy: abnormally small MUAPs with short duration, low amplitude, increased complexity. Attributed to loss of muscle fibers: fewer muscle fibers remain to contribute to the overall potential.

RECRUITMENT AND INTERFERENCE PATTERNS

Recruitment: Ask patient to exert force with muscle being recorded without shortening (isometric). As demand for strength increases, additional motor units become visible in waveform. Firing frequency of first recruited motor unit increases until a second unit is recruited (*recruitment frequency*). Neurogenic disease: abnormally high recruitment frequencies due to loss of motor units. Myopathy: abnormally low recruitment frequencies as motor units are smaller and weaker.

Interference pattern: Overlapping pattern generated by simultaneous activation of large numbers of MUAPs during maximal contraction; normally a dense, broad band of overlapping waveforms. Neurogenic disease: incomplete ("picket fence") pattern due to loss of motor units. Myopathy: early appearance of full interference pattern as many weakened motor units are required to generate even minimal force; total amplitude is low.

TESTS OF NEUROMUSCULAR TRANSMISSION

Repetitive nerve stimulation: series of supramaximal motor nerve stimulations at specific frequency; evaluate for abnormal decreases or increases in consecutive CMAP size.

Postsynaptic neuromuscular junction (NMJ) dysfunction: myasthenia gravis most common cause. Impaired postsynaptic response to acetylcholine, worsened by prolonged exercise. Characteristic decremental response with 2–3 Hz (low frequency) stimulation; transient increase in CMAP size with 15 seconds of intense exercise (post-exercise facilitation); worsening of decrement by exercise at 3 to 4 minutes (post-activation exhaustion).

Presynaptic NMJ dysfunction: impaired release of acetylcholine at rest; incremental response with exercise or rapid rates (10–50 Hz) of stimulation, e.g., Lambert-Eaton syndrome, botulism.

Single-fiber EMG: record action potentials from single muscle fiber in response to nerve stimulation. Sensitive test of NMJ dysfunction, which results in increased "jitter" (variation of time between stimulation and recorded action potential). Not specific. Used to confirm NMJ dysfunction in suspected myasthenia gravis when other tests are equivocal or negative.

TRANSCRANIAL MAGNETIC STIMULATION

Noninvasive method of stimulating electrical activity in cerebral cortex by applying brief, high-intensity magnetic pulse to surface of head. Waveform recordings (motor evoked potential, or MEP) usually obtained from contralateral distal limb muscle.

Used to study conductivity and excitability of the corticospinal system, abnormal cortical circuitry in neurologic diseases, and reorganization of sensorimotor and visual systems after peripheral and central lesions.

Single-pulse TMS: used to calculate central motor-conduction time, prolonged in upper motor neuron disorders.

Paired-pulse TMS: used to assess changes in cortical excitability (e.g., in studies of motor control, movement disorders, nervous system maturation).

Repetitive TMS (rTMS): produces transient changes in cerebral blood flow and cortical excitability. Used in research to study effects of temporary inactivation of cortical regions and to study connectivity among brain regions. Clinical role of TMS (diagnosis, prognosis, treatment) not yet established.

CHAPTER 16 ■ NEUROVASCULAR IMAGING

CT, MRI

See Chapter 13.

CATHETER ANGIOGRAPHY

Intra-arterial injection of iodinated contrast agent. Real-time images of contrast-filled vessels obtained via fluoroscopy. Unsurpassed for detection of stenosis, occlusion, recanalization, ulceration, dissection, aneurysm.

Disadvantages: 0.5–3% risk of embolic stroke; expensive; specialized catheter skills required.

Primary method for preoperative evaluation of intracranial aneurysms or arteriovenous malformation (AVM), especially if interventional catheter therapy is considered.

In many centers, now used only to study intracranial vascular disease not visualized by MRI, MRA, or Doppler.

INTERVENTIONAL TECHNIQUES

Occlusion (using coils, glue) of abnormal vessels and aneurysms, e.g., AVM, aneurysm, fistula.

Under evaluation in clinical trials: direct delivery of thrombolytic agents to intravascular clots; angioplasty or insertion of stent to treat arterial stenosis. See also Chapter 17.

DOPPLER MEASUREMENTS

High-frequency continuous sound wave directed into tissue from crystal probe; signal reflected by flowing blood recorded and processed through loudspeaker (sonography).

Extracranial Duplex Doppler Studies: two crystals in single probe head; one measures blood flow, the other images vessel walls. Commonly used to estimate degree of internal carotid artery stenosis.

Intracranial Doppler Studies: used to determine direction and velocity of arterial flow in major vessels of circle of Willis, distal vertebral, basilar arteries. Advantages: safe, fast, portable.

REGIONAL CEREBRAL BLOOD FLOW

Radioactive xenon (^{133}Xe), inhaled or injected, used to generate map of cortical blood flow. Can be used at bedside, in operating room, or in ICU. Spatial resolution inferior to that of PET or SPECT. Provides no information about subcortical perfusion.

Used with induced hypercapnia or hypotension to test autoregulatory capacity of brain vessels: focal failure of vasodilatory response may indicate reduced perfusion pressure. May also be used to confirm brain death.

STABLE-XENON CT

Inhaled non-radioactive xenon gas used as contrast agent. High-resolution map of cortical and subcortical perfusion, automatically co-registered with baseline CT. Limited by poor signal/noise ratio, physiologic and anesthetic effects of high xenon concentrations required.

SPECT

Maps of photons emitted by injected radioisotopes as they travel through circulation.

Images cerebral perfusion. Examples: (a) measure focal changes in blood flow during seizure; (b) assess cerebrovascular reserve (by comparing SPECT before and after administration of vasodilator, such as acetazolamide) in region downstream of arterial stenosis.

PET

Images physiology based on radioactive compounds.

Imaging brain metabolic activity (FDG-PET): fluoro-deoxyglucose taken up by metabolically active neurons; metabolites do not immediately return to circulation; positron then emitted, indicating location of higher metabolic activity.

Imaging receptor distribution: radioisotope molecule incorporated into receptor-specific binding agent (e.g., raclopride for dopamine receptors).

Imaging particular compound distribution: radioisotope incorporated into compound of choice. Resulting map shows distribution of compound in brain.

Compared to SPECT: not limited to perfusion; more expensive; better spatial resolution; radioisotopes short-lived (must be made in nearby cyclotron); imaging must be performed within minutes of injection.

CHAPTER 17 ■ ENDOVASCULAR SURGICAL NEURORADIOLOGY

Treatment of cerebrovascular disease with minimally invasive intravascular techniques, i.e., introduction of microcatheter via femoral artery.

CEREBRAL ANEURYSMS

Catheter used to place detachable coil (usually platinum wire) inside aneurysm. Occlusion of aneurysm induces local thrombosis followed by healing.

An alternative to craniotomy and surgical clipping of ruptured aneurysms; management of unruptured aneurysms controversial.

ENDOVASCULAR REVASCULARIZATION

Angioplasty: balloon surrounding catheter is temporarily inflated at area of arterial narrowing to expand lumen.
Stent: mesh tube that holds walls of a narrowed blood vessel open.
Extracranial carotid stenosis: surgical carotid endarterectomy is current standard of treatment. Stent angioplasty may be used for patients with contraindications to surgery, restenosis after endarterectomy, radiation-induced stenosis, high cervical stenosis, or contralateral carotid occlusion.
Use of balloon angioplasty for intracranial cerebral revascularization is being explored; experience limited by technical demands and inherent risk.

ACUTE STROKE

Intra-arterial administration of thrombolytics and mechanical thrombectomy within 3 and 6 hours of stroke onset are under investigation.

ARTERIOVENOUS MALFORMATIONS (AVM) AND DURAL FISTULAS

Endovascular AVM embolization prior to surgical resection may reduce surgical morbidity.

Some dural arteriovenous fistulae may be curable with endovascular treatment alone.

PERCUTANEOUS SPINAL INTERVENTION: VERTEBROPLASTY

Injection of cement into vertebral body under fluoroscopic guidance. Stabilizes bone fragments after vertebral compression fracture to palliate back pain.

CHAPTER 18 ■ LUMBAR PUNCTURE AND CSF EXAMINATION

LUMBAR PUNCTURE (LP)

INDICATIONS

See Table 18.1.

CONTRAINDICATIONS

Infection of skin over the spine, at site of planned puncture.

TABLE 18.1

INDICATIONS FOR LUMBAR PUNCTURE

Essential for diagnosis:
  Infections: meningitis (bacterial, fungal, Whipple, Lyme)
  Tumor of meninges (carcinoma, lymphoma, glioma)
  Viral meningitis or encephalomyelitis (for antibodies, PCR)
  Sporadic prion disease (14-3-3 protein test)
  Neurosyphilis
  Intracranial bleeding (if CT negative but suspect
    subarachnoid hemorrhage)

Helpful in diagnosis:
  Ascertain absence of blood before starting anticoagulant
    therapy for stroke
  Disorders of intracranial pressure
  Normal-pressure hydrocephalus
  High-pressure normocephalus (idiopathic intracranial
    hypertension, pseudotumor cerebri)
  Intracranial hypotension
  Peripheral neuropathies (GBS, CIDP, Lyme neuropathy,
    Dejerine-Sottas syndrome)
    MS, transverse myelitis
    Granulomatous angiitis of the brain
    KSS

PCR, polymerase chain reaction.

Mass lesion or edema on head CT. If no evidence of mass lesion or edema on brain imaging, papilledema is not a contraindication to LP.

Platelet count $\leq 50,000/mm^3$: LP only for urgent clinical indications. Platelet count $\leq 20,000/mm^3$ or dropping rapidly: platelet transfusion recommended just before LP.

Patients taking heparin: hold heparin drip for ≥ 1 hour; consider giving protamine. Heparin therapy should not start for at least 1 hour after bloody tap.

Patients taking warfarin: hold warfarin; consider vitamin K or fresh frozen plasma.

COMPLICATIONS

Worsening of brain herniation or spinal cord compression; headache (occurs in about 25%); subarachnoid hemorrhage; diplopia; backache; radicular symptoms.

CSF PRESSURE

Normal lumbar CSF pressure: 60–200 mm H_2O (up to 250 mm in obese people).

Low pressure: recent LP, dehydration, spinal subarachnoid block, CSF fistula.

Increased pressure: brain edema, intracranial mass lesion, infection, acute stroke, cerebral venous occlusion, congestive heart failure, pulmonary insufficiency, hepatic failure.

Benign intracranial hypertension (pseudotumor cerebri), spontaneous intracranial hypotension: see Chapter 50.

CSF ANALYSIS

CSF CELLS

Normal: ≤5 lymphocytes or mononuclear cells/mm^3.

High white cell count (pleocytosis): disease in CNS or meninges (Table 18.2). Includes: brain infarct, SAH, brain tumors, infection/inflammation, MS.

Cytologic studies for malignant cells: for possible CNS tumor.

Aseptic meningitis: CSF pleocytosis with normal CSF sugar; CSF protein high or normal.

BLOOD IN CSF

Corrections for increased white cell count, increased protein: subtract one white cell and 1 mg protein for every 1,000 red cells (if hematocrit normal).

Traumatic LP vs. SAH

Three-tube test: collect CSF in three separate tubes.

Traumatic LP: fluid generally clears between first and third tube, supernatant fluid clear (no hemolysis).

SAH: blood generally evenly admixed in the three tubes.

Xanthochromia: yellow appearance. Due to high CSF protein concentration (≥150 mg/dL), hemolysis. Place tube of CSF upright for 30 minutes; compare supernatant fluid with tap water. Xanthochromic fluid with normal or only mildly increased protein (<150 mg/dL) usually indicates SAH (≥2 to 4 hours earlier).

TABLE 18.2

CSF FINDINGS IN MENINGITIS

Meningitis	Pressure (mm H$_2$O)	Leukocytes (/mm^3)	Protein (mg/dL)	Glucose (mg/dL)
Acute bacterial	Usually high	Several hundred to >60,000; usually few thousand; occasionally <100 (especially meningococcal or early disease); PMNs predominate	Usually 100–500; occasionally >1,000	5–40 in most cases (in absence of hyperglycemia)
Tuberculous	Usually high; may be low with CSF block in advanced stage	Usually 25–100; rarely >500; lymphocytes predominate except in early stages, when PMNs may be 80% of cells	Nearly always elevated, usually 100–200; may be much higher if CSF block	<45 in 75% of cases
Cryptococcal	Usually high	0–800; average 50; lymphocytes dominate	Usually 20–500; average 100	Low in most cases

(*continued*)

TABLE 18.2

CSF FINDINGS IN MENINGITIS (*Continued*)

Meningitis	Pressure (mm H$_2$O)	Leukocytes (/mm^3)	Protein (mg/dL)	Glucose (mg/dL)
Viral	Normal or moderately elevated	5 to few hundred; but may be >1,000, particularly in choriomeningitis; lymphocytes dominate; PMNs in first few days	Frequently normal or slightly high; <100	Normal (reduced in 25% of cases of mumps and herpes simplex)
Syphilitic (acute)	Usually high	Average 500; usually lymphocytes; rarely PMNs	Average 100	Normal (rarely reduced)
Cysticercosis	Often increased; low with CSF block	Increased mononuclear and PMN leukocytes with 2%–7% eosinophilia in about 50% of cases	Usually 50–200	Low in 20% of cases
Sarcoid	Normal or high	0–100 mononuclear cells	Slight-to-moderate elevation	Low in 50% of cases
Tumor	Normal or high	0 to several hundred mononuclear leukocytes plus malignant cells	Elevated, often to high levels	Normal with mass; low in 75% of carcinomatous meningitis

CHARACTERISTICS OF CSF

Total Protein
Normal: 15–45 mg/dL.

High protein content: nonspecific sign of neurologic disease (increased endothelial cell permeability). ≥500 mg/dL: meningitis, bloody fluid, spinal cord tumor with spinal block. 100 to 300 mg/dL: polyneuritis (GBS), diabetic radiculoneuropathy, myxedema.

Low protein content (<20 mg/dL): CSF leak caused by previous LP or traumatic dural fistula; pseudotumor cerebri.

Immunoglobulins
Increased: MS, neurosyphilis.

IgG index: $(IgG_{CSF}/IgG_{serum})/(albumin_{CSF}/albumin_{serum})$. Values >0.65 imply intrathecal synthesis of IgG.

Oligoclonal bands on gel electrophoresis: abnormally increased CSF immunoglobulins. Multiple bands in CSF (and absent in serum) abnormal; present in 90% of MS cases.

Glucose
Normal range may be affected by serum glucose levels. However, values below 40 mg/dL are invariably abnormal.

High glucose: if serum glucose high 4 hours or more prior to LP (diabetes mellitus).

Low glucose (hypoglycorrhachia): hypoglycemia; bacterial or fungal meningitis, or meningeal tumor (gliomatosis or carcinomatosis). Less commonly: mumps, herpes simplex, zoster meningoencephalitis, cysticercosis, amebic meningitis, neurosyphilis, sarcoidosis, SAH (4–8 days after onset). Usually accompanied by increased CSF lactate. Low lactate indicates impaired glucose transport across blood-brain barrier.

MICROBIOLOGIC AND SEROLOGIC REACTIONS

Indication: suspected infection.

Available tests: stains (bacterial, fungal), cultures (bacterial, fungal, viral), antigen detection, treponemal antibody tests for syphilis, polymerase chain reaction.

CHAPTER 19 ■ MUSCLE AND NERVE BIOPSY

Helps in differentiating neurogenic and myopathic causes of limb weakness as well as specific causes of myopathy, peripheral neuropathy.

Indications: syndromes of limb weakness with cause not established by neurologic examination, family history, laboratory tests, CSF, electrodiagnostic studies, or DNA analysis.

Limitations: focal or "skip" lesions may be missed in biopsy; changes too mild to distinguish from normal or too advanced ("end-stage" muscle).

SKELETAL MUSCLE BIOPSY

Open biopsy provides better-quality specimen than needle (percutaneous) biopsy.

May help in evaluation of limb weakness, infantile hypotonia, exercise intolerance, myoglobinuria, cramps.

Identifies muscular dystrophy, polymyositis, inclusion body myositis, congenital myopathy, spinal muscular atrophy; glycolytic or oxidative enzyme defect; myopathies associated with alcohol, electrolyte disturbance, drug toxicity, carcinoma, endocrine overactivity or underactivity, long-term treatment with steroids.

Identifies denervation in motor neuron diseases, neuropathies.

ROUTINE HISTOLOGY

Neuropathy: group atrophy.
Myopathy: necrotic fibers, regenerating fibers, excessive glycogen or fat.
Polymyositis: lymphocytic infiltration.

HISTOCHEMISTRY

Denervation: fiber-type grouping, target fibers.
Congenital myopathy: central cores, nemaline rods.

Metabolic myopathy: excessive sarcoplasmic glycogen, lipid, mitochondria (ragged red fibers).

BIOCHEMICAL ASSAYS

Detect reduction of enzymes of intermediary metabolism (e.g., glycolytic pathway), or mitochondrial enzymes (carnitine palmitoyl transferase, enzymes of oxidative phosphorylation and electron transport chain).

IMMUNOHISTOCHEMISTRY

Absence of dystrophin in Duchenne muscular dystrophy; discontinuities of sarcolemmal dystrophin in Becker muscular dystrophy; lack of sarcoglycans, merosin, emerin, or other proteins in specific muscular dystrophies; abnormal inclusions in inclusion-body myositis; amyloid in amyloid myopathy.

PERIPHERAL NERVE BIOPSY

SURAL NERVE BIOPSY

General indication: seek specific cause of sensory or sensorimotor neuropathy, amyloid periarteritis, infiltration by tumor cells, sarcoid.

Light microscopy: useful in vasculitis, amyloidosis, leprosy, sensory perineuritis, cholesterol emboli, infiltration of nerve by leukemic or lymphoma cells, malignant angioendotheliomatosis (intravascular lymphoma), giant axonal neuropathy, adult polyglucosan body disease.

Special preparations: include semi-thin sections, teased nerve fibers, electron microscopy.

Axonal neuropathy: marked depletion of nerve fibers, interstitial fibrosis, with or without myelin debris or regeneration of axons. Examples: toxic or metabolic disorder (e.g., alcoholism, diabetes), amyloidosis, paraneoplastic syndromes.

Demyelinating neuropathy: segmental demyelination and remyelination, with loss of myelinated fibers and formation of "onion bulbs" (regions of nerve with excessive, irregular myelin layers). Examples: immunologically mediated neuropathy. Demyelination usually variable along nerve in acquired neuropathy, uniform in inherited neuropathy.

Complications: loss of sensation and paresthesias along lateral border of foot in all patients; decreases with time. Causalgia (neuropathic pain) in less than 5%.

SKIN PUNCH BIOPSY

Used to assess cutaneous sensory and autonomic nerves; density of fibers can be quantified at multiple sites to determine course and distribution of peripheral nerve disease.

Indications: suspected pure sensory small-fiber neuropathy (burning feet, painful paresthesias), toxic neuropathy, diabetic truncal neuropathy.

CHAPTER 20 ■
NEUROPSYCHOLOGICAL
EVALUATION

Tests designed to assess cognition, behavior. Helpful in diagnosing and characterizing dementia.

Characteristic patterns of performance support diagnosis of some specific conditions.

Factors that may affect test performance: depression, other psychiatric disorders, medication, motivation.

ABILITIES TESTED IN
NEUROPSYCHOLOGICAL EVALUATION

Intellectual ability: Wechsler Adult Intelligence Scale-III (WAIS-III), Wechsler Intelligence Scale for Children-III (WISC-III): standardized global IQ score with verbal and performance subscores. Mean ± standard deviation: 100 ± 15. Pattern of subtest scores ("scatter") usually of more interest than overall score; identifies specific strengths and weaknesses.

Memory: pattern of memory loss helps in diagnosis of dementia.

Construction: spatial relation abilities.

Language: comprehension, fluency, repetition, naming assessed in spoken and written language (see Chapter 2).

Perception: double simultaneous stimulation in touch, hearing, or sight; stereognosis; graphesthesia; spatial perception; auditory discrimination.

Executive functions: ability to plan, sequence, monitor behavior. Linked to prefrontal cortex. *Wisconsin Card Sort* test: "set switching" (ability to follow new rules without explicit instruction). *Stroop Color-Word* test: "set maintenance" (ability to continue following correct rules despite distractions).

Attention: tasks of reaction-time, mental tracking.

Motor skills, reasoning, personality, emotional state also assessed.

CLINICAL APPLICATIONS

Dementia: (a) detect early changes; (b) differential diagnosis between dementia and non-dementing illness (e.g., depression), or between different forms of dementia (Alzheimer, Lewy body, vascular, frontotemporal); (c) confirm or quantify disease progression.

Epilepsy: presurgical evaluation before temporal lobectomy for intractable epilepsy.

Medication trials: evaluate effects of new drugs on cognition.

Psychiatric disorders: differential diagnosis of psychiatric and neurologic disorders.

Developmental disability: evaluation of learning disabilities, behavioral disorders, attention deficit disorder, autism, dyslexia.

CHAPTER 21 ■ DNA DIAGNOSIS

Several hundred diseases amenable to DNA diagnosis. List is rapidly expanding. Examples provided in chapters on specific inherited conditions.

For further information: **http://www.genetests.org** serves as an online textbook of human genetics and lists laboratories that perform specific genetic tests.

Genetic heterogeneity leads to problems in nomenclature for some conditions:

Allelic heterogeneity: different mutations at the same gene locus cause one phenotype (disease or syndrome).

Allelic affinity: different mutations at the same gene locus produce different phenotypes.

Locus heterogeneity: same clinical syndrome caused by mutations in different genes on different chromosomes.

Section III

Infections of the Nervous System

CHAPTER 22 ▪ BACTERIAL INFECTIONS AND ASEPTIC MENINGITIS

ACUTE PURULENT MENINGITIS

Progression for hours. Polymorphonuclear pleocytosis usually present in CSF.

GENERAL CONSIDERATIONS

Routes of meningeal infection: (a) blood (septicemia or spread from distant sites, e.g., heart, lung); (b) direct extension from local septic focus (e.g., sinusitis, brain abscess); (c) openings in skull (e.g., compound fractures, neurosurgery).

Signs of meningeal irritation: stiff neck; Kernig sign (pain in back or neck as either leg is passively flexed at hip and extended at knee); Brudzinski sign (flexion of legs at hip in response to passive neck flexion). Often absent in newborn, elderly, or comatose patients.

Symptoms and clinical course similar regardless of organism.

Most common organisms differ by age.

Adults: *Streptococcus pneumoniae*, then *Neisseria meningitidis*, then cryptogenic (organism not identified).

Neonates: Group B streptococci, *Escherichia coli* (see Chapter 75).

Children: *Hemophilus influenzae* in past; now very rare due to HIB vaccination.

Evaluation: acute meningeal syndrome mandates emergency lumbar puncture and emergent empiric intravenous antibiotic therapy.

Initial antibiotic therapy: third generation cephalosporin and vancomycin; add ampicillin if *Listeria monocytogenes* is considered. Definitive therapy dictated by organism and identified source of infection.

Mortality of acute bacterial meningitis: 3–21% (depending on organism), mostly in first 48 hours.

MENINGOCOCCAL MENINGITIS

Epidemiology

25% of all bacterial meningitis in United States. Children and young adults predominantly affected. Spread by carriers or infected individuals. Vaccine available against some serogroups.

Symptoms and Signs

Chills and fever, headache, nausea and vomiting, back pain, stiff neck, prostration. Herpes labialis, conjunctivitis, and petechial or hemorrhagic rash common. Characteristic sharp shrill cry in children (meningeal cry). Fever (101–103° F; temperature may be normal with older age, diabetes), tachycardia, tachypnea.

Delirium, stupor, coma. Convulsive seizures frequent. Cranial nerve palsies, focal neurologic signs uncommon early in course.

Laboratory Data

Increased white blood cell (WBC) count; organism may be cultured from nasopharynx, blood, or skin lesions.

CSF: high pressure, cloudy, high WBC count (mostly neutrophils), high protein, low glucose. Gram stain: gram-negative diplococci intra- and extracellular. Culture positive in 90% of untreated cases.

Diagnosis

Diagnosis likely in patient with headache, vomiting, chills and fever, stiff neck, petechial rash. Confirmed by CSF Gram stain and culture. (Rapid bacterial antigen detection in CSF possible, but less sensitive and specific).

Treatment

Initial antibiotics for bacterial meningitis: third-generation cephalosporin (ceftriaxone, cefotaxime) and vancomycin (for cephalosporin-resistant streptococcus). Start no later than 1 to 2 hours after obtaining history and examination consistent with diagnosis.

May change antibiotics to penicillin (chloramphenicol if allergic) after Gram stain or culture confirm organism and sensitivity.

Reexamine CSF after 24 to 48 hours if no dramatic improvement.

Intravenous fluids for dehydration (common), heparin for disseminated intravascular coagulation, anticonvulsants for seizures.

Consider corticosteroids (see below). Prophylactic rifampin for people in intimate contact with patient.

Prognosis
Overall mortality rate about 10%.

Complications and Sequelae
Neurologic: convulsions, cranial nerve palsies (including deafness), focal cerebral lesions, damage to spinal cord or nerve roots, hydrocephalus.

Systemic (if other body sites infected): panophthalmitis, arthritis, purpura, pericarditis, endocarditis, myocarditis, pleurisy, orchitis, epididymitis, albuminuria or hematuria, adrenal hemorrhage, disseminated intravascular coagulation.

HEMOPHILUS INFLUENZAE MENINGITIS

Rare in United States and other countries with vaccination. More frequent in adults in these countries; infancy, early childhood elsewhere.

Pathology, symptoms, signs, and CSF and other laboratory abnormalities: as in other acute purulent meningitis.

Risk factors: acute sinusitis, otitis media, skull fracture, autumn or spring season. Associated with immunodeficiency, diabetes, and alcoholism.

Diagnosis: CSF culture or detection of capsular antigens in CSF (more rapid but less sensitive and specific).

Treatment: initially as in other acute purulent meningitides; add ampicillin to cover *Listeria* in neonates and others at risk (see below). Continue antibiotics for 12 to 15 days. Corticosteroids (given in first 2 to 4 days) reduce frequency of sequelae in children with *H. influenzae* or streptococcal meningitis. Role in adults not established.

Course and prognosis: Duration 10 to 20 days; occasionally fulminant. Mortality >90% in untreated infants, 10% with treatment. Sequelae: mental retardation, seizures, blindness, ocular palsies, deafness, hemiplegia. Suspect subdural effusion (most common with *H. influenzae*) in children with persistent vomiting, bulging fontanelles, convulsions, focal neurologic signs, persistent fever. Treat effusion by needle aspiration.

PNEUMOCOCCAL MENINGITIS
Organism: *Streptococcus pneumoniae.*
Sources: otitis media, sinusitis, skull fracture, upper respiratory infection, lung infection.

Risk factors: alcoholism, asplenism, sickle-cell disease, age
(<1 year or >50 years).

Treatment: as for *H. influenzae* meningitis. Eradicate primary
infection, surgically if necessary. Close persistent CSF fistula
by suturing dura.

Prognosis: mortality 20% to 30%. Good prognostic factors:
meningitis after skull fracture or with no known infection.
Poor prognostic factors: pneumonia, empyema, lung abscess, endocarditis.

Meningitis Due to Other Streptococci

Less than 5% of all meningitis. Always secondary to septic
focus elsewhere.

Clinical manifestations, laboratory findings, and treatment: similar to pneumococcal meningitis.

Group B streptococcus most common cause of meningitis
in neonates (see below).

STAPHYLOCOCCAL MENINGITIS

Relatively infrequent.

Sources: furuncles on face, cavernous sinus thrombosis, epidural or subdural abscess, intraventricular shunts, endocarditis.

Clinical features: as in other acute meningitis.

Treatment: initially as described above. When staphylococ-
cal species identified, change to penicillinase-resistant penicillin; add vancomycin if resistance is likely (e.g., if noso-
comial). Treat for 2 to 4 weeks. Eradicate source of
infection.

ACUTE MENINGITIS CAUSED BY OTHER BACTERIA

Gram-Negative Bacilli

E. coli is second most common cause of meningitis in neonates
(after Group B strep). Often accompanies septicemia. Clinical
syndrome: irritability, lethargy, bulging fontanelle.

Also occurs in adults with immunosuppression, chronic
illness, diabetes, penetrating head injury, neurosurgery.

Treatment: third-generation cephalosporin (ceftazidime if
Pseudomonas aeruginosa suspected) and aminoglycoside.
Mortality 40–70%.

Listeria Monocytogenes

At risk: neonates; adults with chronic disease. Diagnosis: "diphtheroids" in CSF Gram stain. May cause prominent brainstem signs (rhomboencephalitis).

Treatment: ampicillin (add to initial regimen if suspected, as it is cephalosporin-resistant). Mortality 30% to 60%.

Acute Purulent Meningitis of Unknown Cause
Usually syndrome as above but with atypical CSF findings (moderate pleocytosis; normal or slightly decreased glucose). May be due to partial treatment: insufficient antibiotic dose or duration. Treatment is as for other acute purulent meningitis.

Recurrent Bacterial Meningitis
Recurrence usually due to immunosuppression or breach of dura mater (congenital defect, trauma, penetrating injuries, neurosurgery). Organism typically *S. pneumoniae*.

Diagnosis: seek CSF leak as rhinorrhea or otorrhea (check for high glucose concentration in escaping fluid); CT with intrathecal iodinated contrast agent.

Treatment: treat episodes as for any acute bacterial meningitis. Pneumococcal vaccine. Consider prophylactic penicillin therapy. Close CSF fistula if identified.

SUBACUTE MENINGITIS

Usually caused by tubercle bacilli or mycotic organisms.

TUBERCULOUS MENINGITIS

Differs from other bacterial meningitis: subacute course (days to weeks), higher mortality, less CSF pleocytosis, higher risk of sequelae despite treatment.

Symptoms and Signs
Prodrome: headache, vomiting, fever, irritability, insomnia for 2 to 3 weeks. Then progressing headache, stiff neck, seizures (especially in children), cranial nerve syndromes (late), stupor, coma.

Fever (initially may be low-grade), irritability, stiff neck, Kernig and Brudzinski signs, papilledema, cranial nerve abnormalities (especially third nerve palsy), other focal signs. Later apathy, confusion, lethargy, stupor.

Laboratory Data

CSF: increased pressure, slightly cloudy, moderate pleocytosis (25–500 cells/mm^3, mostly lymphocytes), increased protein, decreased glucose (20–40 mg/dL), negative VDRL test and cryptococcal antigen, no growth on routine CSF cultures.

Diagnosis

CSF profile usually suggestive. Confirm by CSF: (1) stained smear identifying acid-fast bacilli (sensitivity 20–30% with single test, up to 75% with multiple tests); (2) PCR for mycobacterial DNA (rapid; highly sensitive and specific); or (3) mycobacterial culture (may take weeks).

Tuberculin skin test, chest X-ray, other tests for primary TB focus.

Differential diagnosis: acute purulent meningitis (higher cell count, positive routine cultures), syphilitic meningitis (normal CSF glucose, positive VDRL), cryptococcal meningitis (positive CSF cryptococcal antigen), viral meningitis (normal CSF glucose), carcinomatous meningitis, sarcoid meningitis.

Treatment

Four oral drugs (rifampin, isoniazid, pyrazinamide, ethambutol). Multidrug resistance increasing. Treat for 18–24 months. Consider steroids in early phase. Pyridoxine given to prevent isoniazid-induced peripheral neuropathy.

Prognosis and Course

Mortality: nearly 100% in 8 weeks if not treated; 10% with treatment. Poor prognostic factors: advanced age, cranial nerve abnormalities, confusion, lethargy, high CSF protein content, late therapy.

Sequelae occur in 25%: seizures, deafness, blindness, hemiplegia, paraplegia, quadriplegia.

SUBDURAL AND EPIDURAL INFECTIONS

See Chapter 23.

LEPROSY

Chronic disease caused by *Mycobacterium leprae*. Skin, peripheral nerves affected. Lepromatous, tuberculoid types.

Epidemiology: tropical and subtropical climates; estimated 10 to 20 million infected worldwide; South and Central America, China, India, Africa.

Etiology: acid-fast, rod-shaped bacillus. Transmitted by prolonged direct contact.

Symptoms and signs. Skin: erythematous macule, then annular macule. Nerve: nodules or fusiform swelling, especially ulnar, great auricular, posterior tibial, common peroneal, fifth and seventh cranial nerves. Attacks of neuralgic pain; then distal weakness, sensory loss. Other signs: anhidrosis (no sweat), cyanosis of hands and feet; trophic ulcers of knuckles and soles; arthropathies; resorption of distal bones of fingers.

Laboratory data: false-positive serologic tests for syphilis in 33%. Slightly increased CSF protein.

Diagnosis: examine cutaneous and nerve biopsy specimens for acid-fast bacilli.

Course and prognosis: death in 10–20 years in cutaneous form (primarily lepromatous). Better prognosis for neural form (primarily tuberculoid).

Treatment: tuberculoid form: dapsone and monthly rifampin, at least 6 months. Lepromatous form: Add clofazimine, treat for at least 2 years.

INFECTIVE ENDOCARDITIS

Risk factors: rheumatic heart disease, prosthetic valve, intravenous drug use, degenerative cardiac disease, congenital heart disease.

Neurologic complications: 20% to 40%: embolic cerebral infarct, intracranial hemorrhage (mycotic aneurysms), brain abscess, meningitis, encephalopathy. *Staphylococcus aureus* and *S. pneumoniae*: high risk of CNS complications.

Diagnosis: serum ESR, blood bacterial cultures, CSF analysis, CT or MRI, transesophageal echocardiogram.

Treatment: prolonged antibiotics; sometimes replace infected valve. Mycotic aneurysms not easily clipped.

RICKETTSIAL INFECTIONS

Obligate intracellular parasites; pathogenic forms in humans replicate in arthropods.

ROCKY MOUNTAIN SPOTTED FEVER

Acute endemic febrile illness caused by *Rickettsia rickettsii*. Transmitted by wood tick in Rocky Mountain and Pacific states, dog tick in East and South.

Epidemiology: 1,000 cases annually in the United States; almost all states, especially rural. Peak incidence: late spring, early summer.

Systemic symptoms and signs: known tick bite 3–12 days before symptoms in 80%. Abrupt onset: headache, fever, chills, myalgia, arthralgia, prostration. Rose-red maculopapular rash on wrists, ankles, palms, soles, and forearms; spreads proximally, becomes petechial.

Neurologic symptoms and signs: Common, headache, restlessness, insomnia, stiff back. Others: delirium or coma alternating with restlessness, abnormal movements, seizures, visual and auditory symptoms.

Laboratory data: proteinuria, hematuria, and oliguria. CSF: slight lymphocytic pleocytosis and protein elevation.

Treatment: tetracycline or doxycycline (chloramphenicol preferred in children). Preventive measures: in tick-infested areas, avoid skin exposure, yearly vaccination for people with occupational risk.

Course and prognosis: fever subsides in 2–3 weeks. Residual neurologic signs for several months. Mortality 20% untreated.

TYPHUS FEVER

Epidemic typhus (*Rickettsia prowazekii*): spread by body louse; Balkans, Middle East, North Africa, Asia, Mexico, Andes.

Brill-Zinsser disease: recrudescence of epidemic typhus occurring years later.

Murine typhus (*Rickettsia typhi*): transmitted by fleas. Southeastern and Gulf states, especially late summer and fall.

SCRUB TYPHUS

Caused by *Rickettsia tsutsugamushi*; transmitted by mites.

Epidemiology: eastern, southeastern Asia, India, northern Australia.

Symptoms and signs: 10- to 12-day incubation, then fever, chills, headache. Primary skin lesion (eschar) at site of mite attachment. Macular rash on trunk spreading to limbs, lymphadenopathy, deafness, apathy. Delirium, restlessness, coma in severe cases.

Diagnosis: Weil-Felix test; antibody detection by immunofluorescence.

Treatment: similar to Rocky Mountain spotted fever.

Course and prognosis: 2- to 3-week course. Complications: bronchitis, pneumonia, myocardial degeneration, gangrene of skin or limbs, thrombosis of large abdominal, pulmonary, or cerebral vessels.

HUMAN EHRLICHIOSIS

Classification of organisms and pathogenesis unknown; apparent leukocyte infection.

Two forms: Human monocytic ehrlichiosis (HME) and human granulocytic ehrlichiosis (HGE).

Probably transmitted by ticks.

Epidemiology: HME, southern and southeastern United States. HGE: Midwest, New England, New York state.

Symptoms and signs: fever, myalgia, headache. Rash in 20%. Encephalopathy and ataxia may occur.

Diagnosis: lymphopenia (HME), neutropenia (HGE), elevated hepatic enzymes. CSF: pleocytosis, elevated protein. Confirm with antibody titers or detection of intracellular organisms by immunofluorescence.

Treatment: doxycycline.

Course and prognosis: both HME and HGE may be fatal. Good prognosis with antibiotic treatment.

OTHER BACTERIAL INFECTIONS

BRUCELLOSIS

Infection by gram-negative rods of genus *Brucella*.

Transmitted from cattle and swine. At risk: slaughterhouse workers, livestock producers, veterinarians, and people who ingest unpasteurized milk or milk products.

Symptoms and signs: chills, sweats, fever, malaise, headache. Approximately 20% progress to chronic localized infection.

Neurologic involvement rare; usually meningitis, sometimes brain abscess.

Laboratory tests: CSF, increased pressure, lymphocytic pleocytosis, increased protein, decreased glucose, increased gamma globulin.

Diagnosis: clinical syndrome, culture of organism from blood or CSF, serologic tests.

Treatment: doxycycline or other tetracycline (or trimethoprim-sulfamethoxazole) plus an aminoglycoside.

MYCOPLASMA PNEUMONIAE INFECTION

Pneumonia caused by *M. pneumoniae* may be complicated by meningitis, encephalitis, postinfectious leukoencephalitis, acute cerebellar ataxia, transverse myelitis, ascending polyneuritis, radiculopathy, cranial neuropathy, and acute psychosis. Meningitis with encephalopathy most common of these.

CSF: leukocytosis (neutrophils or mononuclear cells), mildly elevated protein, normal glucose. Cultures negative. Confirm diagnosis by rise in serum antibody titer or detection of mycoplasma PCR in blood or CSF.

Treatment: doxycycline and erythromycin.

LEGIONELLA PNEUMOPHILA INFECTION

Acquired by inhaling contaminated aerosols or dust from air-conditioning systems, water, or soil.

Pneumonia due to *L. pneumophila* may be complicated by acute encephalomyelitis, pronounced cerebellar deficit, chorea, and peripheral neuropathy. Common symptoms: confusion, delirium, and hallucinations. Organism difficult to culture; diagnosis made by rise in specific antibody titer.

Treatment: erythromycin or azithromycin.

MISCELLANEOUS

See respective chapters for: neurosyphilis (28), leptospirosis (29), Lyme disease (30), Whipple disease (35).

ASEPTIC MENINGITIS

MENINGISM

Headache, neck stiffness, Kernig sign, and, rarely, delirium, seizures, or coma coinciding with onset of any acute febrile illness in child or young adult.

CSF: increased pressure; no cells; protein sometimes reduced; normal glucose.
Treatment: single LP often relieves symptoms. Syndrome resolves spontaneously in few days.

ASEPTIC MENINGEAL REACTION

CSF pleocytosis without bacterial infection.

Causes
Parameningeal infection: associated with infection, tumor, infarct, or other CNS lesion or morbid process in the skull or spinal cavity.
Foreign substance in subarachnoid space: air, dyes, drugs, blood.
Connective tissue disorders: systemic lupus erythematosus, periarteritis nodosa, Sjögren syndrome.
Medications: trimethoprim-sulfamethoxazole; nonsteroidal anti-inflammatory agents; IVIG.

CSF Findings
Increased pressure, pleocytosis, mildly increased protein, normal glucose, absence of organisms on smear or culture.

VOGT-KOYANAGI-HARADA SYNDROME

Rare. Cause unknown. Chronic uveitis, retinal hemorrhages and detachment, depigmentation of skin and hair, CNS signs.
Neurologic symptoms due to arachnoiditis. Headache (common), deafness, hemiplegia, ocular palsies, psychosis, meningeal signs.

CSF: increased pressure, moderate lymphocytic pleocytosis, normal or slightly increased protein, normal glucose.
Course: 6–12 months; sometimes recurs years later. No proven therapy. Corticosteroids may help.

MOLLARET MENINGITIS

Episodic benign aseptic meningitis of unknown cause, with attacks of headache, neck stiffness, and fever lasting 2 to 3 days at a time.

CSF: pleocytosis and slightly increased protein during acute episode. No effective therapy. Course usually 3 to 5 years.

BEHÇET SYNDROME

Inflammatory disorder of unknown cause. Relapsing uveitis, recurrent genital and oral ulcers.

Epidemiology: common in Japan, Turkey, Israel. Male > female, especially young men. Neurologic symptoms in 10%.

Systemic symptoms and signs: ocular signs present in 90%; include keratoconjunctivitis, iritis, hypopyon (pus in aqueous humor of eye, forms visible white layer between cornea and iris), uveitis, vitreous hemorrhage. Recurrent painful oral or genital ulcers in most. Arthritis in 50%. Low-grade fever common during exacerbations. Erythematous pustule at site of needle puncture a pathognomonic sign.

Neurologic symptoms and signs: any part of nervous system may be involved. Cranial nerve palsies common. Also papilledema, seizures, encephalopathy, aphasia, limb weakness, peripheral neuropathy.

Laboratory data: leukocytosis, high ESR, high serum gamma globulin. CSF: increased pressure, pleocytosis, increased protein, normal glucose, increased gamma globulin. MRI may show high T2-signal white matter lesions.

Course: remissions and exacerbations for years. Poor prognosis with neurologic and posterior uveal tract lesions.

Treatment: no proven therapy. Consider immunosuppressive therapy.

CHAPTER 23 ■ FOCAL INFECTIONS

MALIGNANT EXTERNAL OTITIS

Infection in external auditory canal; spreads to soft tissues to cause cellulitis and abscess.

Risk factors: diabetes in almost all patients; also advanced age, HIV infection.

Etiology: *Pseudomonas aeruginosa, Aspergillus fumigatus.*

Symptoms: facial nerve palsy (30%), otalgia, purulent otorrhea, hearing loss, painful swelling of surrounding tissues, mastoid tenderness.

Investigations: elevated ESR, sometimes mild leukocytosis; MRI findings; CT to detect bony erosion.

Treatment: ceftazidime or ciprofloxacin alone for small lesions; antipseudomonal penicillin plus aminoglycoside or third-generation cephalosporin for more extensive disease or drug resistance. Mortality 10–20% with treatment. Cranial nerve lesions imply poor prognosis.

Complications: osteomyelitis of skull base, abscess, meningitis, death.

OSTEOMYELITIS OF SKULL BASE

Rare complication of malignant external otitis, chronic mastoiditis, or paranasal sinus infection.

Etiology: *P. aeruginosa* most common.

Symptoms: headache, otalgia, hearing loss, otorrhea. Later, cranial nerve lesions. Fever frequently absent. Usually starts weeks or months after taking antibiotics for otitis.

Investigations: slight leukocytosis, high ESR, head CT.

Treatment: antipseudomonal penicillin or cephalosporin plus aminoglycoside. Mortality up to 40%. Poor prognostic factors: intracranial extension, cranial nerve involvement.

BRAIN ABSCESS

Encapsulated or free pus in brain parenchyma.

Incidence
Less than 2% of all intracranial surgery. Highest incidence before age 30 (25% before age 15).

Etiology
(1) Direct extension from cranial infection (mastoid, teeth, paranasal sinuses, osteomyelitis of skull). (2) Infections after skull fracture or neurosurgery. (3) Metastasis from infection in other organs (risk factors: congenital heart defects, pulmonary AVM, subacute infective endocarditis).

25–30% of brain abscesses have no obvious source.

Most common organisms: *Staphylococcus aureus*, streptococci, *Enterobacteriaceae*, *Pseudomonas*, anaerobes (e.g., *Bacteroides*). Gram-negative organisms most frequent in infants. Consider opportunistic organisms (e.g., *Toxoplasma*, fungi, *Nocardia*) in immunosuppressed patients.

Pathology
(1) Early cerebritis: patchy or nonenhancing hypodensity on imaging (days 1–3). (2) Late cerebritis: central necrosis, edema, ring enhancement on imaging (next 2 weeks). (c) Capsule formation.

Symptoms and Signs
Headache, nausea, vomiting, seizures. Fever in <50%. Focal signs in 50%.

Sudden worsening of preexisting headache with new stiff neck heralds rupture into ventricles; high mortality.

Investigations
Leukocytosis, high ESR, positive blood cultures: all may be absent. CT or MRI with contrast typically shows ring-enhancing mass with surrounding edema.

LP contraindicated if symptoms of increased intracranial pressure (risk of transtentorial herniation).

Treatment
CT-guided needle aspiration for diagnosis and therapeutic drainage; add antimicrobial drugs. Open craniotomy for multiloculated abscesses or resistant pathogens such as fungi or *Nocardia*.

Initial therapy based on presumed source: (a) Extension of sinus infection: intravenous high-dose penicillin G (10–20 million units per day), or cefotaxime, and metronidazole. (b) Dental procedure or dental abscess: cover *Actinomyces*. (c) Otogenic source: also cover *Enterobacteriaceae* and

P. aeruginosa. (d) Neurosurgical procedures: vancomycin to cover *S. epidermidis.*

Duration of antibiotic therapy: parenteral for 6–8 weeks followed by oral for 2–3 months.

Short course of high-dose corticosteroids for life-threatening cerebral edema or impending herniation. Phenytoin or carbamazepine for seizure prophylaxis (occur in 50%).

Prognosis
Mortality nearly 100% untreated, up to 30% with treatment. Poor prognostic factors: depressed consciousness, immunosuppression, primary infection in lungs, intraventricular rupture. Sequelae: abscess recurrence, residual focal signs (30–56%).

SUBDURAL EMPYEMA

Pus in subdural space (between dura and arachnoid). Rare.

Etiology
Usually contiguous spread from paranasal sinusitis; incubation period 1–2 weeks. Most frequent organism: Streptococcus; also staphylococci, gram-negative enteric organisms, anaerobes.

Risk factors: infection of middle ear, nasal sinuses, or meninges, compound skull fractures, young age, male sex.

Symptoms and Signs
Chills, fever, focal headache, stiff neck. Later confusion, stupor. Focal deficits or focal seizures in 80–90%. Course acute or subacute.

Investigations
Marked leukocytosis. CT: crescent-shaped hypodensity at brain periphery; contrast enhancement of adjacent brain, mass effect. MRI with contrast is diagnostic test of choice.

LP contraindicated if clinical picture and imaging studies suggest diagnosis (risk of transtentorial herniation).

Treatment
Surgical evacuation of pus. Antibiotics (initial empiric therapy similar to brain abscess, see above) for 3–4 weeks after surgery. Anticonvulsants frequently required.

Complications and Sequelae

Short-term: cerebral edema, septic cortical-vein thrombosis, fulminant meningitis, brain abscess.

Long-term: seizures, hemiparesis, other focal deficits.

Mortality 25–40%. Usually attributable to delay in diagnosis.

INTRACRANIAL EPIDURAL ABSCESS

Almost always with overlying cranial bone infection (e.g., chronic sinusitis, mastoiditis).

Symptoms and signs: headache, fever, malaise, symptoms referable to initial site of infection. Focal neurologic signs rare.

Diagnosis by CT or MRI: extradural lens-shaped defect between skull and brain. CSF findings nonspecific; cultures negative.

Treatment: surgical drainage. Antibiotics as for subdural empyema.

SPINAL EPIDURAL ABSCESS

Collection of pus outside dura mater and within spinal canal. One of every 20,000 hospital admissions in United States. All ages susceptible.

Etiology

Route: (a) extension from infection in adjacent tissue (most common route), such as decubitus ulcer, carbuncle, perinephric abscess; (b) metastasis through blood from infection elsewhere; (c) perforating wounds, spinal surgery, LP.

Risk factors: chronic illness, diabetes, immunosuppressive therapy, heroin abuse.

Organisms: *S. aureus* (50–60%), *Escherichia coli*, other gram-negative organisms, hemolytic and anaerobic streptococci.

Symptoms and Signs

Sudden back pain, malaise, fever, stiff neck, headache, radicular pain; progressing to paraparesis with sensory level if spinal cord compression develops. Tenderness on percussing spine; erythema and swelling at site.

Sudden flaccid paraplegia if spinal artery thrombosis.

Chronic cases: symptoms of epidural spinal tumor. Fever rare.

Investigations

Diagnosis by CT or MRI (MRI most sensitive); differentiate from tumor.

Differential diagnosis: acute or subacute meningitis, acute poliomyelitis, infectious polyneuritis, acute transverse myelitis, MS, and epidural hematoma. Clinical and imaging findings usually differentiate these conditions.

Chronic epidural abscess may be confused with chronic adhesive arachnoiditis or epidural tumors. Granulomatous abscess diagnosed at surgery.

Treatment

Prompt surgical drainage by laminectomy; aerobic and anaerobic cultures obtained at operation.

Antibiotics administered before and after operation. Initial broad-spectrum coverage with third-generation cephalosporin plus vancomycin; consider adding metronidazole (for anaerobic coverage) if abscess due to local extension.

Course and Prognosis

Without treatment, complete or partial transection of spinal cord. Mortality: 30% in acute cases; 10% in chronic cases.

Total recovery possible if paralysis not total, or surgery performed within 36 hours of onset of weakness.

CHAPTER 24 ■ VIRAL INFECTIONS

After viral multiplication in extraneural tissues, dissemination to CNS occurs by hematogenous route or spread along nerve fibers.

GENERAL COMMENTS

CNS VIRAL SYNDROMES

Meningitis: headache, photophobia, stiff neck; no brain symptoms; usually self-limited.

Encephalitis: brain parenchyma involved with seizures, impaired consciousness, focal signs.

Myelitis: spinal cord inflammation.

CSF findings similar in all 3 syndromes: increased pressure, lymphocytic pleocytosis, moderate increase in protein content, normal glucose content.

Biologic properties differ: myxoviruses attack ependymal cells; herpes simplex produces latent infection, preference for frontal and temporal lobes; enteroviruses, togaviruses epidemic.

Diagnostic clues: epidemics, seasonal occurrence.

Diagnosis: virus isolation, antibody tests, polymerase chain reaction for viral nucleic acids. Some viruses (e.g., mumps) can be isolated from CSF; others (e.g., poliovirus, herpes simplex virus [HSV] type 1) rarely recovered.

Serology: antibodies rise 4-fold from first few days to convalescent phase (3–5 weeks).

If brain biopsy done: immunostaining, electron microscopy, injection of tissue into susceptible animals or cultured cell lines.

TREATMENT

Specific antiviral agents: acyclovir for HSV; acyclovir, famciclovir, foscarnet for varicella-zoster virus (**VZV**); ganciclovir, foscarnet for cytomegalovirus (**CMV**); reverse transcriptase, protease inhibitors for human immunodeficiency virus (**HIV**).

Immunization available for rabies, poliomyelitis, hepatitis A and B, mumps, influenza, rubella, measles, chickenpox (varicella), smallpox.

Vector control, mass immunization: most practical means of control.

ACUTE VIRAL INFECTIONS

HERPESVIRUS INFECTIONS

HSV type 1, HSV type 2, VZV, Epstein-Barr virus, CMV, human herpes virus (HHV)-6, HHV-7, HHV-8 (also known as Kaposi sarcoma herpes virus). All cause neurologic disease. Occur sporadically or as opportunistic infection in immunocompromised people.

Herpes Simplex Encephalitis

Epidemiology: most common cause of fatal sporadic encephalitis in United States. Early diagnosis crucial because antiviral treatment is available and usually effective. Mostly caused by HSV-1.

Clinical findings: fever, headache, altered consciousness and personality, usually abrupt onset; sometimes seizures, meningism. Behavioral changes vary from withdrawal to agitation with hallucinations. Course progressive for hours to days, with increasing obtundation, focal signs. Herpetic labial lesions in few cases.

CSF: increased pressure, lymphocytic pleocytosis, red blood cells (typical of herpes but not diagnostic), usually normal glucose. First CSF sample normal in 5% to 10%. Detection of viral DNA by PCR is diagnostic.

EEG abnormal in 80%: diffuse slowing or focal changes over temporal areas; periodic complexes against slow-wave background.

Imaging. CT, low-density abnormality (temporal lobe), mass effect, or linear contrast enhancement in 90%. Often normal in first week of disease. MRI: focal abnormalities often present in first week.

Treatment: if clinical picture suggests HSV encephalitis, start intravenous acyclovir immediately after CSF sent for HSV PCR. Continue for 14 days unless initial PCR negative. Treat brain edema with corticosteroids.

Prognosis: mortality 70–80% without treatment; 28% with treatment. Outcome depends on patient's age, level of consciousness, prompt treatment.

Herpes Zoster (Shingles)

Inflammatory lesions in dorsal root ganglia due to VZV. Often seen with systemic illness or immunosuppression.

Neuralgic pain or dysesthesia in distribution of affected root. Followed in 3–4 days by characteristic vesicular rash in same distribution. Resolves in 10–14 days. Simultaneous painless adenopathy. Spinal ganglia most often affected; cranial ganglia in 20%. Almost always unilateral.

Ophthalmic zoster: ophthalmic division of trigeminal ganglion. Complications: permanent eye changes after panophthalmitis or corneal scarring; temporary or permanent paresis of ocular muscles.

Geniculate herpes: otic zoster with involvement of geniculate ganglion (Ramsay Hunt syndrome); facial paralysis, loss of taste over anterior two thirds of tongue. Rash confined to tympanic membrane and external auditory canal.

Treatment: systemic acyclovir (oral or intravenous) or newer formulations (famciclovir, valacyclovir), depending on severity; analgesics, nonspecific topical medications for rash. Postherpetic neuralgia difficult to treat: amitriptyline, anticonvulsants (carbamazepine, phenytoin, gabapentin). Refractory to usual analgesics.

CYTOMEGALOVIRUS INFECTION

Congenital CMV infection: *In utero* infection may result in stillbirth or prematurity. Features of CNS infection: granulomatous encephalitis with extensive subependymal calcification, hydrocephalus, hydranencephaly, microcephaly, cerebellar hypoplasia, other developmental brain abnormalities. Seizures, focal neurologic signs, mental retardation common in infants who survive. Jaundice with hepatosplenomegaly, purpura, hemolytic anemia in some. High mortality in neonatal period.

CMV infection in adults: Mononucleosis-like syndrome. CNS lesions unlikely unless immunocompromised. Subacute encephalitis (possibly fatal); clinically indistinguishable from HIV encephalitis. Diffuse or focal white matter abnormalities on MRI in about 25% of cases. Subacute polyradiculomyelopathy, multifocal neuropathy seen only in AIDS. Ganciclovir, foscarnet reported beneficial.

Epstein-Barr Virus Infection
CNS rarely involved; encephalitis, meningitis. Prognosis excellent.

PICORNAVIRUS (ENTEROVIRUS) INFECTIONS

Poliovirus: acute destruction of motor cells in cord and brainstem; flaccid paralysis (poliomyelitis). Nearly nonexistent where vaccination available.

Coxsackieviruses: aseptic meningitis; rarely, paralytic disease or acute cerebellar ataxia.

Echoviruses: aseptic meningitis with gastroenteritis, respiratory infection, macular exanthema, petechial rash. Children affected more than adults.

Enterovirus 70: acute hemorrhagic conjunctivitis. Polio-like syndrome: flaccid, asymmetric, proximal leg paralysis with severe radicular pain.

Enterovirus 71: hand-foot-and-mouth disease. CNS affected in 25%; aseptic meningitis, cerebellar ataxia, poliomyelitis. Most cases in Europe and Asia.

Hepatitis A virus: encephalitis.

ARBOVIRUSES

Transmitted by arthropods. Moderate or severe encephalitis. Peak incidence late summer, early fall.

Equine Encephalitis
3 types in the U.S., all transmitted by mosquitoes.

Eastern equine encephalitis (EEE): Atlantic and Gulf coasts, Great Lakes areas. Short prodrome (about 5 days): fever, headache, malaise, nausea, vomiting. Then confusion, drowsiness, stupor, coma, seizures, stiff neck. Cranial nerve palsies, hemiplegia, other focal signs. Mortality 50%.

Western equine encephalitis (WEE): throughout United States. Mortality 10%.

Venezuelan equine encephalitis (VEE): Central and South America, southern half of United States. Mortality <0.5%.

Other Arbovirus Infections

St. Louis encephalitis: birds, humans intermediate hosts. Transmitted by mosquitoes. Primarily affects elderly. Acute course (2–3 weeks). Hyponatremia (due to syndrome of inappropriate ADH secretion) in 25–33%. Mortality 2–20%.

West Nile virus encephalitis: syndrome very similar to St. Louis encephalitis, including hyponatremia. Diagnosis: virus-specific IgM in serum or CSF; PCR in CSF.

Japanese encephalitis: major problem throughout Asia; up to 10,000 cases annually. Transmitted by mosquitoes. Most common in children. Mortality 50%. Severe neurologic sequelae common.

California (La Crosse) encephalitis: transmitted by mosquitoes. Mortality less than 1%. Most common in children.

Colorado tick fever virus: transmitted by wood ticks in Rocky Mountains. Abrupt febrile illness with headache, myalgia, retro-orbital pain, photophobia. Aseptic meningitis in 20%.

Tick-borne encephalitis: transmitted by wood ticks. Siberia, northern Europe.

RUBELLA (GERMAN MEASLES)

Congenital rubella encephalitis: acquired if mother infected during pregnancy. Lethargy, hypotonia, followed by restlessness, head retraction, opisthotonus, rigidity. Seizures and meningitis-like illness may occur. Vaccine given to all children between 1 year of age and puberty. Chronic condition discussed later in chapter.

MYXOVIRUS INFECTIONS

Mumps

Mild meningitis or encephalitis in small percentage of all cases. Resolves in few days. Unilateral deafness most common sequela.

Post-Infectious (Subacute) Measles Encephalitis

Opportunistic infection in immunosuppressed or immunodeficient patients (mostly children). Follows measles exposure by

1–6 months (vs. subacute sclerosing panencephalitis discussed below).

Seizures, focal signs, mental deterioration leading to coma and death in weeks to months. Routine CSF tests normal. Measles antibody often absent at onset. Intravenous ribavirin treatment may lead to temporary improvement.

RHABDOVIRUS INFECTION

Rabies
Acute CNS infection transmitted by bite of infected animal. Virus travels to CNS along sensory and motor nerves by axonal transport.

Incubation period 1–3 months. Hyperexcitability, muscle twitching, generalized convulsions. Delirium, hallucinations, bizarre behavior, profuse salivation. Spasmodic contractions of pharynx and larynx precipitated by attempt to swallow, violent refusal to accept liquids ("hydrophobia"). Frequent progression to generalized paralysis, coma.

Treatment: immune globulin infiltrated into wound and intramuscularly (passive immunization), followed by vaccination. Mortality >90%.

ARENAVIRUS INFECTIONS

Lymphocytic choriomeningitis: <0.5% of all cases of viral meningitis. Mice are a major reservoir. Most common in winter when mice move indoors.

Complete recovery in 1–4 weeks; low mortality rate.

ADENOVIRUSES

Respiratory, gastrointestinal routes. Mostly in children. CNS rarely involved: encephalitis or meningoencephalitis. Mortality up to 30%.

ACUTE DISSEMINATED ENCEPHALOMYELITIS (ADEM)

May occur with diverse infections, in the past particularly childhood exanthematous diseases (e.g., measles, rubella); or after vaccination. Most common causes now: VZV, nonspecific respiratory infections.

Symptoms/signs: meningism plus variable neurologic signs. May be followed by encephalitis, cranial nerve palsies (especially optic neuritis), cerebellar dysfunction. Spinal cord involvement (multifocal or as acute transverse myelitis) more common than brain.

Investigations: CSF, mild lymphocytosis, protein normal or slightly elevated, normal glucose. MRI: multiple lesions with increased T2 signal in white and deep gray matter.

Differential diagnosis: acute or subacute encephalitis, other CNS infections, acute diffuse MS.

Course and prognosis: mortality 10–30% in encephalitis from measles, rubella, or after rabies vaccination with old rabbit cord vaccine. Few deaths with acute cerebellar ataxia or only peripheral neuropathy. In survivors, complete recovery in 90%. Exception: measles sequelae in 20–50% (seizures, hemiparesis).

Treatment: intravenous corticosteroids may reduce severity of neurologic deficits.

CHRONIC VIRAL INFECTIONS

SUBACUTE SCLEROSING PANENCEPHALITIS (SSPE)

Progressive encephalitis with onset months to years after measles infection.

More than 50% of patients had acute measles infection before age 2 years. Children younger than 12 years predominantly affected; boys more often than girls; more frequent in rural than urban settings.

Symptoms and signs: gradual onset without fever. Forgetfulness, decline in school work, restlessness. Followed by incoordination, ataxia, apraxia, loss of speech, seizures, dystonic posturing. Terminal stage: rigid quadriplegia. Characteristic noise-induced myoclonus, prolonged relaxation phase ("hung-up" myoclonus).

Investigations: high titer measles antibody in serum, CSF. EEG: slow wave complexes every 4–20 seconds, may be synchronized to myoclonus. CT, MRI: cortical atrophy and focal or multifocal low-density white matter lesions.

Course: progressive, eventually leading to death over months to years; spontaneous long-term improvement or stabilization in 10%.

PROGRESSIVE RUBELLA PANENCEPHALITIS

Onset in second decade of life with dementia, cerebellar ataxia, followed by pyramidal tract signs, optic atrophy, or retinopathy.

Course protracted over 8–10 years.

RETROVIRUSES

HIV infection: see Chapter 25.

HTLV-associated myelopathy (HAM; tropical spastic paraparesis): HTLV = Human T-lymphotrophic virus. See Chapter 118.

Progressive multifocal leukoencephalopathy (PML): See Chapter 25.

ENCEPHALITIS LETHARGICA

Epidemic encephalitis of 1917–1928. Unknown cause. Diffuse brain involvement; sequelae in many survivors. Now rare or non-existent.

Acute or subacute onset of fever, headache, lethargy, abnormal eye movements, motor symptoms of basal ganglia disease.

Most notable sequela: postencephalitic parkinsonism. Distinguished from idiopathic parkinsonism by early onset, grimaces, torticollis, torsion spasms, myoclonus, oculogyric crisis (involuntary persistent deviation of both eyes, usually upwards), facial and respiratory tics, bizarre postures and gait.

CHAPTER 25 ■ AIDS

Dementia, myelopathy due to HIV infection are AIDS-defining illnesses.

CNS PATHOGENESIS

HIV enters CNS in primary infection. May produce no symptoms, acute self-limited syndrome, or chronic disorder.

Possible causes: HIV itself, secondary opportunistic infections or neoplasia, metabolic abnormalities, complications of drug therapy, nutritional.

CNS invasion and injury: mechanism not known. In brain, virus infects only microglial cells and macrophages, not neurons, although designated "neurotropic virus" because neurologic disorders are frequent.

Neurologic disorders affect 70% of patients with AIDS; first manifestation of AIDS in 10–20%.

CLINICAL SYNDROMES

HIV-RELATED NEUROLOGIC SYNDROMES IN EARLY INFECTION

Indistinguishable from CNS infection by other viruses: aseptic meningitis, encephalopathy, leukoencephalitis, seizures, transverse myelitis, cranial or peripheral neuropathy, polymyositis, myoglobinuria. Course self-limited, often full neurologic recovery.

CSF abnormalities (pleocytosis up to 200 cells/mm^3, oligoclonal bands) differentiate HIV from postinfectious disorders. HIV antibody test sometimes negative because symptoms may precede seroconversion by weeks. Consider p24 antigen and viral load assay if serology negative.

HIV-RELATED NEUROLOGIC SYNDROMES IN CHRONIC INFECTION

AIDS Dementia Complex (ADC)

Other terms: HIV encephalitis, HIV encephalopathy.

Severe dementia, behavioral changes; motor disorder. Myelopathy and peripheral neuropathy in 25%. In HIV-positive people, these syndromes are diagnostic of AIDS.

Usually progressive; may be static.

Symptoms

Early: apathy, social withdrawal, diminished libido, slow thinking, poor concentration, forgetful. Psychiatric syndromes: psychosis, depression, mania.

Motor signs: slow movements, leg weakness, gait ataxia.

Advanced stage: akinetic mutism; immobile; global cognitive impairment, urinary incontinence.

Encephalopathy in children: may be static or progressive. Intellectual deterioration, microcephaly, delayed developmental milestones; pseudobulbar palsy; spastic quadriparesis (see also Chapter 168).

Investigations

CSF: normal or mild pleocytosis, high protein content, oligoclonal bands.

CT, MRI: Adults: cerebral atrophy, leukoencephalopathy. Children: also basal ganglia calcification. Pathology: microglial nodules, giant cells, focal perivascular demyelination, gliosis, neuronal loss in frontal cortex. Severity of pathology not always correlated with severity of dementia.

Treatment

Zidovudine (AZT), selegiline, nimodipine: mixed results. Improve, slow dementia, or no effect.

Predictors of dementia: CD4+ count <100 cell/μL, anemia, or AIDS-defining infection or neoplasm (19% to 25% risk in 2 years).

Stroke Syndromes

0.5–8% of patients with AIDS. Causes: secondary infection, neoplasm, HIV-related vasculitis, cardiogenic emboli, thrombogenic conditions, disseminated intravascular coagulopathy, or lupus anticoagulant. Cerebral hemorrhage may occur with thrombocytopenia or toxoplasmosis.

Seizures
Any stage of HIV infection; focal or generalized. Secondary pathogens in 53%; HIV encephalopathy in 24%.

Leukoencephalopathy
Acute fulminating fatal leukoencephalitis; multifocal vacuolar leukoencephalopathy with rapid dementia; relapsing-remitting disease, may simulate MS.

Chronic Progressive Myelopathy
Progressive spastic, ataxic paraparesis with bowel and bladder disorders. MRI: myelitis.

Peripheral and Autonomic Neuropathy
Several types: mononeuritis multiplex, chronic inflammatory demyelinating polyneuropathy, distal symmetric polyneuropathy, ganglioneuritis.

Distal sensorimotor neuropathy: most common neuropathy of AIDS.

Clinical features: painful, burning dysesthesias in soles of feet, stocking-glove sensory loss, muscle wasting, weakness, loss of ankle jerks.
Conduction studies: mixed axonal and demyelinating sensorimotor neuropathy.
CSF: normal or mild pleocytosis and elevated protein content.
Pathology: axonal degeneration, loss of large myelinated fibers, inflammatory cells.
Treatment: pain syndrome tricyclic antidepressants, anticonvulsants, nonsteroidal anti-inflammatory drugs (NSAIDs), narcotics.

Myopathy
Uncommon. Proximal limb weakness, mild CK elevation, myopathic features on EMG.

Differential diagnosis: AZT myopathy (see below).

Steroids sometimes help.

OPPORTUNISTIC INFECTIONS AND NEOPLASMS

Meningitis
Viruses (herpes group, hepatitis B); **fungi** (*Cryptococcus*, *Histoplasma*, *Coccidioides*, *Candida*); **bacteria** (*Listeria*, *Treponema pallidum*, pyogenic bacteria, *Salmonella*, *Staphylococcus*

aureus, atypical or conventional mycobacteria); **neoplasm** (lymphoma).

Cryptococcal infection: most common meningitis in AIDS, 6% to 11%. Diagnosis by finding cryptococcal antigen in serum or CSF, or by CSF culture. Treatment: fluconazole, itraconazole, amphotericin B.

Neurosyphilis: course may be altered by concomitant HIV infection. CSF VDRL test may be nonreactive. Intravenous penicillin therapy for documented neurosyphilis (see Chapter 28). Relapse more common in HIV-infected people.

Tuberculosis: meningitis, atypical mycobacterial infection of brain, tuberculomas with HIV infection (see also Chapter 61).

Encephalitis

Herpes group (CMV most common), *Mycobacterium avium intracellulare*, toxoplasmosis, lymphoma.

Most common cause of intracranial mass lesion in AIDS; chronic progressive focal signs, seizures.

CT or MRI: multiple enhancing lesions with mass effect, typically involve basal ganglia. Anti-toxoplasma antibodies: 95% sensitive. CSF not diagnostic, toxoplasma PCR diagnostic in only 40–80%.

Differential diagnosis: lymphoma. Brain biopsy if no clinical or radiographic response after anti-toxoplasma therapy for 1 week.

Progressive Multifocal Leukoencephalopathy (PML)

Subacute demyelinating disease caused by opportunistic papovavirus (JC virus). Occurs in 1–5% of patients with AIDS.

Clinical features: subacute to chronic onset; multiple progressive focal signs; dementia in advanced stages.

Pathology: multiple, partly confluent, areas of demyelination, most prominent in subcortical white matter. Eosinophilic intranuclear inclusions (virus particles) in oligodendroglial cells at lesion periphery.

Investigations: CT, MRI: nonenhancing multiple confluent lucencies in cerebral white matter. Antibodies not specific. May detect JC virus in CSF by PCR; brain biopsy sometimes necessary if PCR negative.

Course, prognosis, treatment: approximately 80% die in 9 months. No definite treatment. Spontaneous improvement rare.

Primary CNS Lymphoma
Primary CNS neoplasm in AIDS.
    0.6–3% of patients before introduction of highly active anti-retroviral therapy (**HAART**); much lower incidence now with effective immune reconstitution therapy.

Clinical signs nonspecific: CT normal or hypodense lesions, single or multiple, nodular enhancement.
Diagnosis: brain biopsy.
Natural history: poor prognosis, death usually within 6 months. Response to radiotherapy, chemotherapy improved by HAART. Treat coexistent opportunistic infections.

Spinal Cord Infection
Herpes viruses (herpes simplex virus, CMV, varicella-zoster virus); mycobacteria; pyogenic bacteria; toxoplasmosis.
    Spinal cord biopsy for definite diagnosis.

Polyradiculopathy, Cauda Equina Syndrome
Sometimes CMV infection.

DRUG-INDUCED AND NUTRITIONAL SYNDROMES

Chronic AZT therapy: mitochondrial myopathy with ragged red fibers.

    Nucleoside antiretroviral drugs cause severe dose-related, painful sensory neuropathy.

Nutritional deficiency: thiamine, vitamin B12, folic acid, glutathione; may lead to encephalopathy, dementia, neuropathy, spinal cord disorders (see Chapter 154).

TREATMENT

Combination antiretroviral therapy (highly active antiretroviral therapy, or HAART) transformed AIDS from fatal disease to chronic illness in industrialized countries. Some neurologic complications respond to antiretroviral treatment.

CHAPTER 26 ■ FUNGAL AND YEAST INFECTIONS

CNS fungal infection: meningitis, meningoencephalitis, abscess, granuloma, arterial thrombosis. Subacute meningitis, meningoencephalitis most common. Lungs, skin, hair usually primary sites.

Pathogenic fungal infections (occur in normal host): histoplasmosis, blastomycosis, coccidiomycosis, paracoccidiomycosis.

Opportunistic infections (immunocompromised host): aspergillosis, candidiasis, cryptococcosis, mucormycosis, nocardiosis.

CRYPTOCOCCOSIS

Most common mycotic infection directly involving CNS. Major cause of morbidity and mortality among immunosuppressed patients. May simulate tuberculous meningitis, brain tumor, encephalitis, psychosis.

Pathogenesis: respiratory tract usual portal of entry. Associated with debilitating disease in 30–60%. CNS infection may occur with or without systemic disease. At diagnosis of systemic cryptococcosis, 70% have neurologic disease.

symptoms and signs: subacute onset of meningeal symptoms; occasionally prominent focal signs or mental symptoms. Large granulomas in cerebrum, cerebellum, or brainstem cause clinical syndromes characteristic of location.

Investigations. CSF, increased pressure, moderate pleocytosis, increased protein, decreased glucose. Detection of cryptococcal antigen in serum, CSF; positive culture from urine, blood, stool, sputum.

Treatment: fluconazole given until CSF sterile for 3 months. Alternative therapies: amphotericin B, flucytosine. Side effects of amphotericin B: thrombophlebitis, nausea and vomiting, fever, anemia, hypokalemia, uremia.

Course: usually fatal in few months if untreated.

MUCORMYCOSIS

Phycomycetes fungi (usually *Rhizopus* species). Acute, rarely curable. Usually complication of diabetes mellitus or blood dyscrasia, particularly leukemia.

Pathogenesis: fungi enter nose to cause sinusitis and orbital cellulitis. Spread via blood vessels and local invasion to ocular, cerebral, pulmonary, intestinal, and disseminated infection.

Symptoms and signs: proptosis, ocular palsies, hemiplegia common. Organisms may cause meningitis or extend into brain to cause encephalitis.

Diagnosis: examination of sputum, CSF, or exudate from nasal sinuses.

Treatment: amphotericin B, control predisposing factors (e.g., diabetes), local drainage, early surgery of necrotic tissue.

Prognosis: survival rate 73%.

CHAPTER 27 ■
NEUROSARCOIDOSIS

Granulomatous multisystem disease of unknown cause, sometimes involving CNS, peripheral nerves, or muscle.

EPIDEMIOLOGY

Prevalence 3–50 per 100,000 population worldwide. More frequent in African Americans than others in United States. Onset age 30–60.

PATHOLOGY

Granulomas like those of tuberculosis but without tubercle bacilli or caseation; commonly affect lung, lymph nodes, skin, bone, eyes, salivary glands.

Nervous system involved in 5% of patients: typically basal meninges, causing secondary cranial nerve infiltration and obstructed CSF flow. Granulomas may spread to CNS parenchyma (often hypothalamus). Also peripheral neuropathy, myopathy.

SYMPTOMS AND SIGNS

Cranial neuropathy (53%); CNS parenchymal disease (48%); aseptic meningitis (22%); sensorimotor peripheral neuropathy (17%); myopathy (15%); hydrocephalus (7%).

INVESTIGATIONS

CT, MRI: CNS granulomas, meningeal enhancement, hydrocephalus, lesions in spinal cord, cauda equina, or optic nerves.

CSF: lymphocytic pleocytosis, high protein, low glucose, elevated IgG and IgG index, oligoclonal bands. Elevated angiotensin-converting enzyme (ACE); value uncertain. Lymphocytosis, low glucose important but also seen in tuberculous and fungal meningitis.

Supportive studies: chest X-ray or CT (hilar adenopathy or fibronodular disease), pulmonary function studies, bronchiolar lavage for lymphocytes, serum and urinary calcium (hypercalcemia), serum γ-globulin.

DIAGNOSIS

Requires tissue biopsy: lymph node, lung lesion, salivary gland, skin, conjunctiva, or brain.

COURSE AND TREATMENT

Self-limited monophasic illness in two-thirds; chronic remitting-relapsing in others.

Prednisone may reduce granuloma size and ameliorate symptoms; affect on natural history unclear.

Short-term steroid therapy for aseptic meningitis or isolated facial palsy; long-term treatment often given for intraparenchymal lesions, hydrocephalus, optic or other cranial nerve lesions, peripheral neuropathy, or symptomatic myopathy. Immunosuppressive treatment (azathioprine, methotrexate, cyclophosphamide) for refractory patients. Radiation therapy of uncertain benefit.

CHAPTER 28 ■ SPIROCHETE INFECTIONS: NEUROSYPHILIS

DEFINITION

Infection of brain, meninges, or spinal cord by *Treponema pallidum*.

Required: (a) syndrome consistent with neurosyphilis (meningitis, meningoencephalitis, meningomyelitis, cerebral infarcts, dementia paralytica, tabes dorsalis, congenital neurosyphilis, asymptomatic neurosyphilis); (b) abnormal blood titer of treponemal antibody test; (c) positive nontreponemal antibody test in CSF.

EPIDEMIOLOGY

Incidence declined following introduction of penicillin, then increased with AIDS epidemic.

10% of untreated patients with early syphilis develop neurosyphilis. Of HIV-positive patients, 15% have concomitant serologic evidence of syphilis; 1% have neurosyphilis.

PATHOLOGY

Early neurosyphilis: mononuclear cell infiltration of meninges, extending to cranial nerves (causing axonal degeneration) and endothelial proliferation with vessel occlusion (focal ischemic necrosis in brain and spinal cord).

Dementia paralytica: inflammation around small cortical vessels provokes loss of cortical neurons and glial proliferation. Spirochetes in cortex.

Tabes dorsalis: degeneration of posterior roots and posterior fiber columns of spinal cord.

INVESTIGATIONS

Serology

Nontreponemal antibody tests: VDRL, RPR. Both performed on serum; VDRL suitable for testing CSF.

Fluorescent treponemal antibody (FTA-ABS) titer: highly sensitive and specific. Performed as confirmatory test if RPR or VDRL is positive.

CSF

CSF pleocytosis best measure of disease activity. CSF protein usually increased. Glucose low or normal.

DIAGNOSIS

Diagnosis of neurosyphilis requires positive serology in serum (RPR, VDRL or FTA-ABS), reactive CSF VDRL, and CSF pleocytosis.

CLINICAL SYNDROMES

Most common syndromes presently: asymptomatic, meningeal, vascular, mixed "meningovascular" form.

Parenchymal forms (dementia paralytica, tabes dorsalis) almost never seen now.

ASYMPTOMATIC NEUROSYPHILIS

Abnormal serology and CSF findings in absence of symptoms; may show meningeal enhancement on MRI.

MENINGEAL AND VASCULAR NEUROSYPHILIS

Meningeal
Within 1 year after primary infection.

Malaise, fever, stiff neck, headache; sometimes cranial nerve abnormalities (especially facial diplegia, hearing loss). CSF pressure may be increased; WBC may rise to several hundred; glucose may be low but usually >25 mg/dL. Protein may exceed 100 mg/dL. Findings may subside spontaneously. Complications: hydrocephalus, cerebral infarct.

Cerebrovascular
Onset of symptoms typically 5–10 years after primary infection.

Cerebral infarct syndromes similar to those of more common causes, but often follow subacute encephalitic prodrome.

Check serum RPR in all stroke patients with young age or risk factors for venereal disease.

Meningovascular Syphilis of Spinal Cord (Meningomyelitis)
Sensory and motor pathways, bladder control usually affected. Different from tabes, a parenchymal infection now almost unseen (see below).

PARENCHYMATOUS NEUROSYPHILIS

Symptom onset typically >20 years after primary infection.

Paretic Neurosyphilis
Also called dementia paralytica, general paresis of the insane, syphilitic meningoencephalitis.

Loss of memory, poor judgment, emotional lability, sometimes psychosis and seizures; progresses to severe dementia, quadriparesis in late stages. Fatal in 3–5 years if untreated.

Tabes Dorsalis
Lancinating or lightning pains, progressive ataxia, loss of tendon reflexes, loss of proprioception and vibratory sense in legs, dysfunction of sphincters, impaired sexual function in men.

Irregular or unequal pupils in most patients; Argyll Robertson pupils (react to accommodation but not to light) in 48%.

Complications: Charcot joints (loss of pain perception leads to repeated joint trauma, chronic joint inflammation, enlargement), cranial nerve palsies, autonomic dysfunction.

CONGENITAL NEUROSYPHILIS

Transmitted between fourth and seventh months of pregnancy. Now rare in United States. Clinical types similar to those in adults. Additional features: hydrocephalus; Hutchinson triad (interstitial keratitis, deformed teeth, hearing loss).

TREATMENT

Early Syphilis

Standard treatment: a single intramuscular injection of 2.4 million units of penicillin G benzathine. Serologic testing repeated at 3, 6, 12 months.

Re-treatment is indicated if: clinical signs persist or recur, VDRL titer increases fourfold, or VDRL titer fails to decline fourfold within 6 months.

Neurosyphilis

Intravenous aqueous penicillin G, 12–24 million units daily for 10–14 days, or intramuscular aqueous penicillin G, 2.4 million units daily with 2 g probenecid given orally each day. Blood serology determined at 3-month intervals; should show decline in titer.

CSF examined every 6 months until cell count normal. Re-treatment is indicated if CSF cell count has not declined at 6 months, or if CSF remains abnormal at 2 years. After 3 years, if patient has improved and is clinically stable, and if CSF and serologic tests are normal, discontinue neurologic and CSF examinations.

NEUROSYPHILIS AND AIDS

15% of HIV-positive people co-infected with syphilis. Syphilis may be more aggressive in HIV, with more rapid and more severe course.

Frequency of neurosyphilis in HIV-positive population: <2%. No need for special treatment regimen for syphilis in HIV-infected people. However, serum RPR 1:32 and blood CD4 T-cell count <350 cells/μL are risk factors for developing neurosyphilis and need close follow-up.

CHAPTER 29 ■ SPIROCHETE INFECTIONS: LEPTOSPIROSIS

Epidemiology: hosts include humans, wild animals, domestic animals (cats, dogs, cattle). Humans infected via exposure to infested animal tissue or urine, or contaminated ground water, soil, vegetation. Swimming in contaminated water special risk.

Clinical features: acute phase: chills, fever, myalgia, headache, stiff neck, confusion 1–2 weeks after infection. Gastrointestinal and cardiac (including severe bradycardia, hypotension) complications, hepatosplenomegaly, lymphadenopathy, acute renal failure. Second phase of symptoms may occur after resolution of the first; likely immune-mediated.

Investigations: CSF, lymphocytic pleocytosis (more prominent in second phase), increased protein (may be >100 mg/dL). Cultures positive early. Serologic studies in second phase.

Treatment: high-dose penicillin or tetracycline.

Prognosis: young patients may recover spontaneously. Symptoms may recur. Mortality >50% after age 50.

CHAPTER 30 ■ SPIROCHETE INFECTIONS: LYME DISEASE

EPIDEMIOLOGY

Borrelia burgdorferi spirochete transmitted to humans by ixodid ticks (which in the United States infest deer, mice). Usually in wooded areas of United States; peak disease incidence from May to September.

SYMPTOMS AND SIGNS

First Stage
Erythema chronicus migrans (ECM): migrating erythematous circular rash, with appearance of "bull's-eye," or "target," 3 to 30 days after tick bite. Headache, myalgia, stiff neck, cranial nerve palsies (almost always seventh nerve) may occur. CSF usually normal.

Second Stage
Several weeks after onset of ECM.

Heart conduction defects; meningism, often afebrile; radiculitis (multiple or isolated, root pain or focal weakness). Seventh cranial nerve frequently involved, usually bilateral. Polyneuritis or mononeuritis multiplex. Decreased concentration, irritability, emotional lability, memory, sleep disorders.

Neurologic disease may occur without previous ECM or recognized tick bite, but then diagnosis difficult to prove.

Third Stage
Usually months after original infection.

Chronic encephalomyelopathy, manifesting as cognitive dysfunction together with progressive long tract dysfunction. Polyneuropathy (mainly sensory) may develop. Chronic arthritis in patients with HLA-DR2 antigen.

INVESTIGATIONS

CSF: normal pressure, lymphocytic pleocytosis, increased protein, oligoclonal bands, normal glucose; may be normal. Diagnosis supported by finding spirochete-specific antibodies in serum or CSF, in context of clinically appropriate history. Usefulness of CSF Lyme PCR still uncertain.

DIFFERENTIAL DIAGNOSIS

Other viral infections; sarcoidsis (facial dysplasia); chronic fatigue syndrome; somatoform disorder.

TREATMENT

Oral doxycycline or amoxicillin commonly used to treat early (stage 1) Lyme disease. Cefuroxime, erythromycin may also be used. All usually prevent later stages.

Intravenously administered third-generation cephalosporins (ceftriaxone or cefuroxime) standard treatment of disease with neurologic symptoms, typically leading to reversal of acute symptoms. Motor signs last 7 to 8 weeks with or without antibiotic therapy. Even after successful treatment, symptoms may continue for months: memory, emotional, cognitive problems. Length of treatment uncertain; 4 weeks required for most cases. Efficacy of prolonged treatment not established.

Oral antibiotic doses appropriate for ECM are sufficient to treat isolated nerve palsies associated with high spirochete-antibody levels.

Prevention: avoidance of tick-infested areas; appropriate clothing and repellants, tick checks after exposure.

CHAPTER 31 ■ PARASITIC INFECTIONS

Major public health problem in tropical and less developed countries. Predisposing factors: poor living conditions; appropriate climate for vectors to facilitate transmission; immunosuppression. Diseases caused by worms (helminths), protozoa.

HELMINTHIC INFECTION

Frequent systemic allergic responses (e.g., eosinophilia). Nervous system involvement more often focal than diffuse.

CYSTICERCOSIS

Encystment of larvae of *Taenia solium* (pork tapeworm), in tissues. Acquired by ingestion of ova by: (a) fecal contamination of food; (b) autoinfection via anal-oral transfer; (c) reverse peristalsis of proglottids into stomach. Ingestion of infected pork results in adult tapeworm infection, not in cysticercosis.

Epidemiology
Most common parasitic infection of CNS. CNS involved in 50–70% and in virtually all symptomatic patients.

Common in Mexico, Central and South America, Southeast Asia, China, India. Increasing in the United States.

Symptoms and Signs
Depend on cyst location. Common: seizures (cerebral cortex), headache (increased intracranial pressure due to edema), meningitis (meningeal spread). Also: obstructive hydrocephalus (third or fourth ventricle), stroke (cerebral vessels).

Investigations
CT, MRI: hydrocephalus; cyst (MRI) or cyst calcification (CT); enhancement of cyst with intravenous contrast.

Plain radiographs of thighs and calves: multiple cigar-shaped calcifications.

CSF: normal or moderate pleocytosis, elevated pressure. Meningeal form: hundreds to thousands of white blood cells (WBCs) (usually mononuclear), high protein, low glucose.

Antibody to tapeworm usually positive in serum, CSF.

Treatment

Hydrocephalus: ventricular shunting. Seizures: anticonvulsants. Intractable seizures: consider surgical removal of cysts. Meningitis: corticosteroids used, but benefit not proven.

Eradication of infection: albendazole, with corticosteroids during first week of treatment to reduce inflammation due to dying cysts. Indications for eradication of infection ocontrversial.

ECHINOCOCCOSIS (HYDATID CYSTS)

Caused by larvae of *Echinococcus granulosus* (dog tapeworm). Most common in children in rural areas in countries where herd dogs assist in sheep and cattle raising.

Cysts most common in liver, lungs. Brain involved in 2% of cases. Neurologic symptoms may develop with cysts in skull or spine. Cerebral cysts usually single. Most common in cerebral hemispheres.

Symptoms and Signs

Dictated by location of cyst. Seizures, increased intracranial pressure may also occur.

Investigations

CT, MRI: single, nonenhancing cyst of CSF density. Needle biopsy avoided; may cause anaphylaxis from cyst rupture. In spinal disease, vertebral collapse common. Eosinophilia uncommon except after cyst rupture. Liver enzymes usually normal. Serologic tests positive in 60–90% of infected people.

Treatment

Complete surgical removal without puncturing cyst. Albendazole used to: 1) reduce cyst size; 2) prevent secondary hydatidosis at time of surgery. Albendazole alone sometimes curative.

SCHISTOSOMIASIS (BILHARZIASIS)

Schistosoma japonicum: cerebral hemispheres; *S. haematobium*, *S. mansoni*: more often spinal cord.

Epidemiology

Affects >200 million people worldwide. *S. japonicum*: Asia and Pacific tropics. *S. mansoni*: Caribbean, South America, Africa, Middle East. *S. haematobium*: Africa, Middle East.

Syndromes

Symptom onset may be delayed for 2 years. May relapse. CNS involved in 3% to 5% with *S. japonicum.*

Acute cerebral schistosomiasis: diffuse fulminating meningoencephalitis with fever, headache, confusion, lethargy, coma. Focal or generalized seizures, hemiplegia, other focal signs also common.

Chronic cerebral form: localizing signs, increased intracranial pressure with papilledema.

Granulomatous masses in spinal cord: acute onset; signs and symptoms of incomplete transverse lesion. Conus most common site of cord involvement; also granulomatous root lesions.

Investigations

Blood: leukocytosis, eosinophilia. CSF: may be normal; pressure may be increased; slight or moderate pleocytosis (sometimes with eosinophils); increased protein. CT, MRI: cerebral or spinal lesions.

Treatment

Praziquantel. Oral steroids may help. Anticonvulsants for seizures. Surgery for large granulomatous lesions.

PARAGONIMIASIS

Lung flukes (*Paragonimus westermani, P. mexicanus*). Common in China, Korea, Japan, Southeast Asia, South Pacific areas, Africa, India, Central and South America.

Acquired by eating uncooked or inadequately cooked fresh water crustaceans. Most common symptoms pulmonary, intestinal.

CNS involvement: in 10–15% of patients. Fever, headache, meningoencephalitis, focal and generalized seizures, dementia, hemiparesis, visual disturbances, other focal manifestations.

Syndromes: acute and chronic meningitis, acute purulent meningoencephalitis, infarction, epilepsy, subacute progressive encephalopathy, chronic granulomatous disease (tumor form), late inactive forms (chronic brain syndrome).

Blood: anemia, eosinophilia, leukocytosis, elevated erythrocyte sedimentation rate and γ-globulins.

CSF: may observe increased pressure, pleocytosis (polymorphonuclear acutely, lymphocytic chronically), eosinophils, red blood cells, increased protein, decreased glucose.

CT, MRI: acute disease, grape-like clusters of ring-enhancing lesions with edema; Chronic disease: ventricular dilation, intracranial calcifications (characteristic "soap bubble" appearance).

Diagnosis: ova in sputum, stool. Serologic, skin tests available. CSF antibody tests diagnostic but not sensitive.

Treatment: praziquantel or bithionol for acute and subacute meningoencephalitis; surgery for chronic tumor form. Mortality 5–10%.

TRICHINOSIS (TRICHINELLOSIS)

Acute infection caused by roundworm *Trichinella spiralis*. Acquired by eating larvae (in cysts) in raw or undercooked pork. Nervous system involved in 10–25% of symptomatic infections.

Diffuse encephalitis: confusion, delirium, coma, seizures; focal lesions in cerebrum, brainstem, cerebellum. Also possible: edema of optic nerve, meningeal signs, spinal cord syndromes, peripheral neuropathy.

Blood: leukocytosis, eosinophilia; muscle enzymes sometimes increased.

CSF: increased pressure, slight lymphocytic pleocytosis, increased protein. Parasites found in CSF of 30%.

CT: single or multiple small hypodensities in white matter or cortex (75% of cases); contrast enhancement in about half of these.

Prognosis: recovery within days to weeks typical. Mortality 10% to 20% if CNS involved.

Treatment: thiabendazole to kill intestinal worms. Mebendazole to treat tissue larvae. Corticosteroids to reduce inflammation, cerebral edema.

EOSINOPHILIC MENINGITIS

Most commonly caused by rat lungworm, *Angiostrongylus cantonensis*, after ingestion of raw snails, shrimp, crabs, fish. Rarely caused by *Gnathostoma spiginerum*.

Meningitis Due to *A. cantonensis*
Cases reported from Hawaii, Philippines, Pacific Islands, Southeast Asia, Cuba, Africa. Most common in children.

Syndromes: typically, acute meningitis; less frequently, encephalitis, encephalomyelitis, cranial nerves VI and VII. Severe pain in 50%. Neurologic injury attributed to multiple small hemorrhages.
Investigations: eosinophilia in blood present almost invariably. CSF pleocytosis with eosinophils. CT usually normal. Serologic tests available.
Treatment, prognosis: no specific therapy. Usually self-limited.

Meningitis Due to *G. spiginerum*
Cases reported in Europe, Mexico, Central America.
May also cause cranial nerve palsy, radiculomyelitis, encephalitis, subarachnoid and intracranial hemorrhage. CT, MRI usually abnormal. Worse prognosis than with CNS involvement by *A. cantonensis*.

Other Causes of Eosinophilic Meningitis
Other parasites (cysticercosis, schistosomiasis, paragonimiasis), coccidiomycosis, foreign bodies, rug allergies, neoplasms.

TOXOCARIASIS

Caused by larvae of roundworms (ascarids) found in dogs (*Toxocara canis*) and cats (*T. cati*), via ingestion of eggs from feces of infected pets or contaminated soil.

Systemic syndrome: visceral larva migrans (pulmonary symptoms, hepatomegaly, chronic eosinophilia). Ocular involvement more common than CNS invasion.
Symptoms and signs of neurologic syndrome: focal deficits, especially hemiparesis.
Investigations: eosinophils common in blood, rare in CSF. Hypergammaglobulinemia common. Enhancing lesions on CT, MRI.
Treatment: albendazole. Corticosteroids to suppress inflammation.

Similar neurologic syndrome also caused by *Ascaris lumbricoides*.

STRONGYLOIDIASIS

Intestinal infection due to *Strongyloides stercoralis*. Tropical, subtropical regions but also throughout U.S.

CNS involvement (meningitis, encephalopathy, seizures, focal deficits) part of disseminated infection in immunosuppressed host. Eosinophilia infrequent.

Treatment: thiabendazole and ivermectin. Avoid corticosteroids as they may cause dissemination. High mortality from disseminated disease.

PROTOZOAN INFECTION

Single-cell organisms; diffuse CNS disease. No allergic reactions or eosinophilia.

TOXOPLASMOSIS

Toxoplasma gondii. Predilection for eye and brain. Especially common in AIDS.

Acquired by ingestion of oocysts from cat feces, contaminated soil, unwashed vegetables, undercooked meat.

Granulomatous lesions throughout CNS, sometimes meninges.

Clinical Features

Acquired form in immunocompetent patient: usually asymptomatic. Lymphadenopathy, fever. Rarely, meningoencephalitis. Signs of meningeal irritation uncommon.

Acquired form in immunodeficient patients: due to new infection or reactivation. Pneumonitis, myocarditis, myositis, chorioretinitis. Possible manifestations: subacute encephalopathy; seizures; acute meningoencephalitis; focal signs of mass lesion (toxoplasmic abscess); obstructive hydrocephalus due to mass lesion, ependymitis.

Congenital form: inanition, microcephaly, seizures, mental retardation, spasticity, opisthotonos, chorioretinitis, microphthalmos, other defects of eye development. Optic atrophy common. Calcified brain nodules on CT or skull radiographs.

Investigations

CSF: pressure sometimes increased; inconstant pleocytosis; protein generally elevated; glucose normal or mildly reduced.

CT/MRI: low-density focal lesions, usually with ring enhancement. Multiple calcifications in congenital infection.

Diagnosis
Presumptive diagnosis: antibodies. Differentiation from CNS lymphoma may be impossible clinically or by imaging. SPECT helpful. Diagnosis supported by response to treatment. If no clinical response and no improvement of lesion on MRI after 7–14 days, consider brain biopsy.

Course, Prognosis, Treatment
Congenital form: >50% mortality. Frequent neurologic sequelae.

Immunocompetent patient: infection self-limited.
Immunocompromised patients: high mortality.
Treatment: pyrimethamine, sulfadiazine (indefinitely for AIDS patients).

CEREBRAL MALARIA

Endemic in tropical and subtropical areas of Africa, Asia, Central and South America. Seen almost anywhere due to international travel. Transmitted by mosquitos.

CNS involved in 2% of infected patients. Most common: *Plasmodium falciparum*.

Symptoms and Signs
Acute diffuse encephalopathy most common syndrome (headache, photophobia, vertigo, convulsions, confusion, delirium, and coma). Focal signs uncommon. Rare: spinal cord lesions; GBS.

Laboratory Data
Anemia; parasites in red blood cells. CSF usually normal.

Prognosis
Mortality 20–40% overall; 80% if coma and seizures present. Recovery complete in survivors.

Treatment
Cerebral malaria is a medical emergency. Critically ill patients: intramuscular chloroquine and intravenous quinine or quinidine. Less severe cases: chloroquine alone.

If infection occurs in endemic area of chloroquine-resistant falciparum malaria (now most areas of the world): quinine plus pyrimethamine-sulfadoxine (Fansidar), doxycycline, or clindamycin. Other regimens include: quinine plus tetracycline, artesunate (or artemether) plus mefloquine, mefloquine plus doxycycline.

Transfusions for anemia. Anticonvulsants for seizures. Mannitol for life-threatening cerebral edema. Dexamethasone contraindicated.

TRYPANOSOMIASIS

Sleeping Sickness
Trypanosoma brucei (Africa). Transmitted by tsetse fly, mechanical contact. Tremors, incoordination, convulsions, paralysis, confusion, headaches, apathy, insomnia or somnolence, coma. High mortality if untreated. Treatment: melarsoprol.

Chagas Disease
Trypanosoma cruzi (Central and South America). Transmitted by blood-sucking insect ("kissing bug"). Neurologic involvement rare. Meningoencephalitis, miliary granulomas, with diffuse or focal signs. Slowly progressive. High mortality if untreated. Nifurtimox, benzimidazole to treat acute stage. No treatment of chronic form, including CNS component.

PRIMARY AMEBIC MENINGOENCEPHALITIS

Due to free-living amebae. Rare.

Naegleria Infections
Naegleria fowleri: acute illness (primary amebic meningoencephalitis). Usually children or young adults swimming in freshwater lakes or ponds. Entry through olfactory nerves.

Abrupt onset: fever, headache, stiff neck, nausea, disorientation, seizures, increased intracranial pressure, coma, death. Trophozoites recognized in uncentrifuged CSF.

Rapidly fatal: recovery reported with treatment (amphotericin B alone or with rifampin, chloramphenicol, ketoconazole).

Acanthamoeba Infections
Acanthamoeba species: both acute and granulomatous meningoencephalitis. Opportunistic infection in alcoholic and immunocompromised patients. Usually fatal.

CHAPTER 32 ■ BACTERIAL TOXINS

DIPHTHERIA

Diphtheria exotoxin binds to receptors on peripheral nerves, inhibits protein synthesis. Demyelinating neuropathy more likely with severe infection.

Palatal and pharyngo-laryngo-esophageal paralysis early; prominent signs in pharyngeal infection. See also Chapter 106.

TETANUS

Tetanus toxin (tetanospasmin) blocks synaptic release of neurotransmitters at the neuromuscular junction, autonomic terminals, and in the CNS, causing local or generalized muscle spasms.

EPIDEMIOLOGY

Clostridium tetani spores ubiquitous in environment. Entry via puncture wounds, compound fractures, firearms or fireworks wounds, contamination of operative wounds, burns, parenteral injections (particularly in intravenous drug users), through umbilicus of newborn infant.

SYMPTOMS

Incubation period 5–10 days. Localized forms (rare): spasms confined to injured limb or to the head.

Generalized form: jaw clenching (trismus), stiff neck, irritability, restlessness; stiff limbs, opisthotonus. "Risus sardonicus" (forced smiling grimace) due to persistent contraction of facial muscles. Intermittent tonic generalized muscle spasms superimposed on persistent limb stiffness. Fever often present.

Complications: dysphagia, cyanosis/asphyxia, seizures (probably due to anoxia).

COURSE AND PROGNOSIS

Mortality rate >50%, usually due to respiratory compromise. Prompt administration of antitoxin and aggressive management of pulmonary, autonomic dysfunction sometimes lifesaving.

TREATMENT

Admit to ICU. Clean wound surgically.

Human tetanus immune globulin (3,000–6,000 units intramuscularly) neutralizes unbound toxin.

Penicillin G inhibits further growth of organisms. Treat muscle spasms with benzodiazepines. Mechanical ventilation with neuromuscular blockade may be required.

Prevention: childhood immunization with tetanus toxoid (= denatured toxin), with boosters every 10 years.

BOTULISM

Clostridium botulinum toxin blocks acetylcholine release at peripheral synapses, causing muscle weakness and autonomic dysfunction.

See Chapter 123.

CHAPTER 33 ■ REYE SYNDROME

Childhood encephalopathy with fatty changes in viscera. Rarely affects infants or adults.

Epidemiology: linked to ingestion of aspirin-containing compounds to treat childhood fever. Usually associated with influenza A, B, varicella infection. Higher rates in white children in suburban or rural environment than in urban African-American or Hispanic children.

Pathology: likely mechanism: diffuse mitochondrial injury; liver, brain most severely affected.

Clinical features: recurrent vomiting followed by confusion, lethargy, coma; typically 4–7 days after onset of viral illness.

Investigations: elevated blood ammonia, lactate, serum transaminases, and prothrombin time. Brain imaging usually normal; may show cerebral edema. EEG diffusely abnormal.

Differential diagnosis: bacterial meningitis, viral encephalitis, drug intoxication (e.g., aspirin, valproic acid, amphetamines); other metabolic disorders (e.g., inherited defects of fatty acid oxidation, branched-chain amino acid metabolism, or urea cycle). Recurrent attacks of Reye-like syndrome imply underlying metabolic disorder.

Treatment: intensive supportive care; hypertonic glucose to promote anabolic state. Most patients recover within a week.

CHAPTER 34 ■ PRION DISEASES

Human prion diseases: kuru, Creutzfeldt-Jakob disease (**CJD**), variant CJD, Gerstmann-Sträussler-Scheinker syndrome (**GSS**), familial fatal insomnia (**FFI**). All progressive, fatal.

May be sporadic, infectious, or inherited.

Human prion protein (PrP) encoded by gene on chromosome 20. PrP^C: normal cellular form (function unknown). PrP^{Sc} (scrapie type): abnormal form accumulates in neurons in prion diseases.

Transmission of abnormal protein alone (no nucleic acid) causes disease; three-dimensional structure important in pathogenesis.

Familial forms (GSS, FFI, 5–10% of patients with CJD) caused by mutations in prion protein gene (PrP).

Common pathology: spongiform degeneration of brain parenchyma; accumulation of PrP^{Sc} forming aggregates in neurons and extracellular amyloid deposits; no inflammation.

KURU

Affected Fore people of New Guinea. Severe trunk, limb, gait ataxia, involuntary movements, convergent strabismus, dementia. Cerebellum most affected. Fatal in 4–24 months. Disappeared with abolition of cannibalism.

CREUTZFELDT-JACOB DISEASE

Progressive disease of cortex, basal ganglia, spinal cord.

EPIDEMIOLOGY

Occurs worldwide. Incidence 1 case per 1 million people annually. Middle-aged and older people. 5–10% familial. 5–10% iatrogenic (corneal transplant; dural graft; growth hormone from pooled human pituitary glands).

146

CLINICAL FEATURES

Gradual onset of dementia in middle or late life, sometimes with unusual behavior. Rapid progression, with pyramidal tract signs (limb weakness, spasticity, hyperreflexia), extrapyramidal signs (tremor, rigidity, dysarthria, slowness of movement), myoclonus (often stimulus sensitive ["startle myoclonus"]). No fever or other usual signs of infection.

INVESTIGATIONS

Routine CSF tests usually normal. Neuronal protein 14-3-3 found in CSF in up to 96% but non-specific; may be present in herpes simplex encephalitis, acute infarction.

EEG: periodic complexes of spike or slow wave activity at intervals of 0.5 to 2.0 seconds in middle and late stages of disease.

MRI: cerebral atrophy. Increased signal intensity on T2-weighted, FLAIR and DWI images in basal ganglia and cortex ("gyriform" pattern, cortical ribbon).

DIAGNOSIS

Clinical diagnosis strongly suggested by combined findings of dementia, myoclonus, and periodic EEG. CSF 14-3-3 protein supportive but not confirmatory. Brain biopsy may be necessary. DNA analysis available for familial cases.

Differential diagnosis: Alzheimer disease, Pick disease, corticobasal ganglionic degeneration, familial myoclonic dementia, multisystem atrophy, lithium toxicity. Fatal within 1 year in 90% of patients. No specific treatment.

Transmissibility: isolation of Creutzfeldt-Jakob patients not necessary. Special autoclaving or inactivating agents, including sodium hypochlorite (household bleach), required when handling blood, CSF, or tissue from affected patients.

VARIANT CJD

Caused by agent responsible for bovine spongiform encephalopathy ("mad cow" disease); transmitted by ingesting affected beef from the United Kingdom.

Symptom onset before age 40. Ataxia, behavioral changes, followed by rapidly progressive dementia. Myoclonic jerks and characteristic EEG abnormalities of CJD absent. 14-3-3 protein found in only 1/3.

Course slower, up to 22 months. About 150 cases reported, almost all in the United Kingdom.

GERSTMANN-STRAUSSLER-SCHEINKER SYNDROME

Autosomal dominant. Course 2 to 10 years. Onset with ataxia, followed by dementia. Prominent brainstem involvement.

EEG: diffuse slowing.

FATAL FAMILIAL INSOMNIA

Autosomal dominant. Onset: age 18–61 years. Course 7–36 months.

Progressive insomnia, dysautonomia (hyperhidrosis, tachycardia, tachypnea, hyperthermia, hypertension). Pyramidal and cerebellar signs, dementia, myoclonus.

Diverse phenotypic expression, even within a family. Insomnia may be late.

EEG: diffuse slowing. MRI usually normal.

Mutation of PrP gene at codon 178, coupled with methionine at codon 129 (if homozygous for methionine, much more rapid course than if heterozygous). Genotyping critical for confirming diagnosis.

CHAPTER 35 ■ WHIPPLE DISEASE

Caused by bacilliform bacterium, *Tropheryma whippelii* (Actinomycetaceae family). Involves intestinal tract, heart, lungs, liver, kidneys, brain. Rare.

Systemic manifestations: weight loss, abdominal pain, diarrhea, arthritis. Anemia, hypoalbuminemia, steatorrhea.

Neurologic manifestations: CNS symptoms in 6–43% (first symptoms in 5%). Cognitive changes, supranuclear gaze palsy, obtundation; behavioral changes; upper motor neurons signs, hypothalamic manifestations, cranial nerve abnormalities, myoclonus, seizures, ataxia.

Diagnostic triad in 15%: dementia, supranuclear gaze palsy, myoclonus. Pendular vergence oscillations of eyes in synchrony with masticatory or skeletal muscles (oculomasticatory or oculo-facial-skeletal "myorhythmia") in 20%.

Diagnosis: biopsy small intestine to demonstrate periodic acid Schiff–staining macrophages. Polymerase chain reaction for bacillus DNA confirmatory.

Treatment: variable response to antibiotics (tetracycline, penicillin, and trimethoprim-sulfamethoxazole). Fulminant course if untreated; can be fatal within 1 month.

Section IV
Cerebrovascular Diseases

CHAPTER 36 ■ PATHOGENESIS, CLASSIFICATION, AND EPIDEMIOLOGY OF CEREBROVASCULAR DISEASE

DEFINITION AND NOSOLOGY

Stroke: sudden loss of neurologic function (global or focal) due to vascular disruption (infarction or hemorrhage) in CNS.

Transient Ischemic Attack (TIA): clinically identical to stroke but shorter duration (<24 hrs, most <1 hr) and no MRI evidence of infarction.

Stroke types: infarct (ischemic stroke, sometimes with hemorrhagic transformation), hemorrhage (subarachnoid, intracerebral). "Silent" stroke: no clinical manifestations but found on CT, MRI, or autopsy.

Prior TIA in <20% of stroke patients. Focal premonitory symptoms: more frequent with infarct than hemorrhage. Headache, vomiting, seizures, coma more frequent with hemorrhage than infarct.

VASCULAR ANATOMY

ANTERIOR CIRCULATION (CAROTID ARTERY AND ITS BRANCHES)

Common carotid origin: innominate artery on left, aortic arch on right.

Internal carotid branches: ophthalmic, superior hypophyseal, posterior communicating, anterior choroidal. Final bifurcation to anterior cerebral artery (ACA), middle cerebral artery (MCA). Posterior cerebral artery directly from internal carotid in 15% of individuals.

Carotid system territory: optic nerves, retina, anterior portion of cerebral hemisphere (frontal, parietal, anterior temporal lobes).

MCA branches and territories: (a) lenticulostriate penetrators (extreme capsule, claustrum, putamen, most of globus pallidus, part of head and entire body of caudate, superior portions of anterior and posterior limbs of internal capsule; (b) two or three branches (upper, lower, and sometimes middle divisions) reaching most cerebral cortex (including insula, operculum, and cortex of frontal, parietal, temporal, occipital lobes).

ACA: frontal pole, medial and orbital surface of frontal lobe. Largest branch: recurrent artery of Heubner.

POSTERIOR CIRCULATION (VERTEBROBASILAR SYSTEM)

Vertebral artery: arises from subclavian. Branches: anterior and posterior spinal arteries (spinal cord), posterior inferior cerebellar artery (PICA; inferior surface of cerebellum). Lateral medulla: supplied by PICA branches or direct vertebral branches.

Basilar artery: merger of right and left vertebral arteries. Branches: paramedian and circumferential penetrators (brainstem); anterior inferior cerebellar, superior cerebellar arteries (ventrolateral aspect of cerebellar cortex); internal auditory (labyrinthine) artery (direct branch from basilar or from anterior cerebellar artery; cochlea, labyrinth, part of facial nerve). Final bifurcation: left and right posterior cerebral arteries (PCA).

PCA branches: penetrators (posteromedial, thalamoperforates, thalamogeniculate, tuberothalamic; supply hypothalamus, dorsolateral midbrain, lateral geniculate, thalamus). PCA itself supplies inferior surface of temporal lobe and medial and inferior surfaces of occipital lobe, including lingual and fusiform gyri.

OTHER FEATURES

Anastomoses: potential alternate blood routes in case of blockage.

Penetrators: usually end arteries, without anastomoses.

PHYSIOLOGY

Normal total cerebral blood flow: 50 mL/min per 100 g of brain tissue. Adult brain weighs 1500 g.

Cerebral autoregulation: cerebral blood flow maintained constant over range of mean arterial pressure between 60 and 140 mm Hg. Constant flow maintained by cerebral arterioles, which dilate/constrict in response to reduction/increase of partial pressure of carbon dioxide ($PaCO_2$). Changes of partial pressure of oxygen (PaO_2) have the opposite effect.

PATHOGENESIS AND CLASSIFICATION

BRAIN INFARCTION

Sudden interruption of cerebral blood supply: (a) alteration of brain metabolism (after 30 seconds); (b) cessation of neuronal function (1 minute); (c) chain of events leads to infarct (5 minutes; usually irreversible); (d) tissue necrosis and softening (days), then replacement by fluid and gliosis (weeks to months).

Earliest change visualized on MRI: increased water content (diffusion weighted imaging).

Major mechanisms: (a) blood flow reduction (severe arterial stenosis or atherosclerotic occlusion); (b) embolism (thrombus traveling from proximal source to distal cerebral vessel); (c) small-vessel disease (occlusion of penetrating artery).

Less frequent mechanisms: arterial dissection, vasculitis, hypercoagulable states, vasospasm, systemic hypotension, hyperviscosity, moyamoya disease, fibromuscular dysplasia, extrinsic compression of major arteries by tumor, cerebral vein occlusion.

Specific etiologies, syndromes, treatment described in Chapters 37 to 48.

Infarct Subtypes

Atherosclerotic infarction: occlusion by atherosclerotic plaque.

Embolism: cardiac thrombus, fragment of atherosclerotic plaque, air bubbles, fragment of heart valve vegetation, fat particle. Infarct confined to cerebral surface territory of single arterial branch. Propensity to hemorrhagic transformation (see below).

Hemorrhagic infarct: caused by local hemorrhage into necrotic tissue of ischemic infarct. More likely with large infarcts, elevated blood pressure.

Small-vessel lacunar infarction: small zone of ischemia ("lacuna") confined to single vessel territory; usually penetrating artery (see Chapter 42).

Cryptogenic infarction: cause of infarct most often undetermined ("small-vessel lacunar infarction"). Embolism often suspected.

INTRACRANIAL HEMORRHAGE

Classified according to location (extradural, subdural, subarachnoid, intracerebral, intraventricular), nature of ruptured vessel (arterial, capillary, venous), cause (primary, secondary).

Epidural hematoma, subdural hematoma: Chapter 64. Intracerebral, cerebellar hemorrhage: Chapter 40. Subarachnoid hemorrhage: Chapter 46.

STROKE EPIDEMIOLOGY

INCIDENCE, PREVALENCE, MORTALITY

U.S. prevalence: 4 million stroke survivors. Incidence: 100 to 300/100,000 population/year. Mortality 5% per year.

Frequency of Stroke Subtypes

Ischemic stroke: 70% to 80% of all strokes. Of these, subtype is cardioembolic in 15% to 30%, large-vessel atherosclerosis in 14% to 40%, small-vessel lacunar in 15% to 30%, cryptogenic in up to 40%.

Intracerebral hemorrhage: 10% to 30%. Intracerebral 2 to 3 times more frequent than subarachnoid.

Reported frequencies vary with population, geography of study, other factors.

DETERMINANTS OF STROKE

Non-modifiable risk factors: age, male sex, family history of stroke, certain ethnicities (African-American; certain Hispanic populations).

Modifiable risk factors: hypertension, cardiac disease (particularly atrial fibrillation), diabetes, hypercholesterolemia, physical inactivity, cigarette use, alcohol abuse, asymptomatic carotid stenosis, history of transient ischemic attacks.

Most powerful risk factors: age, hypertension.

Potential/unusual risk factors: migraine, oral contraceptive use, drug abuse, snoring, polycythemia, sickle-cell anemia, high white blood cell (WBC) count, fibrinogen, hyperuricemia, hyper-homocystinemia, protein C and free protein S deficiencies, lupus anticoagulant, anticardiolipin antibodies.

OUTCOME

Highest mortality in first 30 days after stroke. 8% to 20% after ischemic stroke, 30% to 80% after intracerebral hemorrhage, 20% to 50% after subarachnoid hemorrhage.

Causes: cardiopulmonary complications (more common), transtentorial brain herniation (less common).

Predictors (at onset) of likely fatality: impaired consciousness, severe initial clinical syndrome, hyperglycemia, advanced age.

Stroke recurrence: greatest risk in first week; 3% to 10% in first 30 days. Highest rate in atherosclerotic infarction; lowest in lacunar. Long-term stroke recurrence 4% to 14% per year. Predictors of recurrence unknown.

CHAPTER 37 ■ EXAMINATION OF THE PATIENT WITH CEREBROVASCULAR DISEASE

GOALS

Immediate information about size, location, etiology of stroke, to guide acute treatment.

Establish site and number of suspected lesions, which may not be visible on initial imaging.

SYNDROMES SUGGESTING SPECIFIC ETIOLOGIES

Wernicke aphasia, homonymous hemianopia, top-of-the-basilar syndrome (cortical blindness, agitation, ocular dysmotility, amnesia): cardiac embolism.

Lateral medullary syndrome (Wallenberg syndrome; see Chapter 39, Table 39.2): vertebral artery thrombosis.

Lacunar syndromes (Chapter 39): lipohyalinosis, fibrinoid necrosis of small deep penetrating arterioles.

Gaze deviation, hemiparesis (opposite to gaze), altered mentation: common manifestation of large infarct. If mentation normal, patient still at high risk of acute worsening during first week with cerebral edema.

Gaze deviation, hemiparesis (same side as gaze): lateral pons.

Aphasia, hemineglect: cortical involvement.

FINDINGS WITH LOCALIZING VALUE

GENERAL EXAMINATION

Temperature: fever (rarely caused by subarachnoid hemorrhage [SAH], brainstem infarction). Fever (of any cause) may exacerbate ischemic brain injury.

Blood pressure (BP): rises acutely in 70% to 80% of strokes; returns to baseline spontaneously in few days. Do not treat hypertension associated with ischemic stroke in acute period, to avoid enlarging infarct (exception: malignant hypertension with encephalopathy). Do treat hypertension in setting of intracranial hemorrhage.

Respiration: see Chapter 4.

Fundi: papilledema (increased intracranial pressure), retinopathy (hypertension, diabetes).

Neck: stiff (subarachnoid hemorrhage), carotid bruit.

Heart: murmurs (valve disease leading to embolism), arrhythmia (atrial fibrillation leading to embolism; neurogenic cardiac changes due to subarachnoid hemorrhage or large infarct). Fever and murmur in setting of stroke: consider bacterial endocarditis.

Lungs: aspiration pneumonia (deep hemispheric, brainstem infarct), pulmonary edema (cardiac disease leading to embolism).

NEUROLOGIC EXAMINATION

Mental Status

Level of consciousness: reduced (brainstem infarction; herniation; extensive hemisphere injury), fluctuating (thalamic hemorrhage). May worsen 3 to 5 days after stroke due to edema. Also consider post-ictal state.

Language: aphasia (cortical lesion on dominant side, Alzheimer disease, thalamus, caudate).

Spatial attention: hemineglect, extinction (cortical lesion on nondominant side).

Memory: short-term (anteromedial thalamus, medial temporal lobe), long-term (may affect orientation).

Cranial Nerves

Homonymous hemianopia (primary visual cortex) homonymous quadrantanopia (optic radiations), sectoranopia (lateral geniculate body).

Gaze palsy: dorsolateral frontal lobe (gaze deviation to opposite side of hemiparesis); lateral pons (gaze deviation to same side as hemiparesis); other brainstem locations (internuclear ophthalmoplegia, vertical gaze palsies, nystagmus, other eye movement problems).

Reflexes
Deeply comatose patient: asymmetry of tendon reflexes may be only sign of unilateral brain injury.

Motor Function
Hypotonia: early after stroke; spasticity: after several days.

Subtle weakness: unilateral flattened nasolabial fold, wide palpebral fissure, pronator drift; one hand or leg drops in posture-holding; arm swing decreased in walking, alternating movements slow.

Weakness of face, arm, leg equally in fully awake patient: small infarct in deep brain region such as posterior limb of internal capsule ("pure motor hemiparesis").

"Fractionated hemiparesis": motor cortex lesion. Examples: face and arm weakness with little or no leg weakness (middle cerebral artery [**MCA**] branch); isolated hand weakness (MCA branch); isolated leg weakness (anterior cerebral artery [**ACA**]; weakness of proximal arm and leg, sparing face ("border-zone" ischemia between MCA and ACA territories, due to hemodynamic failure from high-grade internal carotid artery stenosis).

Sensation
Hemicorporeal sensory loss: thalamic lacunae.

Coordination
Ataxic dysmetria on finger-nose-finger test: ipsilateral cerebellum or cerebellum-brainstem connections.

COURSE OF SYMPTOMS AND SIGNS OF STROKE

Common patterns: fluctuating (atherosclerosis); maximal at onset (embolism); stuttering, stepwise worsening (lacunar).

CHAPTER 38 ■ TRANSIENT ISCHEMIC ATTACK

DEFINITION

TIA: neurologic symptoms of ischemic origin that last less than 24 hours; most 1 to 60 minutes.

POSTULATED MECHANISMS

Transient occlusion: intermittent occlusion by fragment of thrombotic plaque; distal branch occlusion (embolus which then breaks into smaller fragments).

Hemodynamic insufficiency: e.g., arrhythmia; subclavian steal syndrome (arm exercise diverts blood away from vertebrae).

Other: intraparenchymal vascular disease, anemia, polycythemia.

CLINICAL FEATURES

Central retinal artery (internal carotid territory): transient monocular blindness (*amaurosis fugax*). Blurring or darkening of vision, peaking within seconds, sometimes as if a curtain had descended, usually clearing within minutes. Embolic particles (Hollenhorst plaques) may be seen in retinal artery branches on funduscopy.

Carotid territory involving the brain: combinations of limb weakness, sensory loss, aphasia, hemineglect, homonymous hemianopia.

Posterior circulation: cerebrum (visual field defects, cortical blindness), brainstem (cranial nerve and long tract signs), cerebellum (vertigo, gait or limb ataxia).

Recurrent TIAs: usually same pattern of symptoms each time.

DIFFERENTIAL DIAGNOSIS

Migraine, cardiac arrhythmia (when causing lightheadedness, not focal brain ischemia), seizures, hypoglycemia, psychogenic origin.

IMAGING

TIA ischemia usually too brief or incomplete to cause infarct, but old or new infarct often seen on CT or MRI.

PROGNOSIS

TIAs imply increased risk for myocardial infarct, stroke, vascular death for $\geq$10 to 15 years. "Crescendo TIAs": two or more attacks within 24 hours; considered a medical emergency. See Chapter 45.

CHAPTER 39 ■ CEREBRAL INFARCTION

SPECIFIC VESSEL OCCLUSIONS

See Table 39.1. Following are notes on selected features.

MIDDLE CEREBRAL ARTERY (MCA)

UNUSUAL SIGNS OF DOMINANT HEMISPHERE DAMAGE

Apraxia: see Chapter 2.
Gerstmann syndrome: agraphia, acalculia, left-right confusion, finger agnosia; infarct of angular or supramarginal gyrus.

TABLE 39.1
SYNDROMES OF CEREBRAL INFARCTION

Artery occluded	Syndrome
Internal carotid	Ipsilateral blindness Contralateral hemiparesis, hemianesthesia Hemianopia Aphasia (dominant hemisphere), hemineglect (non-dominant)
Middle cerebral Main trunk	Hemiplegia Hemianesthesia Hemianopia Aphasia (dominant hemisphere), hemineglect (non-dominant)
Upper division	Hemiparesis, sensory loss (arm, face more affected than leg) Broca aphasia or hemineglect
Lower division	Wernicke aphasia or nondominant behavior disorder without hemiparesis
Penetrating artery	Pure motor hemiparesis
Anterior cerebral	Hemiparesis, sensory loss (leg more affected than arm) Impaired responsiveness ("abulia," "akinetic mutism"), especially if bilateral infarction Left-sided ideomotor apraxia or tactile anomia
Posterior cerebral	Cortical, unilateral: isolated hemianopia, quadrantanopia; alexia or color anomia Cortical, bilateral: cerebral blindness, with or without macular sparing Thalamic: pure sensory stroke; may leave *anesthesia dolorosa* (spontaneous pain) Subthalamic nucleus: hemiballism Bilateral inferior temporal lobe: amnesia Midbrain: oculomotor palsy, other eye movement abnormalities

UNUSUAL SIGNS OF NONDOMINANT HEMISPHERE DAMAGE

Hemineglect: patient ignores contralateral half of external space or own body, sometimes denies hemiplegia on that side (anosognosia), or cannot recognize affected limb as one's own (asomatognosia); usually parietal lobe lesion.

Altered spatial perception: difficulty copying simple diagrams (constructional apraxia), interpreting maps or maintaining physical orientation (topographagnosia), putting on clothing (dressing apraxia); convexity lesions, especially parietal.

Prosopagnosia: difficulty recognizing faces; bilateral temporo-occipital lesions.

Aprosody: difficulty expressing or recognizing non-propositional (prosodic) aspects of speech (emotional tone, sarcasm, humor); usually due to convexity lesions.

Acute confusional state: typically parietal lesions.

POSTERIOR CEREBRAL ARTERY

Bilateral infarct: (a) cortical blindness, sometimes with denial of blindness (Anton syndrome); (b) tunnel vision (macular sparing); (c) simultanagnosia (inability to synthesize parts of what is normally seen as a whole), poor eye-hand coordination, difficulty coordinating gaze, metamorphopsia (distortion of what is seen), visual agnosia.

    Bilateral involvement of inferomedial temporal lobe or medial thalamus: memory disturbance.

Midbrain damage: (a) bilateral loss of vertical gaze, convergence spasm, retractatory nystagmus, lid retraction (Collier sign), oculomotor palsy, internuclear ophthalmoplegia, decreased pupillary reactivity; (b) lethargy or coma (reticular activating system); (c) contralateral hemiparesis (cerebral peduncle); (d) contralateral ataxia (superior cerebellar peduncle); (e) "peduncular" hallucinosis (formed vivid hallucinations); infarct in thalamus or pars reticulata of substantia nigra.

ANTERIOR CHOROIDAL ARTERY (ACA)

Contralateral hemiplegia, sensory loss, homonymous hemianopia, midbrain peduncle, posterior limb of internal capsule, lateral geniculate body, optic radiations.

INTERNAL CAROTID ARTERY (ICA)

Abrupt cessation of flow (ICA occlusion, hypotension plus stenosis): damage to border zones between arterial territories ("watershed" or "border-zone" infarct). Syncope at onset, focal seizures, transcortical aphasia. Bilateral border-zone infarct: cortical blindness (parietooccipital damage) or bibrachial palsy (bilateral rolandic damage at the MCA-ACA border).

Emboli from atherosclerotic plaques in ICA to retina (via ophthalmic and central retinal arteries): partial or complete visual loss.

VERTEBROBASILAR ARTERIES

See Table 39.2.

Infarct of inferior cerebellum or occlusion of internal auditory artery: syndrome like acute labyrinthitis (vertigo, nausea, vomiting, nystagmus).

Large cerebellar infarct: syndrome like cerebellar hemorrhage (headache, dizziness, ataxia). If cerebellar edema compresses brainstem, may see abducens or gaze palsy, progression to coma and death. Surgical decompression may be indicated.

Bilateral ischemia of pontine or medullary pyramidal tract may cause drop attacks (fleeting loss of strength or muscle tone without loss of consciousness).

Infarct of corticobulbar and corticospinal tracts in basis pontis (sparing tegmentum): "locked-in syndrome" (paralysis of limbs and lower cranial nerves); communication only by preserved blinks or eye movements, proves consciousness intact.

OTHER INFARCT SYNDROMES

Pseudobulbar palsy: bilateral corticospinal reflex signs (with or without major bilateral hemiparesis), supranuclear

TABLE 39.2
SIGNS THAT INDICATE LEVEL OF BRAINSTEM VASCULAR SYNDROMES

Syndrome	Artery affected	Structure involved	Manifestations
Medial syndromes			
Medulla	Paramedian branches	Emerging fibers of 12th nerve	Ipsilateral hemiparalysis of tongue
Inferior pons	Paramedian branches	Pontine gaze center, near or in nucleus of 6th nerve	Paralysis of gaze to side of lesion
		Emerging fibers of 6th nerve	Ipsilateral abduction paralysis
Superior pons	Paramedian branches	Medial longitudinal fasciculus	Internuclear ophthalmoplegia
Lateral syndromes			
Medulla	Posterior inferior cerebellar	Emerging fibers of 9th, 10th nerves	Dysphagia, hoarseness, ipsilateral paralysis of vocal cord; ipsilateral loss of pharyngeal reflex
		Vestibular nuclei	Vertigo, nystagmus
		Descending tract and nucleus of 5th nerve	Ipsilateral facial analgesia
		Solitary nucleus and tract	Taste loss on ipsilateral half of tongue posteriorly
		Descending sympathetic fibers	Ipsilateral Horner syndrome
Inferior pons	Anterior inferior cerebellar	Emerging fibers of 7th nerve	Ipsilateral facial paralysis
		Solitary nucleus and tract	Taste loss on ipsilateral half of tongue anteriorly
		Cochlear nuclei	Deafness, tinnitus
Mid-pons		Motor nucleus of 5th nerve	Ipsilateral jaw weakness
		Emerging sensory fibers of 5th nerve	Ipsilateral facial numbness

Modified from Rowland LP. In: Kandel ER, Schwartz JH, eds. *Principles of neural science*, 3rd ed. New York: Elsevier, 1991.

dysarthria and dysphagia (with impaired volitional movement of soft palate and pharynx but exaggerated gag reflex), emotional incontinence (exaggerated crying or laughing). Two major cerebral infarcts on different sides of brain or numerous bilateral lacunae.

Vascular dementia: see Chapter 107.

CHAPTER 40 ■ CEREBRAL AND CEREBELLAR HEMORRHAGE

INTRACEREBRAL HEMORRHAGE

Blood in brain parenchyma.

ETIOLOGY

Arteriopathy of deep penetrating arteries (arteriolosclerosis): basal ganglia, thalamus, brainstem, cerebellum. Most common type of intracerebral hemorrhage. Greatest risk factor is chronic hypertension. Other risk factors: increasing age, cigarette smoking, alcohol consumption, low serum cholesterol, selected ethnicities (African, Hispanic, Asian origin).

Amyloid angiopathy: recurrent intracerebral hemorrhages, usually after fifth decade, particularly lobar in location. Dementia in 30%.

Other causes: brain tumor, sympathomimetic drugs, coagulopathies, treatment with anticoagulants or fibrinolytic agents, arteriovenous malformations, aneurysms, cavernous angiomas, moyamoya disease, trauma, illicit drug abuse.

CLINICAL FEATURES

Onset gradual (minutes to hours) rather than sudden (as seen with infarct or subarachnoid hemorrhage), because hemorrhage usually starts in small vessels and accumulates over time.

Headache, vomiting often present.

INVESTIGATIONS

CT: high density of acute blood (bright) in brain parenchyma.

SYNDROMES

Progressive for minutes to hours. Vomiting, headache more frequent in hemorrhage than infarct.

Putamen: site most frequently affected. May produce contralateral hemiparesis, hemianesthesia, hemianopia, conjugate horizontal ocular deviation. Aphasia or impaired awareness of deficits (anosognosia) with large hematoma.

Thalamus: hemianesthesia precedes hemiparesis. Upward gaze may be impaired.

Pons: usually coma with quadriparesis and grossly disconjugate eye movements.

Cerebral lobes: usually posterior two thirds of brain. Progressive evolution and vomiting much less frequent. Syndrome determined by affected lobe.

TREATMENT

Airway protection, adequate ventilation, maintenance of mean arterial blood pressure below 130 mm Hg.

Increased intracranial pressure may require osmotherapy, controlled hyperventilation, induced coma. Steroids play no proven role. Treatment with recombinant activated factor VII (rFVIIa) within four hours after symptom onset limits size of hematoma, reduces mortality, and improves functional outcome; small risk of thromboembolic adverse events.

Surgical evacuation commonly performed, but benefit proven only for cerebellar hemorrhage. Intraventricular extension increases likelihood of fatal outcome.

CEREBELLAR HEMORRHAGE

Usually abrupt onset of vomiting and severe ataxia, occasionally with dysarthria, cranial nerve deficit, paralysis of conjugate lateral gaze. Usually no change in consciousness; no focal weakness or sensory loss (vs. brainstem hemorrhage). Lethargy (due to brainstem compression) usually marks irreversibility.

Imperative to consider diagnosis in all patients with this clinical syndrome (or any older person with acute or new difficulty walking). Gait must be tested in all patients with unexplained vomiting.

Treatment: surgical evacuation (within hours) before onset of lethargy. Required in presence of fourth ventricular displacement, lateral ventricular enlargement, cisternal obliteration, or declining level of consciousness.

CHAPTER 41 ■ GENETICS OF STROKE

ISCHEMIC STROKE

Role of genetics incompletely understood in pathogenesis of ischemic stroke; confounded by possible environmental factors.

Documented risk factors of ischemic stroke with strong genetic influence: hypertension, hypercholesterolemia, diabetes, heart disease, obesity.

Single gene disorders rare; account for small proportion of all strokes. See below and Table 41.1.

TABLE 41.1

DISORDERS WITH ISCHEMIC STROKE AND MENDELIAN INHERITANCE

Disorder	Inheritance
Coagulation Disorders	
Protein C deficiency	AD
Protein S deficiency	AD
Activated protein C resistance Leiden type	AD
Antithrombin III deficiency	AD
Sickle cell disease	AR
Connective tissue disorders	
Neurofibromatosis type I	AD
Ehlers-Danlos syndrome type IV	AD
Marfan syndrome	AD
Vasculopathies	
Familial moyamoya disease	Unknown
Metabolic disorders	
Fabry disease	XR
MELAS	AD
Homocystinuria	AR

AD, autosomal dominant; AR, autosomal recessive; XR, X-linked recessive.

CADASIL

Autosomal dominant; mutations in NOTCH3 gene on chromosome 19. Recurrent episodes of subcortical infarcts or transient ischemic attacks; absence of hypertension or other stroke risk factors. Onset age 30 to 50 years old.

Clinical manifestations: stroke, dementia, pseudobulbar palsy, migraine. No specific treatment. Mean survival: 20 years from onset.

MRI: extensive leukoencephalopathy, with deep small infarcts in subcortical white matter, basal ganglia; "U fibers" spared.

Diagnosis: mutation analysis detects up to 95%; skin biopsy with immunostaining for NOTCH3 protein useful in remainder.

Phenotypic variant: familial clusters of hemiplegic migraine (CADASILM; "M" for migraine).

INTRACEREBRAL HEMORRHAGE (ICH)

HEREDITARY CEREBRAL AMYLOID ANGIOPATHY

Dutch and Icelandic forms; autosomal dominant; lobar hemorrhages and premature death in young adults.

Dutch form: mutations in amyloid precursor protein gene. Icelandic form: deletion in cystatin C gene on chromosome 20.

CEREBRAL CAVERNOUS MALFORMATION

Familial forms: autosomal dominant with incomplete penetrance. To date, 3 different loci mapped to chromosomes 3 and 7.

SUBARACHNOID HEMORRHAGE (SAH)

Familial aggregation of SAH, but inheritance mode unclear. First-degree relative with SAH confers 3- to 5-fold increased risk; no specific genes yet identified.

CHAPTER 42 ■ OTHER CEREBROVASCULAR SYNDROMES

LACUNAR STROKES

Small ischemic infarcts due to occlusion of small penetrating arterioles, usually with sustained hypertension. Location: distribution of deep penetrating arteries (basal ganglia, deep hemispheric white matter, brainstem, cerebellum). Often clinically silent.

Pathophysiology: mechanism unknown; pathology described as "lipohyalinosis."

Prognosis usually good, if hypertension is controlled.

LACUNAR SYNDROMES

Certain syndromes characteristic of lacunar stroke. However, these can also be caused by other types of stroke.

Examples

Pure hemiplegia: face, arm, or leg affected, or combination, without sensory loss. Disruption of corticospinal tracts in internal capsule or pons.
Pure hemisensory stroke: numbness or paresthesias of face, arm, leg. Lacunes usually in sensory nucleus of thalamus.
Others: ataxic hemiparesis; dysarthria-clumsy hand syndrome.

HYPERTENSIVE ENCEPHALOPATHY

Encephalopathy with accelerated hypertension. Headache, confusion, drowsiness, blurring of vision, occasional seizures, infrequent focal signs. Attributed to generalized arteriolar constriction, loss of cerebral autoregulation.

Examination: diastolic pressure usually >140 mm Hg (lower in children and postpartum women); papilledema.
Imaging: posterior leukoencephalopathy on MRI.

Differential diagnosis: stroke; systemic disorders (uremia, electrolyte imbalance); cyclosporine toxicity.

Treatment: hypotensive agents (e.g., sodium nitroprusside, labetalol) to reduce mean arterial pressure by 15% to 20%, but not below 125 mm Hg, initially. Sustained hypertension may be life-threatening. However, excessive reduction of blood pressure (BP) may result in watershed infarct. Neurologic symptoms reverse with BP reduction.

FIBROMUSCULAR HYPERPLASIA

Fibromuscular bands of unknown origin cause segmental narrowing in large arteries. Usually middle-aged women.

Manifestations: asymptomatic carotid bruit (most common), TIAs, ischemic infarcts. Hypertension common, with renal artery involvement. Characteristic syndrome: carotid and renal artery bruits, hypertension.

Imaging: "string of pearls" appearance on cerebral angiogram.

Treatment: antiplatelet drugs, anticoagulation, surgical dilation may reduce frequency of TIAs.

MULTI-INFARCT OR VASCULAR DEMENTIA

See Chapter 39.

CEREBRAL AMYLOID ANGIOPATHY

Also known as *congophilic angiopathy*. Symptom onset (usually lobar intracerebral hemorrhage) in late middle age. Recurrence associated with dementia.

ANTIPHOSPHOLIPID SYNDROME

Also known as lupus anticoagulant syndrome, anticardiolipin antibody syndrome. Lupus anticoagulants: anticoagulant activity *in vitro*; however, they are risk factor for thrombosis.

SYNDROMES

Primary antiphospholipid syndrome: recurrent fetal loss, mild thrombocytopenia, false-positive RPR or VDRL.
Secondary antiphospholipid syndrome: with systemic lupus erythematosus, other autoimmune diseases, neoplasm, phenothiazines. Thrombosis both arterial and venous. May be associated with false-positive VDRL test, mild thrombocytopenia.
Sneddon syndrome: antiphospholipid syndrome plus livedo reticularis.

NEUROLOGIC MANIFESTATIONS

Migraine-like headaches, strokes (arterial or venous), encephalopathy with confusion or seizures, retinopathy with amaurosis fugax and acute ischemic neuropathy.

TREATMENT

Long-term anticoagulation; goal International Normalized Ratio (INR) 2.0 to 3.0. Treat primary underlying condition.

HYPERHOMOCYSTEINEMIA

Elevated blood homocysteine levels.
  Causes: low dietary folate intake, renal diseases, inborn errors of metabolism (e.g., homocystinuria), drugs.
  Associated with ischemic stroke, myocardial infarction.
  Reduction of homocysteine does not reduce risk of stroke, myocardial infarction, or death.

CAUSES OF STROKE IN YOUNG ADULTS

Age <45 in 5% to 10% of all strokes. In first year after stroke, mortality 4.5%, recurrence 1.4%.

See Table 42.1. The following are notes on specific conditions.

TABLE 42.1

DIFFERENTIAL DIAGNOSIS OF STROKE IN YOUNG ADULTS

Vascular Diseases
Atherosclerosis
Arteritis
Arteriovenous malformations, telangiectasias, cavernous
  angiomas
Aneurysms
CADASIL (see Chapter 41)
Dissection (traumatic or spontaneous)
Fibromuscular Dysplasia
Migraine
MELAS (see Chapter 97)
Moyamoya syndrome
Oral contraceptive use
Venous occlusive diseases

Cardiogenic Emboli
Anatomic abnormalities: e.g., patent foramen ovale, mitral
  valve prolapse; valvular replacement
Arrhythmias
Cardiomyopathy
Immune complex disorders
Infections: bacterial endocarditis; viral cardiomyopathy;
  rheumatic heart disease
Tumors: atrial myxoma

Blood Elements
Erythrocytes: sickle cell disease; polycythemia vera
Platelets: thrombocytosis; thrombotic thrombocytopenia
  purpura
Proteins: factor V-Leiden mutation; antiphospholipid syndrome;
  Waldenström macroglobulinemia
Coagulation defects: deficiency of Protein C, S, antithrombin III;
  alcohol-induced prothrombotic state; paroxysmal nocturnal
  hemoglobinuria; plasminogen activator inhibitor-1 (PAI-1)
  polymorphism; prothrombin polymorphism

Complicated migraine (migraine with focal neurologic symptoms that persist during headache phase or are prolonged): avoid treatment with vasoconstrictive drugs (triptans, ergot derivatives). Avoid oral contraceptive use if associated with complicated migraine.

Intravenous drug use: strokes due to arteritis, occlusive disease. Bacterial endocarditis poses risk of embolic infarcts, subarachnoid hemorrhage (rupture of mycotic aneurysm).

Patent foramen ovale: venous embolus may reach brain (paradoxical embolus).

Sickle cell disease: see Chapters 44, 147.

Polycythemia vera: TIAs may occur due to hyperviscosity.

CHAPTER 43 ■ DIFFERENTIAL DIAGNOSIS OF STROKE

CLINICAL FEATURES OF STROKE SUBTYPES

Distinction essential in choice of acute treatment of stroke: in first 3 hours, thrombolysis may be indicated in acute infarct; contraindicated in acute hemorrhage. Subsequently, anticoagulation may be indicated for cerebral embolism.

The following clinical features suggest specific stroke subtype but overlap is evident.

INFARCTION

Cerebral embolism. Occlusion usually in distal vessels (e.g., cortex). Sudden onset, isolated cortical signs (aphasia, hemianopia).

Thrombosis. Distal vessel occlusion: often indistinguishable from embolism. Deep penetrating vessel: elementary deficit (weakness, sensory loss, ataxia), often affecting large body regions (arm, face, leg simultaneously), sparing cortical function (language, spatial attention. Proximal occlusion (e.g., MCA stem): severe deficits of entire half of body, often with impaired alertness.

HEMORRHAGE

Characteristically smooth onset. May be indistinguishable from infarction when onset is rapid. CT necessary to rule out hemorrhage.

Epidural hematoma: fracture line passing through groove of middle meningeal artery may be visible on CT (bone windows). Even severe syndrome may be reversible by surgical evacuation.

Subdural hematoma: typically of venous origin. Bleeding may be recurrent. Precipitating trauma often not elicited in history (absent or forgotten).

TRANSIENT ISCHEMIC ATTACK (TIA)

Because subsequent risk of stroke is the same as after stroke, TIA is increasingly managed as it would be for infarction.

UNMASKING PREVIOUS STROKE SYNDROME

Focal deficits similar to those accompanying a previous stroke or TIA can result from generalized metabolic or toxic insult (hypoglycemia, dehydration, systemic infection) or exposure to psychotropic medication. Does not indicate new stroke. Deficits disappear with resolution of systemic stressor.

NONVASCULAR DISORDERS IN DIFFERENTIAL DIAGNOSIS OF STROKE

Characteristic features of stroke: (a) sudden onset; (b) focal signs; (c) presence of vascular disease (e.g., hypertension, cardiac disease, arteriosclerosis) or other risk factors (e.g., co-agulation abnormalities, cardiac disease, certain infections).

DIAGNOSTIC ACCURACY

Emergency room diagnosis of "stroke" 81% accurate in one study. Stroke "mimics" included: seizures, systemic infection, brain tumor, toxic-metabolic encephalopathy.

Less frequent: positional vertigo, cardiac events, syncope, trauma, subdural hematoma, herpes simplex virus encephalitis, transient global amnesia, dementia, demyelinating disease, C-spine fracture, MG, parkinsonism, hypertensive encephalopathy, conversion disorder.

SELECTED STROKE MIMICS

Trauma: brain contusion; usually frontal, temporal, occipital poles. External signs of trauma often present.

Seizures: immediate postictal hemiparesis mimics stroke. Movements at onset (e.g., limb jerking), obtundation, amnesia suggest seizure. Seizure itself may result from infarct (rarely) or hemorrhage.

Migraine: clues include subsequent headache, similar prior attacks, young age, characteristic visual aura at other times. Hemiplegic migraine may be familial.

Tumor, abscess: clues include slow evolution (days to weeks), appearance on imaging.

COMA

Metabolic coma: focal signs occasionally present; usually remit when metabolic cause is reversed.

Barbiturate intoxication: coma may include paralysis of eye movement and flaccid paralysis of limbs with normal pupillary reactions, mimicking brainstem infarct.

Alcohol, drug abuse: exclude subdural hematoma with CT or MRI because of high risk of head injury.

CHAPTER 44 ■ STROKE IN CHILDREN

Important differences from adults characterize childhood stroke: 1) predisposing factors (e.g., cyanotic heart disease) common; 2) clinical evolution (outcome often better in children); 3) anatomic site of pathology (e.g., internal carotid artery occlusions often intracranial rather than extracranial; cerebral aneurysms typically peripheral rather than near circle of Willis).

INCIDENCE

Low overall: annual incidence 2.5/100,000 children in one study.

Groups with increased risk: patients with sickle cell disease (7% to 11% have stroke before age 20 years); premature infants (those <1,500 g in intensive care for >24 hours: 50% incidence of subependymal or intraventricular hemorrhage); children with congenital heart disease.

ETIOLOGY

See Table 44.1. Below are comments on selected causes.

ARTERIAL THROMBOSIS

Arterial compression: trauma, tumor, craniometaphyseal dysplasia, retropharyngeal abscess.

Sickle-cell disease: see Chapter 147.

Extracranial carotid occlusion: usually due to head or neck trauma.

Basal occlusive disease with telangiectasia (*moyamoya*): "puff of smoke" appearance on angiogram; stenosis of arteries at base of brain; often bilateral; prominent telangiectasia. Most are idiopathic. May complicate sickle-cell disease, bacterial or tuberculous meningitis, neurofibromatosis, radiotherapy. Often recurs.

TABLE 44.1

ETIOLOGY OF STROKE IN CHILDREN

Dural Sinus and Cerebral Venous Thrombosis
Infections: face, ears, paranasal sinuses, meninges
Dehydration and debilitating states
Blood dyscrasias: sickle cell, leukemia, thrombotic
  thrombocytopenia
Neoplasm: neuroblastoma
Sturge-Weber-Dimitri syndrome (trigeminal encephaloangiomatosis)
Lead encephalopathy
Vein of Galen malformation

Arterial Thrombosis
Idiopathic
Arterial dissection
Arteriosclerosis: progeria
Cerebral arteritis
Collagen disease: lupus erythematosus, periarteritis nodosa,
  Takayasu arteritis, Kawasaki syndrome
Trauma to cervical carotid or cerebral arteries
Inflammatory bowel disease
Delayed radiation vasculopathy
Sickle-cell disease
Extra-arterial disorders: craniometaphyseal dysplasia,
  mucormycosis, skull base tumors
Metabolic: diabetes mellitus, hyperlipidemia, homocystinuria,
  CDG 1a[a], sulfite oxidase deficiency, molybdenum cofactor
  deficiency
Oral contraceptives
Drug abuse

Arterial Embolism
Air: complication of cardiac, neck, or thoracic surgery
Fat: complication of long-bone fracture
Septic: complication of endocarditis, pneumonia, lung abscess
Arrhythmias
Congenital heart disease
Complication of umbilical vein catheterization

Intracranial Hemorrhage
Premature neonate: subependymal and intraventricular
Full term neonate: subdural
Vascular malformation
Aneurysm
Trauma
Blood dyscrasias
Vitamin-deficiency syndromes
Hepatic disease
Hypertension
Complications of immunosuppressant drugs and anticoagulants
Infarcts of other types
Mitochondrial disease (MELAS)

[a]CDG 1a, congenital disorder of glycosylation 1a.

Treatment

Anticoagulants rarely indicated unless stroke in progress. Parenteral fluids, antibiotics, anticonvulsants as needed. Moyamoya: surgical revascularization procedures improve circulation to ischemic areas; associated with better long-term outcome. Sickle-cell disease: repeated blood transfusion to maintain hemoglobin S <20% reduces risk of future strokes (see Chapter 147).

CEREBRAL EMBOLISM

Usually cardiogenic; echocardiogram should be performed.

Angiography for all children with septic emboli to exclude mycotic aneurysm.

Treatment: anticoagulants for selected cardiac conditions.

INTRACRANIAL HEMORRHAGE

Usually due to trauma or bleeding disorders. Once these excluded, consider ruptured AVM or aneurysm.

METABOLIC DISORDERS

MELAS: see Chapter 97.

Congenital disorder of glycosylation (CDG) 1a (phosphomannomutase deficiency): see Chapter 87. Screening test: serum carbohydrate-deficient transferrin.

Homocystinuria (cystathionine β-synthetase deficiency): autosomal recessive; high serum methionine and homocystine concentrations and excessive urinary excretion of homocystine. High risk of cerebral arterial occlusive disease or venous thrombosis.

CLINICAL EVALUATION

See Table 44.2. Selection of tests guided by clinical situation.

General guidelines: newborn/infant: consider coagulopathy, hypoxia/ischemia. Cardiac anomaly: embolic stroke. Older infants and children: consider vasculitis.

TABLE 44.2

CLINICAL EVALUATION OF CHILD WITH STROKE

Laboratory Studies

Blood
Coagulation profile
Fibrinogen
Protein C
Protein S
Antithrombin III
Factor V Leiden
Prothrombin 20210A
Plasminogen activator inhibitor
Anticardiolipin antibody
Lipid profile
Antinuclear antibody
Anti-dsDNA
ESR
Amino acids
Blood cultures
Toxicology screen
Sickle-cell preparation
Mitochondrial DNA studies

Urine
Amino acids
Organic acids

CSF
Glucose, protein
Cell count, differential
Lactate
Cultures

Imaging

Radiologic
CT head
MRI head
MR angiogram/MR venogram
Cerebral angiogram

Ultrasound
Carotid artery Doppler
Vertebral artery Doppler
Transcranial Doppler
Echocardiogram

Nuclear
SPECT

Other Studies
EEG

COURSE

Infants or young children with new hemiplegia usually recover to point of walking. Children often improve much more than adults with comparable lesions, but up to half will have lifelong disability (hemiparesis, cognitive or social impairment).

CHAPTER 45 ■ TREATMENT AND PREVENTION OF STROKE

ATHEROTHROMBOTIC STROKES AND TIAS

SURGERY

Indications for carotid endarterectomy (CEA): Stenosis $\geq 70\%$ (if patient medically suitable).

Balloon angioplasty, stents (extracranial and intracranial stenosis): under investigation.

MEDICAL THERAPY

Aspirin: 25% stroke recurrence risk reduction. Best dose controversial; 325 mg daily common in U.S.

Clopidogrel: comparable efficacy to aspirin; combined long-term use with aspirin not recommended (increased risk of hemorrhage).

Dipyridamole plus aspirin: may be more effective than aspirin alone.

Anticoagulation with warfarin: no proven benefit for prevention of recurrent stroke beyond that of anti-platelet therapy; increased risk of bleeding.

TABLE 45.1

TISSUE PLASMINOGEN ACTIVATOR (TPA)
CONTRAINDICATIONS

Stroke or head trauma within the preceding three months
Major surgery within the preceding two weeks
History of intracerebral hemorrhage
Systolic blood pressure >185 mm Hg
Diastolic blood pressure >110 mm Hg
Rapidly improving or minor neurologic symptoms and signs
Evidence of subarachnoid hemorrhage
Gastrointestinal or urinary tract bleeding within three weeks
Arterial puncture at a noncompressible site within one week
Seizure at stroke onset
Prothrombin time >15 seconds or INR >1.7
Heparin therapy within two days and elevated PTT
Platelet count < 100,000/mL
Blood glucose <30 mg/dL (2.7 mmol/L) or >400 mg/dL
   (21.6 mmol/L)
Aggressive treatment necessary to lower blood pressure

COMPLETED STROKES WITH FIXED NEUROLOGIC ABNORMALITIES

Intravenous **tissue plasminogen activator (tPA)** if infusion can
be started within 3 hours of onset of symptoms, head CT shows
no hemorrhage and minimal infarction, and no contraindications exist (see Table 45.1).

tPA dose: 0.9 mg/kg: 10% in 1 minute, remainder in 60
minutes.

Better long-term functional disability scores in treated patients.

Incidence of intracerebral hemorrhage in treated patients:
6% in one study (NINDS, 1995).

EMBOLIC STROKES OF CARDIAC AND AORTIC ORIGIN

Indications for **anticoagulation:** atrial fibrillation; presence of
intracardiac thrombus (e.g., post-myocardial infarction, severe
cardiomyopathy). Factors associated with increased risk for
embolization in atrial fibrillation: previous embolization, left

ventricular hypertrophy with reduced ejection fraction, hypertension, congestive cardiac failure, females >age 75.

Infected prosthetic valve: antibiotics; consider valve replacement.

Myxomatous emboli: tumor excision.

Patent foramen ovale: consider aspirin, anticoagulation, surgical repair. No definite guidelines.

Aortic atheroma: benefit of anticoagulation under investigation.

Anticoagulation contraindicated if infarct large.

HEMORRHAGE

Intracerebral: see Chapter 40. Subarachnoid: see Chapter 46.

STROKE REHABILITATION

Multidisciplinary team including physical, occupational, and speech therapists, as well as physicians. Begin physical rehabilitation to maximize functional as soon as possible. Depression frequently accompanies stroke; antidepressant medication may benefit some patients. See Chapter 170.

STROKE PREVENTION

Great overlap with prevention of atherosclerosis.

Treat hypertension (>25% reduction in stroke incidence in past 20 years); control blood cholesterol (increased LDL, reduced HDLs are atherogenic); stop smoking; modify obesity, stress, sedentary lifestyle.

Other measures: control blood glucose in diabetes.

CHAPTER 46 ■ SUBARACHNOID HEMORRHAGE

Acute hemorrhage into space between pia and arachnoid membranes (subarachnoid space). 5% of all strokes; nearly 30,000 cases annually in the United States (annual incidence 1/10,000).

80% due to saccular ("berry") aneurysms. Other causes listed in Table 46.1. Most common at age 40 to 60; women >men.

PATHOLOGY AND EPIDEMIOLOGY OF INTRACRANIAL ANEURYSMS

Saccular aneurysms: prevalence 2% in adults. Uncommon in children. 20% of patients with subarachnoid hemorrhage (SAH) have two or more aneurysms.

Most common sites: junction of posterior communicating and internal carotid arteries ($\approx$ 40%), anterior communicating artery complex ($\approx$ 30%), middle cerebral artery at first major branch point ($\approx$ 20%).

Risk of rupture of asymptomatic intracranial aneurysm: 0.7% per year; of previously ruptured aneurysm after 6 months, 2% to 4% per year.

Major risk factors for aneurysm: increasing age, atherosclerosis, family history of intracranial aneurysm, autosomal dominant polycystic kidney disease (PCKD). Indications for screening for unruptured aneurysms by MRA: PCKD, 2 or more first-degree relatives with intracranial aneurysms (test positive in 10%).

Risk factors for bleeding: previous rupture, large size, cigarette smoking, aneurysm-related headache or cranial nerve compression, alcohol use, family history of SAH, female sex, posterior circulation location, multiple aneurysms, hypertension, cocaine, or amphetamine use.

CLINICAL FEATURES

Explosive ("thunderclap") headache, then stiff neck. Often "the worst headache of my life." Common associated symptoms: loss of consciousness, nausea, vomiting, photophobia, back or leg pain. Focal signs sometimes present.

TABLE 46.1
NON-ANEURYSMAL CAUSES OF SUBARACHNOID HEMORRHAGE

Trauma
Idiopathic perimesencephalic SAH
Arteriovenous malformation
Intracranial arterial dissection
Cocaine and amphetamine use
Mycotic aneurysm
Pituitary apoplexy
Moyamoya disease
Central nervous system vasculitis
Sickle cell disease
Coagulation disorders
Primary or metastatic neoplasm

Neurologic condition on arrival at hospital most important determinant of outcome (Table 46.2).

Prodromal symptoms (headache, stiff neck, nausea, vomiting, syncope, disturbed vision) in 33%. Prodromal headache may disappear for days before onset of full-blown syndrome ("sentinel headache").

Perimesencephalic SAH: blood confined to perimesencephalic cisterns. Normal neurologic examination; benign course; attributed to venous bleeding.

TABLE 46.2
HUNT AND HESS GRADING SCALE FOR ANEURYSMAL SAH

Grade	Clinical findings	Hospital mortality (%)[a]	
		1968	2002
I	Asymptomatic or mild headache	11	7
II	Moderate to severe headache, or oculomotor palsy	26	2
III	Confused, drowsy, or mild focal signs	37	10
IV	Stupor (localizes to pain)	71	35
V	Coma (posturing or no motor response to pain)	100	65
TOTAL		35	20

[a]Data from 275 patients reported by Hunt and Hess in 1968, and 404 patients treated at Columbia University Medical Center between 2000 and 2002.

Signs of unruptured intracranial aneurysm (compression of adjacent neural structures or thromboembolism): oculomotor nerve palsy (posterior communicating artery); deficits of cranial nerves III to VI (intracavernous segment of internal carotid artery).

DIAGNOSTIC STUDIES

CT: sensitivity 90% to 95% within 24 hours; 80% at 3 days; 50% at 7 days.

LP: mandatory with high clinical suspicion and normal CT. Elevated pressure and protein. Large number of red blood cells (RBCs), which does not diminish from first to last collected tube. SAH differentiated from traumatic tap by xanthochromic (yellow-tinged) appearance of centrifuged supernatant; may take 12 hours to appear. High RBCs, xanthochromia disappear in about 2 weeks.

Angiography: defining diagnostic procedure for intracranial aneurysms. If negative, repeat in 2 weeks (except for perimesencephalic SAH).

COMPLICATIONS OF ANEURYSMAL SAH

Rebleeding (if aneurysm not clipped): risk highest in first 24 hours (4%); remains elevated (approximately 1% to 2% per day) for 4 weeks. Cumulative risk in untreated patients: 20% at 2 weeks, 30% at 1 month, 40% at 6 months, then 2% to 4% annually.

Vasospasm: arterial constriction causing cerebral ischemia. Occurs in 70% after SAH; delayed ischemic signs in 20% to 30%. Peak risk: 5 to 14 days after SAH. Never before third day. Risk proportional to amount of blood. Signs: obtundation, focal signs.

Acute hydrocephalus: 15% to 20%. Risk proportional to volume of intraventricular and subarachnoid blood. Signs: lethargy, impaired short-term memory, sixth cranial nerve palsy, limitation of upward gaze, lower limb hyperreflexia.

Delayed hydrocephalus: onset 3 to 21 days after SAH. Syndrome identical to normal pressure hydrocephalus. Improves with ventriculoperitoneal shunting. Overall, 20% of SAH survivors require shunting for chronic hydrocephalus.

Seizures: 5% to 10% during acute hospitalization, another 10% during first year.

Hyponatremia: 5% to 30% of patients. May be due to SIADH (free-water retention) or cerebral salt-wasting (excessive natriuresis and intravascular volume contraction).

Neurogenic cardiac and pulmonary disturbances: transient asymptomatic electrocardiogram abnormalities in 50%. Cardiac enzyme release and reversible neurogenic "stunned myocardium" sometimes lead to reduction of cardiac output. Neurogenic pulmonary edema may occur.

TREATMENT OF ANEURYSMAL SAH

Surgical management: aneurysm clipped within 48 to 72 hours. Benefits of clipping: prevents early rebleeding; permits aggressive treatment of vasospasm. Risk of major surgical morbidity/mortality: 5% to 10% following acute rupture; 2% to 5% for unruptured aneurysm. Highest risk when aneurysm is large or located on basilar artery.

Endovascular therapy: alternative to clipping. Aneurysm packed with thrombogenic platinum coils. Small-neck aneurysms: short-term success rate 80% to 90%; complication rate 9%; long-term effectiveness unknown. (See also chapter 17).

Intensive care management: see Table 46.3 for a suggested algorithm for postoperative management.

OUTCOME AFTER SAH

Mortality: 32%. Permanent disability (primarily cognitive impairment) in 50% of survivors. Depression, anxiety also common.

OTHER KINDS OF MACROSCOPIC ANEURYSMS

MYCOTIC ANEURYSMS

Caused by septic emboli, most often with bacterial endocarditis. Affect distal branches of pial vessels. Found in 10% of endocarditis patients. Rupture fatal in 80%. Cerebral arteriography

TABLE 46.3

COLUMBIA UNIVERSITY MEDICAL CENTER
MANAGEMENT PROTOCOL FOR ACUTE SAH

Blood pressure	Control elevated blood pressure during the preoperative phase (systolic BP <160 mm Hg) with IV labetalol or nicardipine to prevent rebleeding.
IV hydration	Preoperative: Normal (0.9%) saline at 80–100 ml/hr.
	Postoperative: Normal (0.9%) saline at 80–100 ml/hr, and 250 ml 5% albumin every 2 hours if the CVP is ≤5 mm Hg.
Laboratory testing	Periodically check complete blood count; transfuse for hematocrit <24% in stable patients, or <30% in patients with symptomatic vasospasm.
	Periodically check electrolytes to detect hyponatremia.
	Obtain serial ECGs and check admission cardiac troponin I (cTI) level to evaluate for cardiac injury; perform echocardiography in patients with abnormal ECG findings or cTI elevation.
Seizure prophylaxis	Fosphenytoin or phenytoin IV load (15–20 mg/kg); discontinue on postop day 2 unless patient has seized or is unstable.
Vasospasm prophylaxis	Nimodipine 60 mg PO every 4 hours for 21 days.
Physiologic homeostasis	Cooling blankets to maintain T ≤37.5° C
	Insulin drip to maintain glucose ≤120 mg/dl.
Ventricular drainage	Begin trials of clamping external ventricular drain and monitoring ICP on day 3 after placement
Vasospasm diagnosis	Transcranial Doppler sonography every one to two days until the eighth day after SAH.
	CT or MR perfusion on day 4–8 after SAH if high risk.
Therapy for symptomatic vasospasm	Place patient in Trendelenberg (head down) position.
	Infuse 500 ml 5% albumin over 15 minutes.
	If deficit persists, raise the systolic BP with phenylephrine or dopamine until the deficit resolves, up to a maximum of 200–220 mm Hg.
	250 mL 5% albumin solution every 2 hours if the CVP is ≤8 mm Hg or PADP is ≤14 mm Hg.
	If refractory, place pulmonary artery catheter and add dobutamine to maintain cardiac index ≥4.0 L/min/m^2.
	Emergency angiogram for possible cerebral angioplasty unless patient responds well to above measures.

ICP, intracranial pressure; CVP, central venous pressure; PADP, pulmonary arterial diastolic pressure.

indicated if endocarditis accompanied by headache, stiff neck, seizure, focal neurologic symptoms, or CSF pleocytosis. Treatment: surgery.

VASCULAR (ARTERIOVENOUS) MALFORMATIONS (AVMs)

Less than 5% of all SAH. Over 90% asymptomatic throughout life. Bleeding most likely in patients aged <40. Coexist with saccular aneurysms in 7% to 10%.

Risk of bleeding from unruptured AVM 1% to 4% per year. When bleeding occurs: initial mortality 4% to 20%. Early rebleeding uncommon; late rebleeding rate 8% to 18% per year for several years.

Risk factors for bleeding: prior hemorrhage, deep location, small size, single draining vein, high feeding artery pressure, male sex, diffuse nidus.

Diagnosis: MRI to detect AVM; arteriography to delineate blood supply before surgery.

Treatment: surgical resection; endovascular glue embolization; directed beam radiation therapy (linear accelerator or gamma knife). Choice depends on AVM location and size, patient's age and condition.

CHAPTER 47 ■ CEREBRAL VEINS AND SINUSES

Occlusion of cerebral veins and sinuses associated with various disorders (Table 47.1). Lateral, cavernous, superior sagittal sinuses most frequently affected.

LATERAL SINUS THROMBOSIS

Usually due to otitis media, mastoiditis. Infants, children most commonly affected. Septicemia in 50%.

SYMPTOMS AND SIGNS

Fever, headache, nausea, vomiting (increased intracranial pressure). Papilledema (usually bilateral) in 50%. Additionally: drowsiness, coma, seizures, cranial nerve signs; systemic signs of septicemia.

Gradenigo syndrome: lateral rectus weakness (sixth nerve palsy), facial pain (fifth nerve damage).

INVESTIGATIONS

Blood: leukocytosis; cultures positive in 50%. CSF: increased pressure, turbid appearance, leukocytosis.

CT, MRI: clot may appear as linear density ("cord sign"). Magnetic resonance venography (MRV): focal narrowing or nonvisualization of involved portion of sinus.

TREATMENT

Antibiotics for underlying otitis media; surgical drainage; jugular vein ligation. Nonseptic patients: thrombolytic therapy may suffice.

TABLE 47.1

DISORDERS ASSOCIATED WITH CEREBRAL VEIN AND SINUS OCCLUSION

Primary idiopathic thrombosis
Secondary thrombosis
  Pregnancy
  Postpartum
  Oral contraceptive pill
  Trauma: after open or closed head injury
  Tumors
    Meningioma
    Metastatic tumors
Malnutrition and dehydration (marantic thrombosis)
Infection: sinus thrombophlebitis, bacterial, fungal
Hematologic disorders
  Polycythemia
  Cryofibrinogenemia
  Sickle-cell anemia
  Leukemia
  Disseminated intravascular coagulation and other
    coagulopathy
Behçet syndrome

COURSE AND PROGNOSIS

High mortality in untreated cases. Death due to septicemia, meningitis, extension of infection to cavernous or longitudinal sinus, brain abscess.

CAVERNOUS SINUS THROMBOSIS

Usually originates in suppurative disorder of orbit, nasal sinuses, or upper half of face. Unilateral onset with rapid spread to opposite side.

Symptoms and signs: onset of septic thrombosis usually sudden and dramatic: prostration, fever, eye pain, orbital tenderness, proptosis; diplopia (oculomotor nerves); papilledema (occlusion of orbital veins).
Laboratory findings: as in lateral sinus thrombosis.
Treatment: antibiotics, with or without anticoagulation.

SUPERIOR SAGITTAL SINUS THROMBOSIS

Thrombosis less commonly due to infection than in lateral or cavernous. Most common site of nonseptic sinus thrombosis. Predisposing factors include: sinus occlusion by tumor (e.g., meningioma), oral contraceptive use, pregnancy, sickle cell trait, diabetes mellitus. Associated with dehydration and marasmus in infancy.

SYMPTOMS AND SIGNS

Prostration, fever, headache, papilledema, forehead edema, caput medusae (infants; due to engorgement of veins near fontanels).

Clot extension into cerebral veins accompanied by focal neurologic signs due to cortical infarcts and hemorrhage, including seizures.

INVESTIGATIONS

Laboratory findings as in lateral sinus thrombosis. CSF bloody or xanthochromic with hemorrhage.

CT, MRI, MRV: as in lateral sinus thrombosis. Contrast may flow around clot, outlining periphery of sinus and leaving central area dark ("empty delta sign"). MRI may show bilateral hemorrhagic and ischemic lesions.

TREATMENT

Anticoagulation beneficial in some patients. Antibiotics in septic thrombosis.

PROGNOSIS

Guarded in patients with septic thrombosis. Symptomatic improvement over weeks to months. Residual neurologic signs, including seizures, common.

THROMBOSIS OF OTHER DURAL SINUSES

Rarely occurs alone. Thrombosis of great vein of Galen may cause hemorrhages in deep white matter, basal ganglia, lateral ventricles.

DURAL ARTERIOVENOUS MALFORMATIONS

Women > men; posterior fossa > supratentorial. May occur in spinal cord.

Symptoms of cranial nerve involvement (commonly III, VII, VIII, XII), central nervous system manifestations, or (rarely) headache alone. Presumed mechanism: intracranial venous hypertension, decreased CSF absorption, venous sinus thrombosis, subarachnoid hemorrhage.

Diagnosis: cerebral angiography.
Treatment: selective embolization or surgical excision.

CHAPTER 48 ■ VASCULAR DISEASE OF THE SPINAL CORD

BLOOD SUPPLY

Origin: vertebral, subclavian, iliac arteries, aorta. Branches form single anterior median spinal artery, two posterior spinal arteries.

Thoracic region: blood supply relatively sparse. Infarction most likely to occur at T4-T9.

Anterior 2/3, central area of cord supplied by anterior spinal artery; posterior 1/3 from posterior spinal arteries, pial arteriolar plexus.

SPINAL CORD INFARCTION

Anterior spinal artery infarction much more common than posterior because collateral supplies differ; 1% to 2% of stroke admissions.

Common etiologies: atheromatous thromboembolism from aorta; complication of thoracoabdominal aneurysm repair.

Symptoms and signs: onset usually sudden. Transient lancinating or burning, local or radicular back pain; deep aching pain in both legs; burning pain ascends from feet to abdomen. Followed by symmetric leg and (depending on spinal level) arm weakness, urinary and fecal incontinence, sensory level. Proprioception and vibration sensation always spared. Tone flaccid at first, then spastic within weeks. Tendon reflexes decreased at level of lesion, increased below. Bilateral Babinski signs.

Investigations: MRI most sensitive imaging study. CSF: slight protein elevation, normal gamma-globulin (in contrast to MS).

Treatment: supportive care for any patient with quadriplegia or paraplegia. No evidence to support use of antiplatelet or anticoagulant medications.

Prognosis: mortality rate 22%. Of survivors: fully ambulatory (18%), ambulatory with aids (25%), wheelchair-mobile (57%).

VENOUS DISEASE

Rare. Associated with sepsis, systemic malignancy, spinal arteriovenous malformation.

Sudden back pain, then motor, sensory, autonomic dysfunction. Posterior columns not spared.

CSF examination necessary to exclude infectious-inflammatory or neoplastic condition in patients with spinal cord ischemia. CT or MRI necessary to exclude alternative lesions, including vascular malformation.

FOIX-ALAJOUANINE SYNDROME

Subacute or Progressive Necrotic Myelopathy

Spinal cord necrosis and enlarged, tortuous, thrombosed veins. Multiple infarcts and hemorrhages. Thoracolumbar corticospinal tract most often affected, sparing anterior horn cells.

Subacute or progressive leg weakness, incontinence, sensory loss, often preceded by back pain.

CSF: usually marked protein elevation, pleocytosis, red blood cells. Normal angiogram.

No effective treatment.

SPINAL CORD HEMORRHAGE

Rare. May be epidural, subdural, subarachnoid, intramedullary (intraparenchymal).

Associated with leukemia, anticoagulation therapy, arteriovenous malformation, venous spinal cord infarction.

Hematomyelia (hemorrhage into spinal cord parenchyma) usually due to trauma. Non-traumatic causes of spinal cord hemorrhage: coagulopathy, AVM, venous spinal cord infarction, epidural anesthesia.

Signs and symptoms: sudden onset of back or radicular pain. Variable combination of spinal signs (spastic weakness, hyperreflexia, bladder dysfunction, sensory loss) determined by hemorrhage location.

Investigations: CSF bloody or xanthochromic with elevated protein. MRI demonstrates site of hemorrhage. Spinal angiography if spinal vascular malformation is suspected.

Treatment: subdural, epidural hemorrhage: surgical decompression. Prognosis poor with paraplegia, delay in surgical intervention. Fresh frozen plasma and vitamin K if hemorrhage due to coagulopathy or anticoagulant therapy.

Section V
Disorders of
Cerebrospinal Fluid

CHAPTER 49 ■ HYDROCEPHALUS

DEFINITION

Increased CSF volume and dilation of cerebral ventricles.

CLASSIFICATION

Obstructive Hydrocephalus
Due to obstruction of CSF flow out of cerebral ventricles. Sometimes termed "non-communicating" hydrocephalus (CSF does not communicate with subarachnoid space).

Obstruction may occur at foramen of Monro, third ventricle, aqueduct of Sylvius, fourth ventricle, foramina of Luschka and Magendie.

Congenital Malformations and Developmental Lesions
Incidence 0.5 to 1.8/1,000 births.

Nongenetic causes: intrauterine infection, intracranial hemorrhage due to birth trauma or prematurity, meningitis.
Genetic causes: X-linked hydrocephalus, Dandy-Walker syndrome, Arnold-Chiari malformation. Etiology of congenital aqueductal stenosis unclear.

Post-Inflammatory or Post-Hemorrhagic Hydrocephalus
Obstruction of CSF flow by clot in ventricular system or arachnoiditis. Transient or permanent.

Major sequel of intracranial hemorrhage (intraventricular, intraparenchymal, subarachnoid). May follow meningitis, especially at base of brain (syphilis, tuberculosis).

Mass Lesions
Intracranial neoplasms (progressive hydrocephalus); intraparenchymal cerebral or cerebellar hematoma, infarction (acute hydrocephalus).

Communicating Hydrocephalus
Unhindered CSF flow from ventricles to subarachnoid space.

Mechanisms

CSF oversecretion: choroid plexus papilloma. CSF production >1.0 mL/min (normal 0.35 mL/min, or 500 cc/day).

Impaired venous drainage: follows lateral sinus thrombosis (otitic hydrocephalus after ear infection).

Impaired absorption: (a) congenital agenesis of arachnoid villi; difficult to confirm; (b) CSF hyperviscosity: protein content >500 mg/dL (polyneuritis, spinal cord tumor).

Normal Pressure Hydrocephalus (NPH)

Mechanism unknown. May be idiopathic; sequel of head trauma, subarachnoid hemorrhage, meningitis; associated with occult brain tumor. Potentially reversible cause of parkinsonism, dementia.

Hydrocephalus Ex Vacuo

Increase in CSF volume reflecting generalized loss of brain tissue (e.g., Alzheimer disease). Accompanied by widening of cerebral sulci. CSF pressure is normal.

CLINICAL INFORMATION

Signs And Symptoms

Children, before fusion of cranial sutures: skull enlargement, widened fontanels, exophthalmos, sluggish pupillary reaction, impaired upward gaze, impaired lateral gaze, absence of visual fixation or response to visible threat.

Otitic hydrocephalus: fever, listlessness, ipsilateral sixth nerve paralysis, papilledema.

Adults: headache, lethargy, malaise, dementia, lethargy, ocular nerve palsies, papilledema, weakness, ataxia.

NPH: dementia, slowness and unsteadiness of gait, urinary incontinence. Insidious onset, gradual progression. Gait is with feet appearing "stuck" to ground ("magnetic" gait), with tendency to fall backwards ("retropulsed" posture).

EVALUATION

CT, MRI, Ultrasonography: diagnosis of intracranial hemorrhage and monitoring of hydrocephalus in premature infants.

NPH: various approaches used to select patients likely to benefit from CSF shunting. None reliably predicts favorable outcome. Most common: evaluate gait before and after repeatedly removing CSF by lumbar puncture or lumbar drain.

PROGNOSIS AND TREATMENT

Prognosis determined by underlying disease. Progression may arrest spontaneously (benign communicating hydrocephalus of infants).

Progressive infantile hydrocephalus: survival 50% after 15 years; 15% incidence of mental retardation.

Treatment: shunting procedure allows CSF flow from cerebral ventricles to another fluid space (peritoneum, pleura). Success determined by procedures used, patient status, cause and duration of hydrocephalus.

NPH: 1/3 to 2/3 of patients with idiopathic NPH improve with shunting; complications in 1/3, including subdural hematoma, death, persistent disability. Patient selection criteria and success rates vary in different series.

CHAPTER 50 ■ DISORDERS OF INTRACRANIAL PRESSURE

BRAIN EDEMA

DEFINITION

Increased brain volume due to increase in water and sodium content.

MAJOR TYPES OF BRAIN EDEMA

Features of three major forms of cerebral edema (*vasogenic, cytotoxic, interstitial*) summarized in Table 50.1.

OTHER TYPES OF BRAIN EDEMA

Ischemic brain edema: cellular edema in first few minutes to hours, then vasogenic edema (hours to days).

Fulminant hepatic encephalopathy: due to acute hepatocellular failure (acute hepatitis, Reye syndrome). Progressive stupor and coma, severe intracranial hypertension; often fatal. Imaging: global brain edema without contrast enhancement.

Granulocytic brain edema: due to pus accumulation. Seen with brain abscess, purulent meningitis. Simultaneous features of cellular, vasogenic, sometimes interstitial edema.

TREATMENT

Dictated by cause of edema (see Table 50.1).

Glucocorticoids

Reduce vasogenic edema in hours by normalizing endothelial cell permeability; effective for edema of brain tumor, abscess.

Common regimen: dexamethasone 10 mg intravenous starting dose, followed by 4 mg administered four times a day. Gastric hemorrhage most significant complication.

Use in spinal cord injury discussed in Chapter 65.

TABLE 50.1
FEATURES OF VARIOUS TYPES OF BRAIN EDEMA

	Vasogenic	Cytotoxic	Interstitial (Hydrocephalic)
Pathogenesis	Increased capillary permeability	Cellular swelling (glial, neuronal, endothelial)	Increased brain fluid
Location of edema	Chiefly white matter	Gray and white matter	Chiefly periventricular white matter
Clinical disorders	Brain tumor, abscess, infarction, contusion, hemorrhage, lead encephalopathy Ischemia Purulent meningitis (granulocytic edema)	Hypoxia, hypo-osmolality (e.g., water intoxication) Ischemia Purulent meningitis (granulocytic edema), fulminant hepatic encephalopathy	Obstructive hydrocephalus, pseudotumor (benign intracranial hypertension) Purulent meningitis
Clinical manifestations	Focal neurologic deficits, disturbances of consciousness, severe intracranial hypertension	Stupor, coma, asterixis, myoclonus, focal or generalized seizures	Dementia and gait disorder with advanced hydrocephalus
CT, MRI	Abnormal, with contrast enhancement	Often normal, without contrast enhancement	Enlarged ventricles, loss of sulci, periventricular abnormalities
CSF	Increased protein	Normal protein	LP may be contraindicated
EEG changes	Focal slowing common	Generalized slowing	EEG often normal
Therapeutic Effects			
Steroids	Beneficial in brain tumor, abscess	Not effective (except perhaps in fulminant hepatic encephalopathy)	Uncertain effectiveness
Osmotherapy (e.g., mannitol)	Reduces volume of normal brain tissue only, acutely	Reduces brain volume acutely	Rarely useful

Modified from Fishman RA. *Cerebrospinal fluid in diseases of the nervous system.* Philadelphia: WB Saunders, 1992:116–137.

Osmotherapy

Hypertonic parenteral fluids reduce brain volume by creating osmotic gradient between blood and brain.

Effective for edema of any cause. Effect short-lived; osmotic equilibrium reached after few hours. Temporary measure, as with large cerebellar hemorrhage to prevent brain herniation until surgical decompression performed.

Hypertonic mannitol most commonly used. Give intravenously, 100 to 200 mL 20% solution; repeat every 6 hours as needed.

Surgery

Excision or decompression of intracranial mass lesions. Shunting procedures for obstructive hydrocephalus.

Other Therapeutic Measures

Hyperventilation, hypothermia, barbiturates (pentobarbital coma) used, but none proven. Acetazolamide and furosemide may relieve interstitial edema by reducing CSF formation.

General Management

Treatment of intracranial infection. Maintenance of patent airway; avoidance of hypoxia. Maintain blood pressure adequate to sustain mean cerebral perfusion pressure >50 mm Hg.

Hypotonic intravenous solutions contraindicated.

DISORDERS OF INTRACRANIAL PRESSURE

IDIOPATHIC INTRACRANIAL HYPERTENSION (PSEUDOTUMOR CEREBRI)

Increased intracranial pressure without intracranial mass lesion, obstructive hydrocephalus, intracranial infection, or hypertensive encephalopathy. Age 10 to 50 years.

Pathogenesis poorly understood. Most often occurs in isolation. Sometimes with endocrine disorders (obesity, menarche, Addison disease), pregnancy, intracranial venous sinus thrombosis, drugs (vitamin A, lithium, tetracycline), hematologic disorders, high CSF protein content.

Clinical Features

Early symptoms: headache (worse on waking, coughing, straining), visual blurring (papilledema). Brief, fleeting dimming or complete loss of vision (*amaurosis fugax*) indicates vision in jeopardy.

Examination: large blind spots; constricted peripheral fields; central or paracentral scotoma; papilledema; retinal exudates or hemorrhages; diplopia (sixth nerve palsy).

May persist for months or years without serious sequelae. Recurrence rate 5% to 10%.

Laboratory and Imaging Findings

CT, MRI: normal or small (slit-like) ventricles.

CSF: elevated pressure, usually 250 to 600 mm H_2O. Normal upper limit: 200 mm (250 mm in obesity). CSF otherwise normal, protein levels commonly low-normal (<50 mg/dL).

Treatment

Non-surgical: weight reduction, acetazolamide, furosemide.

If vision threatened: CSF shunt or optic nerve decompression (fenestration); mannitol sometimes used while awaiting surgery if vision deteriorating acutely.

SPONTANEOUS INTRACRANIAL HYPOTENSION

Due to spontaneous CSF leaks via dural fistulae adjacent to spinal roots. Likely non-traumatic rupture of arachnoid (Tarlov) cysts on nerve roots. Common sites of leakage thoracolumbar.

Clinical Manifestations

Headache in upright position, relieved by lying down. Some patients headache free. Somnolence, stupor, cranial nerve signs sometimes present.

Laboratory and Imaging

MRI with contrast: diffuse dural enhancement; "sagging" brain appearance (flattened optic chiasm, pons displaced against clivus, descent of cerebellar tonsils below foramen magnum); venous sinus engorgement; enlarged pituitary.

Injection of radioisotope tracers into CSF results in urinary excretion.

Treatment

Usually resolves spontaneously or with bed rest. Large-volume lumbar epidural blood patch, surgical closure of fistula for intractable cases.

CHAPTER 51 ■ SUPERFICIAL SIDEROSIS OF THE CNS

Deposition of hemosiderin on pial surfaces of brain and spinal cord. Evolves for years; caused by chronic, intermittent, or persistent oozing of blood into CSF.

Clinical features: sensorineural deafness, cerebellar ataxia; then myelopathy, anosmia, dementia.
MRI: rims of hypointensity; seen on T2-weighted images; located on cerebral surface, cerebellar vermis, adjacent cerebellar cortical sulci.
CSF: xanthochromic, often with no cells.
Treatment: identify and treat bleeding source: aneurysm, vascular malformation, tumor (particularly ependymoma); repair spinal dural defect. Source of bleeding identified in only 50%.

CHAPTER 52 ■ HYPERGLYCEMIC NONKETOTIC SYNDROME

Definition: serum osmolality >350 mOsm/kg; plasma glucose content >600 mg/dL; depressed consciousness without ketosis.

Comprises 10% to 20% of all cases of severe hyperglycemia. Most common in elderly with mild recent-onset diabetes mellitus. Mortality 40% to 50%.

Average age 60 years. Diabetes often unrecognized; few patients taking insulin.

Often precipitated by *associated illness* (chronic renal insufficiency, gram-negative pneumonia or sepsis, gastrointestinal hemorrhage, myocardial infarction, pulmonary embolism, subdural hematoma, stroke, pancreatitis, burns) or *medical therapy* (diuretic agents, corticosteroids, phenytoin, propranolol, cimetidine, diazoxide, chlorpromazine, loxapine, L-asparaginase, immunosuppressive agents, hyperalimentation, peritoneal dialysis, hemodialysis, cardiac surgery).

CLINICAL FINDINGS

Polyuria and polydipsia for days or weeks; then dehydration, altered mental state.

Also: seizures, hemiparesis, aphasia, hemianopia, visual loss, visual hallucinations, nystagmus, pupillary reflex abnormalities, asymmetric caloric responses, dysphagia, hyperreflexia, myoclonus, Babinski sign, urinary retention, systemic signs of dehydration.

Differential diagnosis: diabetic ketoacidosis, alcoholic ketoacidosis, lactic acidosis, hepatic failure, uremia, hypoglycemia, drug ingestion, stroke.

LABORATORY FINDINGS

Serum glucose level 600 to 2,700 mg/dL. Serum osmolality 325 to 425 mOsm/kg. Mild acidosis with elevated anion gap in 50%. No ketonuria. Plasma sodium concentrations variable (120 to 180 mEq/L after correction for excess glucose). Free water deficit common. Hypokalemia due to sustained osmotic diuresis. Severe prerenal azotemia common.

TREATMENT

Management best in ICU. Aim to replace volume deficits, correct hyperosmolality, normalize plasma glucose, treat underlying illness. Central venous pressure monitoring sometimes useful.

Fluid replacement: normal saline until blood pressure and urine output stabilize; then half-normal saline. Goal: replace 1/2 of estimated fluid deficit in first 12 to 24 hours and remainder over next few days. Serum glucose levels may drop by

25% with fluid replacement alone. Add 5% dextrose once glucose levels fall <200 mg/dL.

Insulin necessary if patient acidotic, hyperkalemic, or in renal failure.

Potassium supplementation early in treatment (patients have total body potassium deficit, and hydration and insulin further depress serum potassium level).

Seizures treated with intravenous benzodiazepines. Phenytoin usually ineffective.

Section VI
Tumors

CHAPTER 53 ■ GENERAL CONSIDERATIONS

EPIDEMIOLOGY

Incidence of symptomatic brain tumors: 12/100,000 population. Approximately 35,000 new patients diagnosed each year in the U.S.

Incidence by age: small peak before age 10 years; gradual increase from 15 years on; highest incidence between 75 and 84 years.

In children: brain tumors are most common form of solid tumor; second most common malignancy overall (after leukemia). Low-grade astrocytoma and medulloblastoma most common tumor types. 70% of all childhood brain tumors infratentorial.

In adults: malignant astrocytoma and meningioma most common.

RISK FACTORS

High-dose irradiation (gliomas, meningiomas, nerve-sheath tumors); immunosuppression caused by HIV or chronic immunosuppressive therapy (primary CNS lymphoma).

Genetic syndromes: NF-1 (gliomas), NF-2 (schwannoma, meningioma), Li-Fraumeni syndrome (autosomal dominant, multiple-cancer syndrome; glioma, medulloblastoma), TS (subependymal giant cell astrocytoma), Von Hippel-Lindau (hemangioblastomas of brain, spinal cord, retina).

Studies inconclusive for chemicals, viruses. No support for environmental electromagnetic radiation or cell phones as risk factors.

CLINICAL DIAGNOSIS IN ADULTS OR CHILDREN

Symptoms and signs due to: brain invasion with destruction of underlying tissue; brain compression by mass and surrounding edema; CSF obstruction leading to hydrocephalus. Symptoms may be focal or generalized (usually due to increased intracranial pressure [ICP]).

Headache: first symptom in 30% to 40%. Usually non-localizing. Features suspicious of raised ICP: (a) early morning headache, awakening patient from sleep; (b) frequency, severity increasing over weeks to months; (c) accompanying nausea and vomiting; (d) associated papilledema or focal cerebral signs.

Seizures: occur in 1/3 of patients. Focal in onset; may generalize. Most common in glioblastoma, astrocytoma, oligodendroglioma.

Focal Symptoms by Tumor Location

Frontal lobe: initially silent; behavior change, dementia, gait disorders, urinary incontinence, hemiparesis, seizures, primitive reflexes (grasp, palmomental), expressive aphasia (dominant hemisphere).

Temporal: seizures (olfactory hallucinations, complex partial seizures), visual field changes, behavioral changes, sensory aphasia.

Parietal: cortical sensory loss, neglect, anosognosia, hemiparesis, visuospatial disturbance.

Occipital: visual field changes.

Pineal: hydrocephalus, Parinaud syndrome (paresis of upgaze, convergence-retraction nystagmus, lid retraction, light-near dissociation of pupil responses), precocious puberty.

Brainstem: cranial nerve symptoms, vomiting, vertigo, hemiparesis, hydrocephalus.

Cerebellopontine angle (8th nerve tumor): ipsilateral deafness and facial numbness, weakness, ataxia.

Cerebellar: headache, ataxia, vertigo, nystagmus, neck stiffness.

Skull base: cranial nerve signs. Meningioma of olfactory groove: anosmia. Optic nerve glioma, meningioma: monocular visual loss. Pituitary tumors: bitemporal hemianopia, panhypopituitarism. Cavernous sinus, brainstem tumors: eye movement abnormalities. Acoustic neuroma: hearing loss. Leptomeningeal metastasis: multiple cranial nerve signs.

False localizing signs: focal signs caused by raised ICP. *Sixth nerve palsy* (nerve vulnerable due to long course); *uncal herniation* causing ipsilateral hemiparesis (compression of contralateral cerebral peduncle against tentorium);

posterior cerebral artery compression causing *occipital infarction* (cortical blindness, hemianopia); *tinnitus.*

Third cranial nerve palsy due to compression (e.g., uncal herniation, aneurysm): dilated pupil almost always accompanies ophthalmoplegia (vs. diabetic third nerve palsy, in which pupil is usually spared).

LABORATORY EXAMINATION

MRI with and without contrast is imaging investigation of choice.

Other Studies

MR spectroscopy: identifies intracellular metabolites characteristic of high-grade tumors.

Functional MRI: sometimes useful in presurgical evaluation to determine resection margins (border between tumor and functional cortex).

PET: may help diagnosis of presumed low-grade glioma when MRI or CT shows nonenhancing mass; also in differentiating tumor recurrence (hypermetabolic) from radiation necrosis (hypometabolic).

SPECT: similar to PET; more readily available but less sensitive or specific.

SYMPTOMATIC MANAGEMENT

Corticosteroids

May provide dramatic, rapid symptom relief by reducing edema around tumor and decreasing intracranial pressure.

Indicated in any symptomatic patient with brain tumor, especially if neuroimaging demonstrates significant edema around tumor.

Dexamethasone commonly used; standard dose is 16 mg/day in 4 divided doses. If expected steroid course is >6 weeks, trimethoprim-sulfamethoxazole given for *Pneumocystis carinii* prophylaxis.

Caution in patients with suspected lymphoma: corticosteroids may cause tumor regression, preventing histologic diagnosis if given before biopsy.

Anticonvulsants

No role for prophylactic anticonvulsants.

Treat any patient who has a seizure. Preferably avoid anticonvulsants that may interact with chemotherapeutic agents by inducing hepatic metabolism (e.g., phenytoin, carbamazepine). Fewer drug reactions with lamotrigine, topiratmate, gabapentin, levetiracetam.

COMPLICATIONS

Deep venous thrombosis (DVT) in at least 25%; pulmonary embolism common. High risk in postoperative period; give DVT prophylaxis with low-molecular-weight heparin and pneumatic compression boots.

In event of thromboembolism: full-dose anticoagulation safe in patients with intracranial neoplasm. May use low-molecular-weight heparin until therapeutic INR is reached on warfarin; common duration of treatment 3 to 6 months.

CHAPTER 54 ■ TUMORS OF THE SKULL AND CRANIAL NERVES

BENIGN TUMORS

OSTEOMA

Benign growth of mature dense cortical bone in paranasal sinuses, cranial vault, mandible, mastoid sinuses. Associated with Gardner syndrome (autosomal-dominant osteoma, colon polyps, soft tissue fibromas).

Usually asymptomatic with slow growth. Sometimes causes local pain, proptosis, headache, recurrent sinusitis.

CT: circumscribed homogeneous bone density.

CHONDROMA

Rare, slow-growing benign tumor; arises from cartilaginous portion of bones of skull base or paranasal sinuses. Often causes cranial nerve palsies.

CT: lytic lesion, sharp margins, erosion surrounding bone, stippled calcification.

HEMANGIOMA

Benign vascular bone tumor of capillary or cavernous vascular channels. More common in vertebral column than cranium.

MRI: flow voids, suggesting vascular lesion.

DERMOID, EPIDERMOID

Cranial vault, paranasal sinuses, orbit, petrous bone. Common in children.

CT: round or ovoid lytic lesions with sharp sclerotic margins; involves all 3 layers of bone. Treatment rarely necessary.

TREATMENT

Treatment for all types (if symptomatic): surgical resection.

MALIGNANT TUMORS

METASTASES TO SKULL BASE

Most common: breast, lung, prostate; head-neck tumors; lymphoma. Local pain, cranial neuropathy.

Lesions usually readily demonstrated on MRI.

Differential diagnosis: leptomeningeal metastasis.

Treatment: palliative radiotherapy.

EXTENSION OF MALIGNANT TUMORS TO SKULL BASE

Squamous cell carcinomas (nasal sinuses, temporal bone), carcinoma of salivary gland, olfactory mucosa, nasopharynx. Local pain, cranial neuropathy.

CT or MRI: soft tissue mass, erosion of skull base. Biopsy often diagnostic.

Treatment: surgical resection if small; usually radical excision plus radiation therapy; prognosis poor.

PRIMARY MALIGNANT TUMORS OF SKULL

Chondrosarcoma: malignant cartilage tumor. Usually in skull base. Most common in men aged 30 to 40.

Chordoma: arises in primitive notochordal tissue at either end of vertebral column or skull base. Locally invasive.

Osteogenic sarcoma (osteosarcoma): most common primary malignant bone tumor. Most frequent in 10 to 20 age group. Risk factors: prior radiation, Paget disease, fibrous dysplasia, chronic osteomyelitis. Prognosis poor.

Fibrous sarcoma: soft tissue tumor arising from bone, periosteum, scalp, dura.

Treatment: radical surgical resection; radiotherapy. Recurrence common despite aggressive therapy. Proton beam radiation effective for skull base chordomas, chondrosarcomas.

GLOMUS JUGULARE TUMORS (PARAGANGLIOMAS)

From chromaffin cells in region of jugular bulb. Invade neighboring temporal or occipital bones; may extend into middle ear and posterior fossa. Highly vascular. Some secrete catecholamines.

Symptoms: tinnitus, audible bruit, deafness, lower cranial neuropathies. Larger tumors: cerebellar and brainstem symptoms.

Seen on MRI or CT with contrast; confirm with angiogram.

Treatment: embolization followed by surgical resection.

NEOPLASTIC-LIKE LESIONS AFFECTING THE SKULL

Hyperostosis: local overgrowth of skull bones. Asymptomatic. Hyperostosis of inner table of frontal bone (hyperostosis frontalis interna) most common in women after age 40.

Fibrous dysplasia: more common in men before age 40. Etiology unknown. Skull base, especially sphenoid wing. Signs:

cranial nerve compression. Treatment: nerve decompression.

Paget disease (osteitis deformans): see Chapter 150.

Mucocele: encapsulated, thick-fluid collection in obstructed nasal sinus. May erode through skull with intracranial compression. Treatment: surgery with reconstruction.

MISCELLANEOUS DISEASES INVOLVING SKULL

Systemic diseases (xanthomatosis, multiple myeloma, osteitis fibrosa cystica), leptomeningeal cysts (growing skull fractures), sinus pericranii, metabolic diseases (hyperparathyroidism, acromegaly), infection, sarcoidosis, histiocytosis X, neuroectodermal dysplasia.

NERVE-SHEATH TUMORS

May occur sporadically (usually single tumor) or as part of genetic syndrome, e.g., neurofibromatosis type 1 or 2 (NF-1, NF-2) (usually multiple tumors).

Eighth cranial nerve most commonly involved within cranium.

Treatment: surgical resection if symptomatic; usually requires sacrifice of involved nerve.

VESTIBULAR SCHWANNOMA (ACOUSTIC NEUROMA)

Benign tumor arising from Schwann cells of vestibular branch of eighth cranial nerve.

5% to 10% of all intracranial tumors; most common tumor of cerebellopontine angle. Peak age: 40 to 60 years.

Bilateral in <5% of patients; defining characteristic of NF-2.

Slow-growing, extends into internal auditory meatus, cerebellopontine angle, displacing cerebellum, pons, fifth and seventh cranial nerves.

Initial symptoms: almost always, progressive unilateral hearing loss. Tinnitus (70%), unsteady gait (70%); vertigo (rarely).

Further growth: facial numbness, loss of taste, otalgia; headache, nausea, vomiting, diplopia, ataxia, symptoms of increased intracranial pressure and hydrocephalus.

Other signs: nystagmus, abnormal eye movements, facial weakness, decreased sensation in trigeminal distribution, decreased corneal reflex.

Imaging: MRI with contrast most sensitive diagnostic test: contrast-enhancing mass, distinguished from meningioma by origin in internal auditory canal.

Treatment: surgical resection often curative; for tumors <2 cm, high chance of preserving intact seventh and eighth nerve function. Radiosurgery is an alternative for tumors <3 cm.

TRIGEMINAL SCHWANNOMA

Rare. Nearly always with numbness and pain in trigeminal distribution but not with specific pain features of trigeminal neuralgia. Chewing weak in <50%.

Diagnosis by MRI or CT with bone windows. Surgical resection usually curative.

CHAPTER 55 ■ TUMORS OF THE MENINGES

GENERAL CONSIDERATIONS

Meningiomas originate in arachnoid coverings of brain; 90% intracranial, 10% spinal.

Comprise 20% of all intracranial tumors. M:F ratio 1:2. Peak age: 50 to 70 years. Rare tumor in children, frequently associated with neurofibromatosis type 2.

Multiple meningiomas (typical of neurofibromatosis): 5% to 15% of patients.

ETIOLOGY

Radiotherapy is only established risk factor. Estrogen, viral antigens, loss of tumor suppressor gene may contribute.

PATHOLOGY

Cells arranged in sheaths separated by connective tissue trabeculae. Whorls of arachnoid cells surround central hyaline material (psammoma bodies). Calcification frequent.

Malignant meningiomas rare but aggressive; may metastasize outside central nervous system.

Risk of recurrence depends on tumor grade: benign (7% to 20%), atypical (30% to 40%), anaplastic (50% to 78%).

Hemangiopericytomas: arise from pericytes (smooth muscle cells of small blood vessels); aggressive.

CLINICAL FEATURES

Dictated by tumor location: seizures, hemiparesis, gait disturbance (convexity, falx); diplopia, visual loss, cranial neuropathies (skull base). Often asymptomatic.

IMAGING

CT: isointense or slightly hyperdense to brain. Smooth; often calcified. Enhancement strong, homogeneous. Margins distinct; tumor arises from dura. Edema in adjacent brain. Hyperostosis in 25%.

MRI: isointense (65%) or hypointense (35%) compared with normal brain on T1- and T2-weighted images. "Dural tail" common but also seen in acoustic neuroma, dural metastasis.

Angiography: mass with vascular "blush."

TREATMENT

Surgery

Surgical resection potentially curative. Operative morbidity 1% to 14%.

Recurrence rate 20% at 5 years, 25% at 10 years.

Radiation Therapy

Indications: residual tumor after surgery; recurrent tumor; malignant histology; surgically inaccessible site.

Malignant meningiomas: 28% 5-year survival after combined surgery and radiation. Recurrence rate 90% after subtotal resection, 41% for resection plus radiation.

Specialized techniques: *proton beam* (highly focal), *radiosurgery* (focused radiation given in one large dose using linear accelerator or gamma rays), *stereotactic radiotherapy* (multiple small fractions for optic nerve tumors, cavernous sinus meningiomas, or those close to brainstem).

SPECIFIC TUMOR LOCATIONS

Convexity: most amenable to surgical resection.

Parasagittal: involvement of superior sagittal sinus may result in venous infarction.

Tuberculum sellae: visual loss, anosmia, headache, hypopituitarism.

Optic sheath: surgery only if visual loss present.

Cerebellopontine angle: hearing loss, facial pain or numbness. Second most common posterior fossa tumor, after acoustic neuroma. May invade bone, cranial nerves, and thus recur.

Clivus: meningioma arises from dura anterior to brainstem. May invade petrous bone, cranial nerves.

Tentorial: headache, cerebellar signs.

Foramen magnum: neck pain, gait difficulties, hand muscle wasting. Resection difficult.

Intraventricular: arise from arachnoid cells. 1% of intracranial meningiomas.

Sphenoid wing: sphenoid hyperostosis, proptosis, visual loss, third nerve palsy.

Spinal: most common in thoracic spine. Paraparesis in 80%.

CHAPTER 56 ■ GLIOMAS

EPIDEMIOLOGY

Most common primary brain tumors. Incidence increases with age. M:F ratio 1:1.6.

Astrocytomas: 25% of all brain tumors. Before age 25, 67% are astrocytomas in posterior fossa; after age 25, 90% supratentorial.

Oligodendrogliomas: Median age at diagnosis, 50. Rare in children.

Ependymomas: More common in children; 10% of all pediatric intracranial tumors.

PATHOLOGY

Gliomas originate from glial cells or their precursors. Include astrocytomas, oligodendrogliomas, ependymomas. Some tumors may have both astrocytic and oligodendroglial features ("mixed" gliomas), or contain foci of different grades.

Highly infiltrative (with exception of pilocytic astrocytoma).

FAMILIAL CONDITIONS

About 5% of gliomas are familial. Due to loss of a tumor-suppressor gene. Syndromes include neurofibromatosis (types 1 and 2), Li-Fraumeni syndrome, Turcot syndrome (includes several disorders with familial polyposis).

CLINICAL FEATURES

Symptoms and Signs
Spectrum similar in all grades of glial tumors: symptoms may be generalized (headache, nausea, vomiting, lethargy, personality or behavioral changes) or focal (seizures, hemiparesis, aphasia, ataxia, cranial neuropathies).

Seizures are presenting symptom in >80% with low-grade glioma; most patients with high-grade glioma present with prominent focal sensory or motor symptoms.

Most common site for ependymoma: fourth ventricle, causing obstructive hydrocephalus.

IMAGING CHARACTERISTICS

Astrocytoma, Oligodendroglioma
Low-grade: non-enhancing, infiltrative mass seen best on T2 or FLAIR MRI. Typically in frontal or temporal lobe.
High-grade: large, contrast-enhancing, with surrounding edema.

Ependymoma
Heterogeneous, well-delineated, contrast-enhancing. Occasionally with hemorrhage, calcification.

TREATMENT AND PROGNOSIS

See Table 56.1.

GLIOMATOSIS CEREBRI

Diffuse infiltration of neoplastic glial cells throughout hemisphere or even entire brain. Occurs in adults. Patients present with personality or cognitive changes. MRI: diffuse, non-enhancing abnormalities in white matter; generalized swelling. Histology: diffuse astrocytoma (rarely, oligodendroglioma), sometimes with anaplastic foci. Variable clinical course, from rapid progression to survival for many years. Treatment: radiotherapy.

NEURONAL AND MIXED NEURONAL-GLIAL TUMORS

CENTRAL NEUROCYTOMAS

Rare, peak incidence between 20 and 40 years. Arise from subependymal matrix cells, usually present as intraventricular mass spanning both lateral ventricles, causing CSF obstruction. MRI: microcystic ("honeycomb"), well-circumscribed lesion with strong contrast enhancement. Treatment: surgery; total resection may be difficult due to location. Radiotherapy if recurrence. Benign course unless leptomeningeal seeding occurs.

TABLE 56.1

GLIAL TUMORS: SUMMARY OF PATHOLOGY, TREATMENT AND OUTCOME

WHO[a] designation	Grade	Pathology	Treatment	Prognosis
Astrocytoma Pilocytic astrocytoma	I	Bipolar, multipolar astrocytes, long processes, microcysts		Occurs in children, young adults; excellent prognosis
Astrocytoma	II	Well-differentiated fibrillary or neoplastic astrocytes with nuclear atypia	Focal radiotherapy; gross total surgical excision. Timing of treatment controversial	Median survival 5 years. Potential for malignant transformation to high-grade tumor
Anaplastic astrocytoma	III	Same as grade II, plus mitoses	Gross total surgical resection followed by focal RT. Adjuvant chemotherapy may prolong survival in some patients.	>80% recur at original site after surgery/RT. Median survival 3 years. Age most important prognostic factor: >65 years, poor prognosis
Glioblastoma multiforme	IV	Same as grade III, plus endothelial proliferation, necrosis	As for grade III	Median survival 1 year

(continued)

225

TABLE 56.1

GLIAL TUMORS: SUMMARY OF PATHOLOGY, TREATMENT AND OUTCOME (Continued)

WHO[a] designation	Grade	Pathology	Treatment	Prognosis
Oligodendroglioma				
Oligodendroglioma	II	Rounded ("fried egg") tumor cells with nuclear atypia, mitoses	Follow clinically and radiologically until significant symptom progression or growth, then surgical resection + RT. RT or chemotherapy for recurrence	Median survival 8–16 years. May eventually develop malignant transformation
Anaplastic oligodendroglioma	III	Same as grade 2, plus microvascular proliferation, necrosis	Complete surgical resection + RT. Chemosensitive, but timing of chemotherapy controversial: may be used before RT, reserving RT for recurrence	Median survival 5 years; longer for tumors with chromosome 1p/19q loss of heterozygosity
Ependymoma				
Ependymoma	II	Perivascular pseudo-rosettes	Gross total excision. RT controversial	Overall 5-year survival 40–80%. Good prognostic factors: young age, infratentorial location, low-grade histology
Anaplastic ependymoma	III	Same as grade II, plus mitoses, microvascular proliferation, necrosis	Gross total excision + focal postoperative RT	

[a]World Health Organization.
RT, radiation therapy.

GANGLIOGLIOMA AND GANGLIOCYTOMAS

Usually slow-growing lesion in children and young adults, most commonly in temporal lobe, causing resistant focal seizures. Excellent long-term survival after surgical resection.

Dysembryoplastic Neuroepithelial Tumor (DNET): low-grade, tumor of mixed glial and neuronal origin, usually in temporal cortex, causing seizures from childhood. Gross total excision often curative; partial resection improves seizure control.

CHAPTER 57 ■ LYMPHOMAS

SYSTEMIC LYMPHOMA

Metastasis to CNS much more common with non-Hodgkin lymphoma (NHL) than with Hodgkin disease.

Nervous system sites involved in NHL: meninges (10%), epidural space (3% to 5%), brain (<1%, vs. primary CNS lymphoma, where >90% have brain parenchyma tumor).

Factors predisposing to CNS involvement: older age, bone marrow or retroperitoneal involvement, high serum lactic dehydrogenase (LDH).

MENINGEAL LYMPHOMA

4% to 11% of patients with NHL.

Clinical features: headache, nausea, vomiting, back pain, confusion, behavioral changes, cranial nerve palsies (commonly 3rd, 6th, 7th), limb weakness, sensory changes.

Diagnosis: MRI; CSF with lymphoma cells or elevated β_2 microglobulin (tumor marker).

Treatment and prognosis: focal radiotherapy and intrathecal chemotherapy. Median survival 4 months; highly variable.

EPIDURAL SPINAL CORD COMPRESSION

5% of NHL patients. Usually direct extension from vertebral body metastases. Thoracic cord most common site; 5–10% have multifocal epidural tumor so entire spine should be imaged (noncontrast MRI sufficient).

Treatment: focal radiotherapy.

PRIMARY CNS LYMPHOMA

IMMUNOCOMPETENT PATIENTS

Epidemiology
3% of all intracranial neoplasms, 7% of all malignant lymphomas. Incidence rising in people >60, peak incidence age 40 to 60; M:F ratio 3:2.

Clinical Features
Behavioral changes and lateralizing symptoms (hemiparesis, aphasia, visual field deficits) common. Occasionally: seizures, ataxia, cranial nerve palsies. 20% have ocular disease (blurred vision, floaters, visual loss due to retinal detachment).

Diagnosis

CT or MRI: single or multiple contrast-enhancing lesions with mild to moderate surrounding edema. (In immunocompetent patients, ring enhancement, calcification, hemorrhage *rare*). Typically periventricular, often frontal. Small number of patients have leptomeningeal disease only. *Differential diagnosis*: high-grade gliomas, metastasis, abscess, sarcoid, TB, active demyelination.

Histological confirmation: stereotactic brain biopsy needed in most; 15% have positive CSF cytology.

Pathology: >98% B-cell tumors, most diffuse large-cell type.

Initial evaluation must include: ophthalmologic examination with slit-lamp, CSF cytology and tumor markers, HIV serology, spine MRI with gadolinium. Requirement for imaging of chest/abdomen/pelvis and bone marrow biopsy depend on individual treatment protocol (<3% of patients have systemic disease).

Treatment

Corticosteroids: avoid use before diagnosis made. Dramatic, temporary resolution of lesion in 60%, may last months after discontinuation of steroids.

First treatment: chemotherapy including high-dose methotrexate; sometimes with whole-brain radiotherapy (RT).

Prognosis

Median survival with combined modality regimens 30 to 60 months (vs. 12 to 18 months with RT alone). 50% relapse, usually within 2 years of diagnosis; 2nd remission achieved in 60% of these patients. Patients >60 years at risk for permanent, severe long-term neurotoxicity following combined therapy with RT and high-dose methotrexate.

IMMUNODEFICIENT PATIENTS

Epidemiology

Immunocompromised states associated with primary CNS lymphoma: HIV infection (most common), renal transplantation, Wiskott-Aldrich syndrome, ataxia telangiectasia, IgA deficiency, rheumatoid arthritis.

Most common brain tumor in patients with AIDS. Usually occurs with marked T-cell depletion (CD4 <50/mm^3); incidence much decreased since advent of highly active antiretroviral therapy (HAART).

Strong association with Epstein-Barr virus (EBV) infection.

Diagnosis

Unlike primary CNS lymphoma in immunocompetent hosts, lesions are almost always multiple and show ring enhancement on CT or MRI. *Differential diagnosis*: toxoplasmosis.

PET or SPECT helps differentiate from toxoplasmosis (tumor is hypermetabolic).

CSF: Positive EBV PCR supports diagnosis of lymphoma. Positive PET or SPECT + positive EBV PCR establishes diagnosis; if both tests negative, diagnosis excluded. If only one test positive, brain biopsy may eventually be necessary (risk of hemorrhage greater in patients with AIDS than immunocompetent patients).

Practical approach in patient with HIV and intracerebral mass: treat with antitoxoplasmosis medication; if no clinical or radiographic improvement after 2 weeks, consider biopsy for definite tissue diagnosis.

Treatment and Prognosis

Standard treatment: whole-brain RT; most patients respond clinically. Some also benefit from high-dose methotrexate. Immune reconstitution with HAART may markedly improve response to treatment.

Good prognostic factors: limited disease (i.e., no meningeal metastasis), good performance status, no coexisting medical conditions, CD4 count >200/mm^3.

Median survival 4 months with RT.

INTRAVASCULAR LYMPHOMA

Also called neoplastic angioendotheliomatosis, angiotropic lymphoma. Form of B-cell NHL; tumor cells grow within and occlude lumen of small blood vessels. Predilection for skin and CNS. Three main forms: cutaneous (mild); progressive disease of skin and viscera; aggressive multiorgan syndrome. M:F ratio 2:1. Median age at onset: 60 years.

Clinical features: progressive dementia and lethargy, waxing and waning multifocal signs. Skin lesions: telangiectasia, hemorrhagic nodules, leg lymphedema.

Laboratory findings: anemia, elevated ESR, elevated lactate dehydrogenase. CSF: elevated protein with or without mild pleocytosis; oligoclonal bands present in 77%, neoplastic cells detected in only 3%.

Imaging: multifocal abnormalities; mass-like lesion with increased signal on T2 (most common); multifocal infarcts with gyriform enhancement; meningeal enhancement. White matter most commonly affected.

Diagnosis: usually requires brain biopsy.

Treatment and prognosis: corticosteroids plus combination of systemic and intrathecal chemotherapy, radiation, plasmapheresis. Median survival 6 months.

LYMPHOMATOID GRANULOMATOSIS

EBV-associated, B-cell lymphoproliferative process preferentially affecting lungs.

Pathophysiology: perivascular neoplastic infiltrate leads to vascular damage, granuloma formation.

CNS involvement in 30% (headache, cranial nerve palsies, multi-infarct dementia); peripheral neuropathy in 25%.

Brain MRI: multiple gray and white matter lesions, with foci of enhancement and hemorrhage, associated with edema.
Prognosis: median survival 2 years.

CHAPTER 58 ■ PINEAL REGION TUMORS

1% of all intracranial tumors; wide variety of cell types.

GENERAL CONSIDERATIONS

Symptoms
Mechanisms of symptoms: (a) increased intracranial pressure from hydrocephalus; (b) direct compression of brainstem, cerebellum; (c) endocrine dysfunction.

Headache most common symptom at onset.

Dorsal midbrain compression: (a) *Parinaud syndrome* (paresis of upgaze, convergence-retraction nystagmus, light-near pupillary dissociation); (b) *Sylvian aqueduct syndrome* (Parinaud syndrome plus paralysis of downgaze or horizontal gaze); (c) lid retraction (*Collier sign*); (d) *ptosis*; (e) fourth nerve palsy (diplopia, head tilt).

Direct cerebellar compression: ataxia, dysmetria.

Endocrine dysfunction rare: diabetes insipidus, precocious puberty in boys.

Diagnosis
Brain MRI with gadolinium.

Additional staging investigations: complete spine MRI, CSF cytology. High levels of α-fetoprotein or β-human chorionic gonadotropin in CSF or serum indicate presence of malignant germ cells.

Surgical excision of tumor for tissue diagnosis, debulking.

Postoperative evaluation for CSF seeding with contrast MRI of whole spine, CSF tumor markers and cytology prior to starting adjuvant therapy.

TUMOR TYPES

GERM CELL TUMORS (GCTs)

1/3 of all pineal tumors. Histologically identical to gonadal GCTs. Arise in midline, in pineal region and suprasellar cistern. Predominantly boys and young men.

2 main categories: germinoma vs. non-germinomatous (embryonal-cell carcinoma, choriocarcinoma, teratocarcinoma, endodermal sinus tumor)

Non-germinomatous tumors highly malignant; more aggressive and more likely to seed CSF than germinomas.

Treatment and prognosis: Benign GCTs (e.g., teratomas, dermoids, epidermoids) generally cured by surgery alone. Germinomas: adjuvant whole-neuraxis radiotherapy; 80% to 90% 5-year survival. Non-germinomatous tumors: radiotherapy plus chemotherapy; relapse common within 2 years.

PINEAL CELL TUMORS

Arise from pineocytes. Range: histologically primitive *pineoblastoma* to well-differentiated *pineocytoma*. Affect children and young adults before age 40; higher grade tumors tend to occur in younger age group.

Treatment: complete resection of pineocytoma requires no additional therapy. Incomplete resection or intermediate-grade tumor: adjuvant radiotherapy. Pineoblastoma: radiotherapy + chemotherapy.

Prognosis: 5-year survival 80% for pineocytomas, 50% for pineoblastomas.

GLIOMAS

1/3 of pineal tumors; invasive; prognosis comparable to brain-stem astrocytomas. 33% low-grade, cystic (better prognosis). Oligodendrogliomas, ependymomas may occur.

Treatment identical to treatment of gliomas elsewhere in CNS (see Chapter 56).

MENINGIOMAS

Higher incidence in middle age and later. Amenable to surgical resection.

METASTASIS AND MISCELLANEOUS TUMORS

Pineal does not have blood-brain barrier; susceptible to metastasis from systemic tumors. Miscellaneous tumors: sarcoma, hemangioblastoma, choroid plexus papilloma, lymphoma, chemodectoma.

PINEAL CYSTS

Often found incidentally on imaging: diameter <2 cm; frequent peripheral enhancement due to compression of normal gland tissue. No surgical treatment required unless cyst grows large enough to cause symptoms (headache, visual disturbance); this is uncommon.

CHAPTER 59 ■ PITUITARY TUMORS

Most are pituitary adenomas. Often asymptomatic. Peak ages 20 to 40.

CLASSIFICATION

Secreting tumors: produce one or more anterior pituitary hormones; prolactinoma most common.
Mixed secretory tumors: 10% of all adenomas.
Non-secreting ("null cell") adenoma: no hormone secretion.

Also divided by size: microadenomas (<1.0 cm in diameter) usually cause symptoms due to excess hormone secretion; macroadenomas (>1.0 cm) cause symptoms due to mass effect.

CLINICAL FEATURES

Symptoms due to either endocrine dysfunction or direct tumor mass effect. Secreting tumors: see Chapter 146.

Non-secreting Tumors

Hypopituitarism (See Table 59.1).
Mass effect: headache; visual field defects (typically, bitemporal hemianopia from upward compression of optic chiasm); may have optic pallor; papilledema rare.
Compression or invasion of cavernous sinus (rare): diplopia; facial numbness.
Suprasellar extension: hydrocephalus, diabetes insipidus, personality changes, dementia, seizures, motor dysfunction, CSF rhinorrhea.
Pituitary apoplexy: hemorrhage or infarction of adenoma; presenting symptoms in 5%. Sudden onset of headache, oculomotor palsies, nausea, vomiting, altered mental state, diplopia, rapidly progressive visual loss. May require emergency surgery.

TABLE 59.1

SYMPTOMS OF PITUITARY FAILURE

Gonadotroph Failure
  Loss of libido
  Impotence

Thyrotroph Failure
  Fatigue
  Malaise
  Apathy
  Constipation
  Weight gain

Somatotroph Failure
  Weight gain
  Depression
  Premature atherosclerosis
  Muscle weakness

Corticotroph Failure
  Fatigue
  Weight gain
  Hypoglycemia

Adenoma may enlarge in pregnancy; increased blood flow requirement may not be met during labor, causing pituitary apoplexy during or after labor (*Sheehan syndrome*).

IMAGING

Microadenoma sometimes difficult to see on MRI; may be inferred from glandular asymmetry, focal sellar erosion, asymmetric convexity of upper margin of gland, displaced infundibulum, reduced contrast enhancement.

Macroadenoma: normal gland may not be visualized; bright signal of posterior lobe may be absent.

TREATMENT

Correct electrolyte dysfunction; replace deficient pituitary hormones; including adequate steroid coverage for situations of physiological stress (e.g., febrile illness, surgery).

Secreting tumors: see Chapter 146.

Non-secreting tumors: surgical reduction (trans-sphenoidal resection) to maintain pituitary function. Subtotal debulking, radiotherapy reduce recurrence, progression.

Asymptomatic adenomas: no intervention; follow with periodic visual field examination and MRI. Indications for treatment: onset of symptoms or growth on MRI.

CHAPTER 60 ■ CONGENITAL AND CHILDHOOD CNS TUMORS

EPIDEMIOLOGY

Primary CNS tumors: 20% of all childhood cancers, second only to leukemia. Incidence 2.8 per 100,000 under 15 years. Relative frequency: see Table 60.1.

Unlike adults, CNS metastasis from solid tumors rare in children.

Most tumors sporadic. Genetic neurocutaneous syndromes include neurofibromatosis (types 1, 2; see Chapter 100), tuberous sclerosis (see Chapter 103), epidermal nevus syndrome, von Hippel-Lindau disease (see Chapter 61).

SYMPTOMS AND SIGNS

Increased intracranial pressure: headache, vomiting, diplopia. Also fatigue, personality change, worsening school performance. Onset may be gradual.

Infants: nonspecific symptoms, including irritability, anorexia, persistent vomiting, developmental delay or regression, macrocephaly, downward deviation of eyes ("sun-setting").

Warning signs: persistent vomiting, recurrent headache (awakening child from sleep), neurologic findings (ataxia,

TABLE 60.1

COMMON CHILDHOOD CNS TUMORS

Tumor type	Percentage of all CNS tumors
Pilocytic astrocytoma	24%
Medulloblastoma	16%
High-grade astrocytoma	14%
Ependymoma	10%
Craniopharyngioma	6%
Germ cell tumors	2.5%

head tilt, visual loss, papilledema), endocrine disturbance (growth deceleration, diabetes insipidus), stigmata of neurofibromatosis.

Childhood CNS tumors equally frequently supratentorial and infratentorial (Table 60.2). Supratentorial tumors: headache, limb weakness, sensory loss, occasionally seizures, deteriorating school performance, personality change. Infratentorial tumors: headache, vomiting, diplopia, imbalance.

CONGENITAL TUMORS

CRANIOPHARYNGIOMA

Originates from remnants of embryonic tissue in Rathke pouch. Vary from small, well-circumscribed solid nodules to large multilocular cysts invading sella turcica. Histologically benign but extensive local invasion may make total surgical removal difficult.

Clinical features: Short stature, hypothyroidism, diabetes insipidus, visual loss, signs of increased intracranial pressure.

Treatment options: (a) cyst drainage, resection of nonadherent tumor, localized radiation therapy (main side effect: cognitive loss in younger children); (b) gross total resection without irradiation (main side effect: lifelong panhypopituitarism). (c) stereotactic radiosurgery ("gamma knife") for small tumors.

Recurrence rates: 20% to 40%.

TABLE 60.2

LOCATION OF CENTRAL NERVOUS SYSTEM TUMORS IN INFANTS, CHILDREN, ADOLESCENTS

Location	Infants	Children	Adolescents
Supratentorial	Teratoma Cerebral astrocytoma Choroid plexus tumor PNET Craniopharyngioma Optic glioma Dermoid	Cerebral astrocytoma Optic pathway/diencephalic glioma Craniopharyngioma Suprasellar germ cell tumor Ependymoma Ganglioglioma	Cerebral astrocytoma Glioblastoma multiforme Pineal germ cell tumor Craniopharyngioma Oligodendroglioma Meningioma Lymphoma Colloid cyst
Infratentorial	Medulloblastoma Ependymoma Astrocytoma	Medulloblastoma Brainstem glioma Ependymoma Cerebellar astrocytoma	Medulloblastoma Cerebellar astrocytoma Ependymoma Epidermoid

EPIDERMOID (CHOLESTEATOMA) AND DERMOID TUMORS

2% of childhood intracranial tumors. Usual locations: suprasellar, skull base, brainstem, cerebellopontine angle, inside ventricle. Encapsulated, sometimes cystic. Young adults. Symptoms dictated by location. Treatment: surgical resection.

TERATOMA

4% of childhood intracranial tumors. Infants, young children. Lobulated and cystic, often contains bone, cartilage, teeth, hair, or intestine. Usually in pineal region; Parinaud syndrome, hydrocephalus. Treatment: resection.

CHORDOMA

<1% of childhood intracranial tumors. From remnants of embryonic notochord. Half sacrococcygeal, 1/3 sphenoid-occipital junction, remainder elsewhere along spinal cord. Locally invasive.

Usually starts in adulthood; visual loss or cranial nerve dysfunction. Can invade nasopharynx, intracranial sinuses, neck.

Grows slowly but may recur after excision. Treatment: resection.

CHOROID PLEXUS TUMORS

Rare. Location: in or near lateral ventricle. Symptoms before age 2 years: macrocephaly, bulging fontanelle, split sutures (hydrocephalus). CSF overproduction to 2,000 mL/d.

Papilloma (2/3): usually not invasive. Surgical resection curative.

Carcinoma (1/3): invasive; nearly half disseminate in CSF. Treatment: resection, followed by chemotherapy and radiotherapy for residual tumor. Median survival 6 months.

COLLOID CYST

Grows in anterior superior portion of third ventricle. Usually in adults with intermittent (sometimes positional) hydrocephalus, due to "ball-valve" obstruction of CSF flow. Treatment: excision.

ASTROCYTOMA

CEREBELLAR ASTROCYTOMA

12% of all childhood brain tumors; 30% to 40% of posterior fossa tumors. Peak incidence in adolescence. May be cystic or solid. Usually histologically benign.

Clumsiness, unsteadiness, intermittent morning headache, vomiting, dysmetria, papilledema.

Juvenile pilocytic variant: cystic tumor with mural nodule on MRI. >90% survival with surgery alone.
Infiltrating variant: hypercellularity or frank anaplasia; brainstem invasion. 30% recurrence-free survival.

BRAINSTEM GLIOMA

10% to 20% of posterior fossa tumors. Peak age 5 to 8 years.

Symptoms: slowly progressive abnormalities of cranial nerves, limb weakness, gait, swallowing, and speech. Vomiting and headache indicate hydrocephalus.
Imaging: focal lesion with little or no enhancement; surrounding edema; compression of surrounding cisterns.
Focal radiation therapy: some benefit.

Surgical resection not warranted in diffuse intrinsic pontine lesions (70%). Monitor for hydrocephalus; CSF diversion by shunting can improve quality of life.

Diffuse intrinsic pontine lesions fatal in 18 to 24 months (worst prognosis of any brain tumor). Better prognosis: primarily exophytic variant, focal midbrain lesions.

DIENCEPHALIC AND OPTIC PATHWAY GLIOMAS

5% of childhood CNS tumors. Onset before age 20 years. Neurofibromatosis type 1 associated with 50% to 70% of isolated optic nerve tumors, 10% to 20% of optic chiasm tumors.

Slowly progressive visual loss, strabismus, nystagmus, developmental delay, visual loss, bitemporal field defects, hemiparesis, endocrine dysfunction.

Main treatment: radiotherapy, chemotherapy. Recurrence common.

CEREBRAL HEMISPHERE LOW-GRADE GLIOMAS

Peak incidence: ages 2 to 4 years, then early adolescence. Symptoms of increased intracranial pressure, developmental delay, growth retardation, plus limb weakness, sensory loss, or visual loss.

Slow-growing; malignant transformation less likely than adult gliomas.

Gross total resection often effective but not curative. Radiotherapy used postoperatively with 5-year survival rates of 75% to 85%. Chemotherapy for younger children with residual or recurrent tumor (vincristine and carboplatin) to defer radiotherapy.

CEREBRAL HEMISPHERE HIGH-GRADE ASTROCYTOMAS

11% of childhood brain tumors. High-grade astrocytomas classified as in Chapter 53. Symptoms: headache, vomiting, seizures, limb weakness, behavioral change, usually <3 months duration.

Treatment: resection improves survival but tumors disseminate in CSF; recur without further therapy. Postoperative irradiation, chemotherapy increase survival.

SPINAL CORD ASTROCYTOMA

4% of childhood CNS neoplasms. Affects any part of cord; solid or cystic. Histologically benign; slow growth.

Symptoms: pain (localized or radicular), limb weakness, spasticity, altered gait, bowel or bladder dysfunction.

Treatment: gross total resection, or partial resection with decompression of cysts and postoperative radiotherapy (or chemotherapy in very young children). Recovery depends on preoperative condition.

Low-grade tumors: 55% survival at 10 years. High-grade: up to 46% progression-free survival at 5 years following chemo- and radiotherapy.

EMBRYONAL TUMORS

PRIMITIVE NEUROECTODERMAL TUMORS (PNET)

Most common malignant CNS tumors of childhood. Most in posterior fossa (medulloblastoma); these comprise 30% of all infratentorial tumors in children. Abnormal chromosome 17 in 33%. Supratentorial PNETs histologically identical; arise in cerebral cortex or pineal region.

Symptoms: increased intracranial pressure, ataxia, diplopia. Median age 5 years. Symptom duration before diagnosis <3 months.

Imaging: homogeneous enhancement; hydrocephalus in >80%. Dissemination to spine in 33%.

Treatment: attempt complete resection, follow with craniospinal irradiation (entire neuraxis at risk for recurrence), chemotherapy. Postoperative complication: posterior fossa syndrome (mutism, pharyngeal dysfunction, ataxia).

Prognosis: overall 5-year disease-free survival 55%. Poorer prognosis if residual tumor, brainstem invasion, meningeal spread, age <3 years.

ATYPICAL TERATOID/RHABDOID TUMORS

Affect infants, toddlers. Usually arise in cerebellum or cerebellar-pontine angle. Mean survival <1 year; high recurrence.

EPENDYMOMA

5% to 10% of all primary childhood brain tumors. Usually within or adjacent to ependymal lining of ventricular system; 60% to 75% in posterior fossa.

Variants: anaplastic ependymoma; subependymoma (lower grade). Ependymoblastoma is a type of PNET.

Symptoms dictated by location: nausea, vomiting, morning headache from obstructive hydrocephalus (ependymoma filling or compressing fourth ventricle); neck pain, cranial nerve palsies (posterior fourth ventricle, extending into lower medulla); seizures, focal sign of supratentorial mass.

Imaging: calcification, variable enhancement.

Prognosis: best predictor of outcome is extent of surgical resection. Total resection: 75% 10-year survival. Subtotal resection: local recurrence common, 10-year survival 15%. Postoperative localized radiation therapy increases survival; adjuvant chemotherapy may improve outcome.

GERM CELL TUMORS

See Chapter 58.

MENINGIOMA

Rare in childhood; association with neurofibromatosis type 2. Usually arises on meningeal surface but (in contrast to adults) may be parenchymal. Enhancement on imaging. Usually benign. Treatment: resection.

Meningeal sarcoma: aggressive, treated with combined radiation, chemotherapy.

LATE EFFECTS OF TREATMENT

RADIATION THERAPY

Cognitive impairment in 2/3 of brain tumor survivors; children under 5 years particularly susceptible.

Also: growth impairment, endocrine dysfunction, neurologic sequelae (hearing loss, blindness, cataracts, motor and coordination problems, seizures).

Increased risk of second tumors after cranial irradiation. See also Chapter 72.

CHEMOTHERAPY

Chronic neurotoxicity: hearing loss (especially cisplatin), peripheral neuropathy (vincristine, cisplatin, etoposide).

Risk of secondary leukemia after treatment with alkylating agents, etoposide.

CHAPTER 61 ■ VASCULAR TUMORS AND MALFORMATIONS

VASCULAR MALFORMATIONS

Most probably congenital, though may enlarge progressively. Some arteriovenous fistulas acquired, follow trauma or arterial or venous occlusion.

ARTERIOVENOUS MALFORMATIONS (AVMs)

Affect brain more than dura, sometimes both.

Incidence approximately 1.5/100,000 population, half diagnosed at time of hemorrhage.

Pathology: tangle of abnormal arteries and veins with interposed sinuses lacking media; no capillaries. Variable location, blood supply.

Major risk is hemorrhage: parenchymal, intraventricular, or subarachnoid. Bleeding risk similar to aneurysms, but morbidity less. Features associated with increased bleeding risk: deep location, presence of deep-venous drainage, associated aneurysm, multiple arterial feeding vessels, small size. Most common in middle life. Less commonly, may cause chronic seizure disorder or headaches.

MRI, magnetic resonance angiogram (MRA) document AVM, prior major hemorrhage, intranidal aneurysms, main source of blood supply. Treatment plan requires conventional angiography.

Treatment: (a) *surgical resection* (most effective); usually preceded by *embolization* using glues, coils, other agents to reduce size and pressure within AVM. (b) Focused-beam radiotherapy (*radiosurgery*) for small (<2.5 cm), deep lesions not suitable for embolization or surgery.

Vein of Galen malformation: special AVM associated with deep venous system, often with marked aneurysmal dilation of vein of Galen. Complex blood supply, including arteries. Symptoms develop in neonatal period or early childhood; severe arterial shunting causes cardiac failure, midbrain compression with subsequent hydrocephalus. Treatment: embolization, occasionally followed by surgery.

VENOUS MALFORMATIONS (DEEP VENOUS ANOMALIES)

No apparent arterial supply. May cause headaches, seizures, or, rarely, hemorrhage. Generally in deep white matter, brainstem, cerebellum.

Often not amenable to safe surgical resection. Generally benign.

CAVERNOUS MALFORMATIONS

Highly focal, usually small clusters of tiny vessels of uniform size. Occur anywhere in CNS.

May cause limited local hemorrhage; may recur. Major bleeding uncommon. Multiple lesions sometimes familial. May cause seizures, headaches.

Not seen on angiogram. Sometimes visible on CT or MRI after asymptomatic hemorrhage. Characteristic "target" appearance on MRI.

Surgery usually recommended after hemorrhage if lesion is readily accessible.

TELANGIECTASIAS

Collections of engorged capillaries or cavernous spaces separated by normal brain tissue. Usually small, poorly circumscribed; propensity for white matter. May be associated with telangiectasia outside CNS (Rendu-Osler-Weber syndrome).

Not visible on angiography or CT. Rarely clinically significant.

STURGE-WEBER-DIMITRI SYNDROME

See Chapter 101.

SINUS PERICRANII

Thin-walled vascular spaces interconnected by anastomoses that protrude from skull and communicate with superior longitudinal sinus.

Evident in infants. Soft, compressible. Size increases when venous pressure in head raised by coughing, straining, lowering head. May enlarge over years.

Usually asymptomatic, except for external swelling. Radiographs show defect of underlying bone.

VASCULAR TUMORS

Intricate vascular network composed of irregular capillaries and intervening stromal cells, with occasional nuclear pleomorphism. Three forms, histologically indistinguishable:

ANGIOBLASTIC MENINGIOMA

Grossly identical to other meningiomas; attached to dura.

HEMANGIOPERICYTOMA

Arises from endothelial elements of blood vessels; may be found elsewhere in body.

HEMANGIOBLASTOMA

Posterior fossa and spinal cord. No dural attachment. Composed of primitive vascular elements. Any age, especially young adults or middle aged.

Symptoms often present one year before diagnosis made. Clinical features dictated by location.

Predominantly cerebellar, often with large cysts. Resembles cyst and mural nodule of cystic cerebellar astrocytoma but distinctive vascular appearance on angiogram. May be multiple. Sometimes with polycythemia.

von Hippel-Lindau disease: hemangioblastoma and multiple angiomatoses of retina, cysts of kidney and pancreas; occasionally, renal cell carcinoma or capillary nevi of skin. Familial in 20% of cases. Pheochromocytoma, syringomyelia may occur.

Treatment: surgical resection. Survival: 85% alive 5 to 20 years after total resection. May recur if tumor only partially removed or tumors multiple.

CHAPTER 62 ■ METASTATIC TUMORS

EPIDEMIOLOGY

Eight times more common than primary brain tumors. 25% of all patients with systemic cancer have intracranial metastases (15% brain, 5% meninges, 5% dura; Table 62.1).

BRAIN METASTASIS

50% of patients have single lesion, 20% have only 2 lesions.

CLINICAL FEATURES

Usually subacute symptom onset (weeks): headache (25%), hemiparesis (25%), cognitive or behavioral change (15%),

TABLE 62.1

PRIMARY TUMORS COMMONLY ASSOCIATED WITH CNS METASTASIS

Parenchyma	Lung, melanoma, breast, renal, gastrointestinal
Meninges	
Dura, subdural	Breast, prostate, melanoma, leukemia, neuroblastoma, lymphoma
Leptomeninges	Leukemia (especially ALL), lymphoma, carcinoma (breast, lung, melanoma)
Perineural (cranial nerves)	Squamous cell carcinoma, basal cell carcinoma, carcinoma of minor salivary glands
Calvarium, skull base	Breast, lung, prostate carcinoma
Spine	Breast, prostate, lung carcinoma

ALL, acute lymphocytic leukemia.

seizures (15%). Acute symptom onset may occur with intra-tumor hemorrhage (melanoma, thyroid, renal cell, choriocarcinoma).

Brain imaging: MRI shows contrast-enhancing lesions: typically spherical, at gray-white matter junction, with significant surrounding edema. Large lesions may show ring enhancement (due to central necrosis).

In patient with suspected brain metastases and unknown primary tumor: assess with thorough physical examination (breast, prostate, testicular, rectal lesions); check stool for occult blood; image with either CT of chest, abdomen and pelvis or total body PET scan with fluorodeoxyglucose to try to locate primary site.

Differential diagnosis: brain abscess, multifocal gliomas, demyelinating disease (occasionally large enhancing lesions), delayed radiation necrosis, stroke.

TREATMENT

Corticosteroids reduce edema of tumor, radiation. Administer for at least 48 hours prior to starting radiotherapy.

Radiotherapy (RT): effective palliative treatment. Whole-brain RT relieves symptoms in 80% of patients, but median survival only 4 to 6 months (approximately half die from progressive CNS disease, half from systemic disease).

Stereotactic radiosurgery (gamma knife, linear accelerator): increasingly used as initial treatment, may also be considered at recurrence after whole-brain RT. Most effective for lesions <3 cm. Median survival after radiosurgery: 1 year.

Surgery: treatment of choice, with or without postoperative radiotherapy, for accessible single lesions. Partial resection (debulking) for symptoms of mass effect.

Chemotherapy: limited role; usually used only at recurrence once other treatment options exhausted. Metastases from some primary tumors may be chemosensitive: breast, small-cell lung cancer, choriocarcinoma.

DURAL METASTASIS

Usually from direct extension of calvarial metastasis.

Symptoms: painless, growing skull lesions, seizures, headaches, hemiparesis.

Imaging: MRI appearance may be identical to meningioma. For tumors near vertex, MRV helps to assess patency of superior sagittal sinus.

Treatment: focal radiotherapy.

MENINGEAL METASTASIS

Pathogenesis: hematogenous spread, spread from bone metastases via venous sinuses or brain metastases via CSF, seeding of subarachnoid space during surgical resection.

Clinical features: multilevel symptoms and signs affecting 3 main areas: (1) cranial nerves; (2) spinal roots and cord; (3) cerebrum (see Table 62.2).

INVESTIGATIONS

CSF: elevated pressure (50%), pleocytosis (60%), elevated protein (80%), low glucose (25%). Demonstration of tumor cells in CSF confirms diagnosis: positive cytology found in 50% of patients after first lumbar puncture, 90% after third.

TABLE 62.2
CLINICAL FINDINGS IN MENINGEAL METASTASIS

Site	Symptoms/signs
Cerebrum	Mental status change (50%), difficulty walking (45%), headache (40%), seizures (15%), nausea and vomiting (12%)
Cranial nerves	Diplopia (30%), facial weakness (25%), hearing loss (20%), trigeminal neuropathy (12%), optic neuropathy (2%)
Spinal cord and roots	Limb weakness (78%), reflex asymmetry (60%), radicular pain (25%), paresthesias (10%), sphincter dysfunction (2%)

MRI: sensitivity approximately 70%. Definite findings, confirming diagnosis: contrast enhancement of sulci, cranial nerves, subependymal; enhancing subarachnoid tumor nodules (e.g., on cauda equina). Other imaging findings suggest leptomeningeal metastasis (indicating need for CSF examination): communicating hydrocephalus, multiple metastases on brain surface, intraventricular nodules. Entire neuraxis should be imaged.

TREATMENT AND PROGNOSIS

Palliative. Radiotherapy for symptomatic sites (e.g., brain for cranial neuropathies) or sites of bulky disease.

CSF shunt may be necessary to relieve hydrocephalus.

Intrathecal chemotherapy: methotrexate, cytosine arabinoside, or thiotepa. Ventricular injection preferred to lumbar injection. Complications: aseptic meningitis (43% with intraventricular route), myelosuppression, chemotherapy-related leukoencephalopathy.

Median survival 4 to 6 months. Treatment may prevent neurologic deterioration. Prognosis worse with widespread systemic disease, CSF block, coexistent bulky CNS metastases.

EPIDURAL SPINAL METASTASES

Most commonly lung, breast, prostate cancer.

Epidural cord compression occurs in 5% of patients with cancer; usually associated with known bone metastases. 70% thoracic, 20% lumbar, 10% cervical.

Pain first symptom in 97% (local or radicular, often aggravated by movement or supine position). Limb weakness in 76%; autonomic symptoms (57%), sensory loss (51%). Urinary incontinence occurs late. Location often indicated by sensory level.

Noncontrast MRI of entire spine preferred for epidural tumors. Severe or rapidly progressive symptoms: neurologic emergency.

Treatment: goals are preserving neurologic function (steroids, radiation), relieving pain (analgesics, steroids, radiation). Early recognition and treatment crucial. Surgery (laminectomy for posterior tumor; vertebral body resection for anterior tumor) considered in appropriate patients (see Chapter 63).

Most important prognostic factor: neurologic state at time of treatment. Survival depends mostly on control of underlying malignancy.

CHAPTER 63 ■ SPINAL TUMORS

Cell types similar to intracranial tumors. Arise from cord parenchyma, nerve roots, meninges, intraspinal blood vessels, sympathetic nerves, vertebrae.

Intramedullary (10%), extramedullary (90%; intradural or extradural). Intramedullary more common in children; extramedullary in adults.

Most common primary tumors with spine metastases: lung, breast, prostate.

TABLE 63.1
RELATIVE FREQUENCY OF DIFFERENT TYPES OF SPINAL TUMORS

Type	Percent
Neurofibroma	29
Meningioma	26
Ependymoma	13
Miscellaneous	12
Astrocytoma	7
Metastatic and other	13
Total	100

FREQUENCY

Much less prevalent than intracranial tumors (1:4). Relative frequency of tumor types: see Table 63.1. Most in young or middle-aged adults. Meningioma more common in women; ependymoma in men. Most common site: thoracic.

PATHOPHYSIOLOGY

Extramedullary: compression of nerve roots or spinal cord, occlusion of spinal blood vessels. Intramedullary: direct interference with intrinsic structures (mass effect, edema, syringomyelia).

CLINICAL MANIFESTATIONS

Extramedullary Tumors
Either intradural or extradural (= epidural). Usually involve multiple adjacent segments.

Nerve root compression: focal pain, paresthesias followed by sensory loss, weakness, atrophy in distribution of affected roots.

Spinal cord compression: usually late syndrome. Pathways at cord periphery affected first. Early findings: (a) spastic weakness below lesion; (b) impaired cutaneous and proprioceptive sensation below lesion; (c) urinary incontinence; (d) overactive tendon reflexes, Babinski signs, loss of abdominal reflexes. If untreated, syndrome may progress to complete transection of spinal cord: wasting and atrophy of muscles at level of lesion with paraplegia or quadriplegia below.

Spinal vessel occlusion: myelomalacia, cord necrosis; symptoms similar to those of intramedullary lesion.

Anterior spinal artery occlusion: segmental lower motor neuron signs at level of occlusion; bilateral loss of pain and temperature sensation and upper motor neuron signs below. Posterior columns spared.

SPINAL METASTASIS

Epidural Spinal Cord Compression

Onset: neck or back pain; relentless, persists when patient supine. Limb weakness, paresthesias in distribution of nerve root, sphincter dysfunction: neuro-oncologic emergency.

Primary tumor: lung or breast >50% of cases. Also gastrointestinal system, prostate, melanoma, lymphoma.

Treatment of Epidural Metastatic Disease

Usually palliative. Management individually for patient's specific clinical situation.

Loss of bowel or bladder function, rapidly progressive paraparesis usually irreversible. Conversely, 94% of patients treated while still walking remain ambulatory.

Radiation: treatment of choice for most patients with spinal metastases. Goals: relieve pain, prevent or reverse neurologic impairment.

Indications for surgery: radioresistant tumor (e.g., melanoma), recurrent tumor at site of prior radiotherapy, spinal instability, unknown tissue diagnosis, rapid progression. Contraindication: advanced systemic disease.

Intramedullary Metastasis

Most common primary tumors: lung, breast cancer.

Early diagnosis crucial for reversal or stabilization of neurologic signs. Survival: only 20% at 3 months.

PRIMARY INTRAMEDULLARY TUMORS

Usually extend over many segments. Ependymoma, astrocytoma most common.

Signs, symptoms vary more than in extramedullary tumors.

Central cord (crossing pain fibers): loss of pain and temperature only in affected segments.

Central gray matter (anterior horn cells): weakness, atrophy.

Peripheral spread (spinothalamic tracts): lose pain and temperature below affected segments. Normal pain and temperature perception in sacral segments (sacral sparing) because spinothalamic fibers from sacral cord run laterally at cord surface in thoracic and cervical regions.

INTRADURAL TUMORS

Neurofibroma, schwannoma, meningioma most common. Enhance brightly on MRI.

Meningeal "drop" metastases of intracranial tumors also intradural. Appear as small nodules on cord surface or cauda equina roots.

REGIONAL SYNDROMES

Foramen Magnum Tumors

May extend up into posterior fossa or down into cervical region. Signs and symptoms of cranial nerves 11, 12 (rarely, 9, 10).

Ventrolateral meningioma: loss of position, vibratory, light touch perception, more prominent in arms than legs. Upper motor neuron signs in all four limbs.

Cervical Tumors

Pain or paresthesias in occipital or cervical region, stiff neck, weakness, and wasting of neck muscles. Spastic tetraplegia or hemiplegia, with or without reduced sensation, below lesion.

Characteristic findings at different levels (Table 63.2). T1 lesions rarely cause motor symptoms. Nystagmus may be present, attributed to involvement of median longitudinal fasciculus descending into cervical cord. Horner syndrome with intramedullary lesions affecting descending sympathetic pathways.

Thoracic Tumors

Clinical localization by sensory level. Abdominal skin reflexes absent below lesion.

TABLE 63.2
FEATURES LOCALIZING UPPER LEVEL OF CERVICAL SPINAL TUMORS

Level	Paralysis and atrophy	Sensory deficit	Reflexes	Special features
C4	Diaphragm			
C5	Deltoid, biceps, supinator longus, rhomboid, spinati	To outer arm surface	Absent biceps, supinator	Upper arms hang limply at side
C6	Triceps, wrist extensors	Line running down middle of arm slightly to radial side	Triceps reflex lost	Forearm held semiflexed; partial wrist drop
C7	Wrist flexors, finger flexors and extensors	As in C6, but slightly more to ulnar side of arm		Efforts to close hands result in wrist extension and slight finger flexion (preacher's hand)
C8	Small muscles of hand	Inner aspect of arm; fourth, fifth fingers; ulnar aspect of middle finger		Clawhand (*main en griffe*), Horner syndrome

Lumbar Tumors

Localized by levels of sensory loss and weakness, but need CT or MRI for precise diagnosis.

L1, L2 segments alone: lose cremasteric reflexes. Abdominal reflexes, knee and ankle jerks preserved.

L3, L4 segments, sparing cauda equina: quadriceps weakness, absent patellar reflexes, hyperactive Achilles reflexes.

Tumors of Conus and Cauda Equina

First symptom: pain in back, rectal area, or both legs, followed by loss of bladder function, impotence. Later, flaccid leg paralysis, atrophy of leg muscles, foot drop, fasciculations. Saddle area sensory loss.

Papilledema, other symptoms or signs of raised intracranial pressure with ependymomas of this region if CSF protein content >100 mg/dL, attributed to interference of viscous solution with absorption of CSF.

DIAGNOSIS OF SPINAL TUMORS

MRI most useful test. CT more limited for imaging soft tissue, but demonstrates bony changes. Spinal angiography helpful for vascular malformations. Radiography alone may provide useful information if CT or MRI not available.

Differential diagnosis: transverse myelitis, MS, syringomyelia, combined system disease, syphilis, ALS, primary lateral sclerosis, anomalies of cervical spine and skull base, cervical spondylosis, adhesive arachnoiditis, radiculitis of cauda equina, hypertrophic arthritis, ruptured intervertebral discs, vascular anomalies, epidural lipomatosis.

TREATMENT OF PRIMARY SPINAL TUMORS

Surgical removal whenever possible. Emergency surgery indicated if neurologic disorder rapidly progressing. Best results if signs and symptoms due solely to compression by benign encapsulated tumor (e.g., meningioma).

Postoperative results depend on severity of preoperative disability.

Radiotherapy not indicated for most intradural extramedullary tumors (usually benign); rarely used after partial removal of intramedullary tumor.

After radical and extensive spinal surgery for tumors, vertebral deformities requiring fixation may develop, especially in children.

Section VII
Trauma

CHAPTER 64 ■ HEAD INJURY

Focus of chapter is on craniocerebral trauma, also referred to as traumatic brain injury (TBI).

EPIDEMIOLOGY

2 million patients annually in the United States.

200,000/year die or permanently disabled.

Peak ages 15 to 24. Leading cause of death before age 24 years. Four times more common in men than women.

Major causes: motor vehicle accidents, personal violence (including guns).

PATHOLOGY AND PATHOPHYSIOLOGY OF CRANIOCEREBRAL TRAUMA

SKULL FRACTURES

Linear (nondisplaced): 80% of skull fractures. Most common site: temporoparietal, where skull thinnest. CT otherwise normal. Generally, surgery not needed.

Open (compound): scalp lacerated over fracture.

Depressed: fragments of bone displaced inward, compress brain.

Comminuted: multiple shattered bone fragments.

About 85% depressed fractures open and liable to infection or CSF leak. Even if closed, most depressed or comminuted fractures provide indication for surgical exploration to debride, elevate bone fragments, repair dural lacerations. Underlying brain often injured.

Complications: tearing, compression, thrombosis of nearby venous dural sinuses.

Basilar skull fractures: linear, depressed or comminuted. Identified by CT with "bone windows." May injure cranial nerves or tear dura tear leading to delayed meningitis. Hemotympanum, tympanic perforation, hearing loss, CSF otorrhea, peripheral facial nerve weakness, ecchymosis around mastoid process (Battle sign) raise suspicion of petrous bone fracture. Anosmia, bilateral periorbital ecchymosis, CSF rhinorrhea suggest possible fracture of sphenoid, frontal, ethmoid bones.

Prognosis depends on nature and severity of brain injury.

CEREBRAL CONCUSSION AND AXONAL SHEARING INJURY

Violent acceleration-deceleration of head with stretching and shearing of axons, even without impact (e.g., forceful shaking). See Table 64.1.

Concussion: "dazed" state or unconscious for <6 hours without clinical evidence of brain injury.

Diffuse axonal injury (DAI): term sometimes used to describe traumatic coma lasting >6 hours. Refers to presumed mechanism of coma, i.e., shearing injury to axons from rotational forces.

CT, MRI usually normal.

Autonomic dysfunction (e.g., hypertension, sweating, fever) common with acute severe DAI. Coma may persist for days, months, years. Cognitive impairment, spasticity, ataxia common in survivors.

BRAIN SWELLING AND CEREBRAL EDEMA

Brain swelling after head injury poorly understood. Diffuse or focal after any type of head injury.

Mechanisms: abnormal vasodilation (increased cerebral blood volume); increased extravascular brain water (cerebral edema, which may be cytotoxic, vasogenic, or interstitial).

PARENCHYMAL CONTUSION AND HEMATOMA

Cerebral contusion: focal parenchymal hemorrhage after "scraping" or "bruising" brain as it moves across inner surface of skull. Usually superficial (affecting cortex). Inferior frontal and temporal lobes most commonly affected, because of irregular protuberances at base of skull.

Usually small and multiple; at site of impact ("coup lesions"), or at opposite pole as brain contacts skull ("contrecoup lesions"). Frequently enlarge for 12 to 24 hours; may appear 1 or more days after injury.

Prognosis: excellent if contusions small and DAI absent.

TABLE 64.1
CLINICAL CHARACTERISTICS AND OUTCOME OF DIFFUSE BRAIN INJURIES

| | Mild concussion | Cerebral contusion | Diffuse axonal injury | | |
			Mild	Moderate	Severe
Loss of consciousness	None	Immediate	Immediate	Immediate	Immediate
Length of unconsciousness	None	<6 hr	6–24	>24 hr	Days–weeks
Decerebrate posturing	None	None	Rare	Occasionally	Present
Posttraumatic amnesia	Minutes	Minutes-hours	Hours	Days	Weeks
Memory deficit	None	Mild	Mild-mod.	Mild-mod.	Severe
Motor deficits	None	None	None	Mild	Severe
Outcome at 3 months (%)					
Good recovery	100	95	63	38	15
Moderate deficit	0	5	15	21	13
Severe deficit	0	0	6	12	14
Vegetative	0	0	1	5	4
Death	0	0	15	24	51

Adapted from Gennarelli TA. Cerebral concussion and diffuse brain injuries. In: Cooper PR, ed. *Head injury*, 3rd ed. Baltimore: Williams & Wilkins, 1993:140.

Hematoma: focal collection of blood clot displaces brain. Caused by tearing of blood vessel by rotational forces. Usually in deep white matter. May require surgery.

SUBDURAL HEMATOMA

Blood between arachnoid membrane and dura mater. Due to rupture of veins traversing subdural space.

Causes: trauma, spontaneous (especially in elderly, alcoholics), coagulation disorder (including treatment with anticoagulants).

Most common over lateral cerebral convexities. Sometimes no overt head trauma in elderly or alcoholic patients with cerebral atrophy.

CT: crescent-shaped collection between skull and brain across entire hemisphere, crossing skull suture lines. High density (bright; acute hematoma); isodense (gray; subacute to chronic); low density (dark; chronic).

Acute subdural hematoma: symptomatic within 72 hours of injury. More common after falls or assaults. Three fourths patients lose consciousness before arriving in ER. Half of those who awake lose consciousness again after "lucid interval" of minutes to hours, as hematoma grows. Common manifestations: ipsilateral pupillary dilation and contralateral hemiparesis. "False localizing signs": contralateral pupillary dilation, ipsilateral hemiparesis common.

Chronic subdural hematoma: symptoms persist or start after 21 days. Incidence higher after age 50. No recognized head trauma in 25% to 50%. Risk factors: alcoholism, epilepsy, ventriculoperitoneal shunts, bleeding disorders, anticoagulant therapy.

Symptoms and signs: altered mental status, sometimes mistaken for dementia.

Treatment: surgical evacuation if mass effect present (focal neurologic deficit, seizures). Observation alone may be appropriate (small, nonexpanding, or chronic hematoma). Reoperation for acute subdural hematoma needed in 15%.

EPIDURAL HEMATOMA

Generally injury of middle meningeal artery; less frequently (15% of cases) dural sinus. About 75% with skull fracture.

Clot increases until ruptured vessel compressed or occluded by hematoma.

Locations: hemisphere convexity in middle cranial fossa (most frequent; usually middle meningeal artery); occasionally, anterior fossa (possibly anterior meningeal artery); rarely, posterior fossa (tear of torcula). Almost always ipsilateral to impact.

Course in one third of patients: immediate loss of consciousness (concussion), then "lucid interval" (no neurologic symptoms), followed by relapse into coma with hemiplegia as hematoma expands. Dilated, fixed ipsilateral pupil indicates transtentorial herniation. "False localizing signs" occur.

Cerebellar signs, stiff neck, drowsiness, occipital bone fracture suggest posterior fossa hematoma.

CT: "bulging" convex (lens-shaped) hyperdensity, does not cross skull sutures.

Herniation and death occur rapidly if bleeding arterial. Mortality near 100% if untreated, 5% to 30% otherwise. The shorter the interval between injury and surgery, the better the survival. Sequelae depend on severity of brain damage.

Treatment: surgical evacuation; occasionally, observation alone suffices (e.g., small venous hematoma).

SUBARACHNOID HEMORRHAGE (SAH)

Usually small, clinically unimportant after head trauma. In larger hemorrhage, blood distributes over hemispheres; contrasts with aneurysmal SAH with blood in basal cisterns.

Delayed complications of aneurysmal SAH (hydrocephalus, vasospasm) rare after traumatic SAH.

INITIAL ASSESSMENT AND STABILIZATION

Immediate management goals: (a) assess and stabilize airway, breathing, circulation; (b) judge severity of head injury (Table 64.2); (c) rule out cervical spine fracture (see below); (d) identify extracranial injuries. For moderate- and high-risk patients, CT to rule out fracture or intracranial bleeding.

Glasgow Coma Scale (GCS; Table 64.3): measures severity of brain injury; guide to prognosis (Table 64.4). Coma: GCS <8.

TABLE 64.2

RISK STRATIFICATION OF PATIENTS WITH HEAD INJURY

Risk category	Characteristics
Mild	Normal neurologic examination
	No concussion
	No drug or alcohol intoxication
	May complain of headache and dizziness
	May have scalp abrasion, laceration, or hematoma
	Absence of moderate or severe injury criteria
Moderate	Glasgow coma score of 9–14 (confused, lethargic, stuporous)
	Concussion
	Posttraumatic amnesia
	Vomiting
	Seizure
	Signs of possible basilar or depressed skull fracture or serious facial injury
	Alcohol or drug intoxication
	Unreliable or no history of injury
	Age <2 years, >65 years
Severe	Glasgow coma score of 3–8 (comatose)
	Progressive decline in level of consciousness ("talked and deteriorated")
	Focal neurologic signs
	Penetrating skull injury or palpable depressed skull fracture

Adapted from Masters SJ, McClean PM, Arcanese MS, et al. 1987.

Imaging: see below.

Coma or clinical signs of herniation: emergency measures to reduce intracranial pressure (ICP; Table 64.5).

DIAGNOSIS

HISTORY

Trauma, loss of consciousness, previous medical problems; alcohol, drug use.

EXAMINATION

Quick assessment on arrival, more detailed examination after stabilization. Palpate skull for fractures, inspect entire body for trauma, inspect head for bloody or CSF discharges. Evaluate

TABLE 64.3

GLASGOW COMA SCALE

Activity/response	Score[a]
Eye opening	
Spontaneous	4
To voice	3
To pain	2
None	1
Best motor response	
Obeys commands	6
Localizes to pain	5
Withdraws to pain	4
Flexor posturing	3
Extensor posturing	2
None	1
Best verbal response	
Conversant and oriented	5
Conversant and disoriented	4
Inappropriate words	3
Incomprehensible sounds	2
None	1

[a]Total score, sum of the score for each of the three components.
From Teasdale G, Jennett B, 1974.

mental state: especially attention, concentration. Pupils, eye movements, motor functions important.

RADIOGRAPHY AND IMAGING

Imaging: CT, including "soft tissue" windows (acute blood, contusion, edema), "bone" windows (fractures), "blood" windows (subdural hematoma).

All patients except asymptomatic patients in low-risk group (Table 64.2): lateral cervical spine x-ray or CT to rule out unstable fracture before removing cervical collar. CT more sensitive for fractures of upper 3 vertebrae.

MANAGEMENT

Admission to hospital: criteria in Table 64.6. Low-risk and moderate-risk patients (Table 64.2) with GCS score of 15 and normal head CT may be sent home. After severe head injury, admit to ICU to minimize secondary brain injury (e.g., increased ICP).

Surgery: debride wound and fracture, elevate depressed fracture, evacuate hematoma (epidural, subdural, parenchymal).

TABLE 64.4

ESTIMATED MORTALITY BASED ON VARIOUS FEATURES OF HEAD INJURY

	Mortality (%)
Glasgow Coma Scale score	
15	<1
11–14	3
8–10	15
6–7	20
4–5	50
3	80
Age, among comatose patients	
16–35	30
36–45	40
46–55	50
≥56	80
CT abnormalities, among comatose patients	
None	10
Intracranial pathology without diffuse swelling or midline shift	15
Intrcranial pathology with diffuse swelling (cisterns compressed or absent)	35
Intracranial pathology with midline shift (>5 mm)	55
Intracranial pressure, among comatose patients	
<20 mm Hg	15
>20 mm Hg, reducible	45
>20 mm Hg, not reducible	90
Pathologic entity	
Epidural hematoma	5–15
Gunshot wound	55
Acute subdural hematoma	
Simple	20–25
Complicated	40–75
Bilateral	75–100

Percentages are adapted from several sources and have been rounded.
From Greenberg J, Brawanaki A. Cranial trauma. In: Hacke W, *Neurocritical care*. New York: Springer-Verlag; 1994:705; Vollmer DG, Torner JC, Jane LA, et al. *J Neurosurg* 1991;75 (Suppl 1):S37–S49; Marshall LF, Gautille T, Klauber MR, et al. *J Neurosurg* 1991;75 (Suppl 1):S28–S36; Miller JD, Becker DP, Ward JD, et al. *J Neurosurg* 1977;47:503–516.

TABLE 64.5

EMERGENCY MEASURES FOR ICP REDUCTION IN AN UNMONITORED PATIENT WITH CLINICAL SIGNS OF HERNIATION

1. Elevate head of bed 15–30 degrees
2. Normal saline (0.9%) at 80–100 mL/hr (avoid hypotonic fluids)
3. Intubate and hyperventilate (target $P_{CO_2} = 28$–32 mm Hg)
4. Mannitol 20% 1–1.5 g/kg via rapid i.v. infusion
5. Foley catheter
6. Neurosurgical consultation

ICP, intracranial pressure.

ICU MANAGEMENT

Indicated for severely head-injured patients.

ICP management: ICP monitor for all comatose head-injured patients (GCS score <8). Cerebral perfusion pressure (CPP) = blood pressure – ICP. Goals: ICP <20 mm Hg, CPP >70 mm Hg (Table 64.7). Mannitol, hyperventilation only after sedation and CPP management fail to reduce ICP to normal. Hypertonic saline may be considered instead of mannitol if patient is hypotensive. High-dose barbiturate therapy with pentobarbital ("pentobarbital coma") if previous steps fail. Hypothermia may be considered if ICP elevation is refractory to pentobarbital. Mortality after head injury with increased ICP refractory to pentobarbital: over 90%.

Seizure control: nonconvulsive seizures and status epilepticus occur in 10% of comatose patients with TBI; associated with poor outcome. Detectable only with continuous EEG monitoring. Generally warrant aggressive treatment.

TABLE 64.6

CRITERIA FOR HOSPITAL ADMISSION AFTER HEAD INJURY

- Intracranial blood or fracture identified on head CT
- Confusion, agitation, or depressed level of consciousness
- Focal neurologic signs or symptoms
- Posttraumatic seizure
- Alcohol or drug intoxication
- Significant comorbid medical illness
- Lack of a reliable home environment for observation

TABLE 64.7

STEPWISE TREATMENT PROTOCOL FOR ELEVATED ICP (>20 mm Hg FOR MORE THAN 10 MIN) IN A MONITORED PATIENT

1. Consider repeat CT and surgical removal of an intracranial mass lesion or ventricular drainage.
2. I.V. sedation to attain a motionless quiet state.
3. Pressor infusion if CPP <70 mm Hg, or reduction of blood pressure if CPP remains >120 mm Hg.
4. Mannitol 0.25–1 g/kg I.V. every 2–6 h as needed.
5. Hyperventilation to Pco_2 levels of 28–32 mm Hg.
6. High-dose pentobarbital therapy (load with 5–20 mg/kg, maintain with 1–4 mg/k/h).
7. Systemic hypothermia (T $\leq 33°C$).

CPP, cerebral perfusion pressure.

Fluids, nutrition: Negative fluid balance associated with poor outcome. Early enteral feeding (day 1) associated with improved outcome.

Other goals: serial neurologic evaluation; management of airway, ventilation, blood pressure; sedation; temperature control (fever exacerbates TBI); nimodipine for subarachnoid hemorrhage.

ACUTE COMPLICATIONS OF HEAD INJURY

CSF fistula: 3% of patients with closed head injury, 5% to 10% of those with basilar skull fracture. Prophylactic antibiotics often used for dural leaks.

Pneumocephalus (air in intracranial cavity): usually asymptomatic, resorbs spontaneously.

Carotid-cavernous fistula: pulsating exophthalmos, ocular chemosis, orbital bruit. Laceration of internal carotid artery in cavernous sinus. Treat with: endovascular balloon.

Vascular injury and thrombosis: (a) dissection of extracranial or intracranial internal carotid or vertebral arteries, ischemic stroke from distal thromboembolism; (b) thrombosis of adjacent dural sinus; (c) cerebral infarction from compression of ipsilateral anterior cerebral artery against falx, or contralateral posterior cerebral artery against tentorium.

Cranial nerve injury: frequent complication of skull base fracture, especially facial nerve (see Chapter 68).

Infections: extradural (osteomyelitis), subdural (empyema), subarachnoid (meningitis), intracerebral (abscess). See Chapters 22, 23.

OUTCOME

Depth of coma (GCS score), CT findings, age predictive of late outcome (Table 64.4). In Traumatic Coma Data Bank (746 patients), 33% died, 14% became vegetative, 28% remained dependent with severe disability, 18% regained independence with moderate disability; only 7% made full or near-complete recovery.

About 50% of adults and 60% of children comatose for 30 days recover consciousness within 1 year (vs. 15% of patients in coma from non-traumatic causes).

Common permanent sequelae: impaired memory, attention, concentration; slow psychomotor functions; personality change; motor deficits.

In patients with moderate or severe injuries, only 46% working 2 years later; only 18% financially independent.

POST-CONCUSSION SYNDROME

Persistent headache, dizziness, fatigue, insomnia, irritability, restlessness, inability to concentrate.

Depression occurs in about 40% of patients with minor or severe head injury.

Prognosis uncertain. May last days to years. Treatment: psychotherapy, cognitive and occupational therapy, vocational rehabilitation, antidepressant or anti-anxiety drugs.

SEIZURES AND POST-TRAUMATIC EPILEPSY

Immediate seizures (within 24 hours): rare but risk factor for further early, not late, seizures.

Early seizures (first week): 3% to 6% of patients with head injury admitted to hospital. Risk factor for late seizures.

Late seizures (after first week; post-traumatic epilepsy): 5% after closed head injury; 30% with intracranial hemorrhage or depressed skull fracture; 50% of patients with early seizures. Therapy discussed in Chapter 141.

PEDIATRIC TRAUMA

Brain injury most common cause of pediatric traumatic death.

BIRTH INJURIES

Common lesions: skull fractures, subarachnoid hemorrhage, hematoma (epidural, subdural, intracerebral). Surgical evacuation of hematoma sometimes used.

LEPTOMENINGEAL CYSTS

Rare complication of head injury, most common under age 2 years. Cyst between pia and arachnoid, typically with dural tear. Treatment: excision of cyst and repair of dural defect.

CHILD ABUSE

Frequent features: delay in seeking medical care; history of multiple previous injuries; incomplete or inconsistent history; bruises or injuries in unusual locations (between shoulder blades, circumferentially around arm, behind legs). Skeletal survey may reveal multiple healed fractures. See also Chapter 168.

Shaken baby syndrome: retinal hemorrhages, subdural hematoma frequent. MRI may show intracranial lesions of varying age.

NEUROLOGY OF PROFESSIONAL BOXING

Chronic traumatic encephalopathy (previously also referred to as dementia pugilistica) is highly prevalent among boxers, who achieve points and victory based on infliction of repeated head trauma, with or without concussion (knock-out). Syndrome may include parkinsonism, dementia, seizures.

CHAPTER 65 ■ SPINAL INJURY

EPIDEMIOLOGY

Annual incidence of spinal injury: 15 to 50/1,000,000. Prevalence about 900/1,000,000.

Mortality >50% at scene of accident; about 13% at one year for those who survive acute hospital care.

Peak incidence at age 20 to 24 years, during summers and weekends. M:F ratio 4:1.

Most common level of injury C5, followed by C4 and C6.

ETIOLOGY

Most common causes: road accidents (48%), falls (21%; especially in elderly), sports (13%), industrial (12%), violence (16%).

MECHANISM OF INJURY

Most common: indirect force to vertebral column (e.g., sudden flexion, hyperextension, vertebral compression or rotation of vertebral column).

Secondary injury: ongoing injury after initial insult. May continue for years. Mechanism poorly understood.

PATHOLOGY

Hyperemia, edema, inflammatory exudate within first few hours. Resolves in weeks or months. Hemorrhage may occur (hematomyelia).

Cavity (syringomyelia) or area of tissue softening (myelomalacia) may form in months, with slowly progressive neurologic deterioration.

NEUROLOGIC ASSESSMENT AND CLASSIFICATION

ASIA/IMSOP Impairment Scale
Published by the American Spinal Injury Association (ASIA) and International Medical Society of Paraplegia (IMSOP).

A. **Complete:** No motor or sensory function in sacral segments S4/S5.

B. **Incomplete:** Sensory but not motor function preserved below level, extending through sacral segments S4/S5.

C. **Incomplete:** Motor function preserved below neurologic level; key muscles below level have power grade <3.

D. **Incomplete:** Motor function preserved below neurologic level; key muscles have power grade >3.

E. **Normal:** Motor and sensory function normal.

CLINICAL PATTERNS

Cauda equina lesions: flaccid, areflexic paralysis, sensory loss in area of affected roots, paralysis of bladder and rectum.

Conus medullaris lesions: urinary and fecal incontinence, failure of erection and ejaculation, paralysis of pelvic floor muscles, sensory impairment (frequently dissociated in saddle region). Tendon reflexes frequently preserved.

Mixed cauda-conus lesions: both frequently injured together.

Spinal cord concussion: transient neurologic symptoms below level of blow, recovery in minutes or hours.

Spinal shock: after abrupt lesion of cord. Immediately, complete paralysis and anesthesia below lesion, hypotonia, areflexia. Plantar responses inconsistent. Hyperreflexia and spasticity supervene in 3 to 4 weeks.

Complete cord transection: permanent motor, sensory, autonomic paralysis below lesion.

Brown-Séquard syndrome (cord hemisection): Ipsilateral paresis, ipsilateral corticospinal signs, contralateral loss of pain and temperature sensation, ipsilateral impairment of vibration and joint position sense.

Central cervical cord syndrome: weakness (arms > legs), urinary retention, patchy sensory loss below lesion. Pain and temperature sensation more affected than vibration or proprioception.

Anterior cord syndrome: immediate complete paralysis, mild-to-moderate impairment of pinprick and light touch below injury; position, vibration preserved.

Posterior cord syndrome: Pain and paresthesias in neck, upper arms, trunk.

Spinal cord concussion: transient neurologic symptoms with recovery in minutes or hours.

Spinal shock: seen after abrupt injury to spinal cord. Complete paralysis, anesthesia below level of lesion, with hypotonia, areflexia, potentially life-threatening autonomic disturbances. Plantar response may be extensor, flexor, or absent. After 3 to 4 weeks, syndrome pyramidal signs appear.

COMMON LEVELS OF INJURY

Clinical patterns in Chapter 63 (Table 63.2).

DIAGNOSIS

Lateral x-rays of the cervical spine encompassing the lower cervical region are mandatory.

CT to evaluate uncertain findings on plain films; also detect bone pathology.

MRI for soft tissue imaging.

Neurophysiology: sensory and motor evoked responses.

COURSE AND PROGNOSIS

Factors affecting long-term survival include level and extent of lesion, age, availability of special treatment by multidisciplinary personnel.

Mortality higher for cervical injury. Causes of death in chronic phase include pneumonia, cardiac dysfunction, septicemia, pulmonary emboli, suicide, accidents.

TREATMENT

Before hospital: blood pressure support, oxygen, spine immobilization, communication with physicians at trauma center.

Emergency management within 8 hours of injury: methylprednisolone (before imaging studies; bolus injection of 30 mg/kg, then 5.4 mg/kg/h for 23 hours); control blood pressure, body temperature; intermittent catheterization.

Immediate surgery for cord compression, selected cases of unstable spine injury.

Correct misalignment or instability of spine: external skeletal traction (cervical fracture-dislocation) or surgical stabilization (Harrington rods).

Long-term care and rehabilitation to maximize functional recovery and minimize complication rate.

COMPLICATIONS

Dysautonomia: peak occurrence in first few days. Sudden tachycardia and hypertension may be triggered by pain, fecal impaction, abdominal distension, voiding. Attention to bowel, bladder function therefore important.

Pulmonary dysfunction: a leading cause of morbidity and mortality, especially with cervical lesions. Focus on prevention of atelectasis, aspiration, deep vein thrombosis, pulmonary embolism.

Bladder: intermittent catheterization superior to indwelling catheters in reducing complications and developing bladder training. Cystitis, pyelitis respond to antibiotics.

Bowel training: laxatives, digital removal of feces for first few weeks. Laxatives, glycerin suppositories for bowel training.

Pressure sores: eliminate pressure points by padding, frequent change of position, keep bed scrupulously clean. Use sheepskin, alternating pressure mattresses.

Nutritional deficiency: diet high in protein, calories, vitamins.

Muscle spasms: baclofen (oral or intrathecal), diazepam, dantrolene, injections of botulinum toxin.

Sexual dysfunction: for men, consider sildenafil (Viagra), vacuum device, injection of vasoactive agents into corpora cavernosa, implantable prosthesis. Women: dysfunction also present, but treatment little investigated.

Pain: treatments include spinal anesthesia, posterior rhizotomy, sympathectomy, cordotomy, posterior column tractotomy, transcutaneous electrical stimulation. Narcotic analgesics avoided.

REHABILITATION

Multidisciplinary approach, including physical, occupational, and psychological therapy, can be critical in maximizing maintenance of preserved function, and in enabling adaptive/compensatory strategies to regain function in the face of fixed deficits.

CHAPTER 66 ■ INTERVERTEBRAL DISCS AND RADICULOPATHY

PATHOGENESIS

Displaced disc material bulges beneath annulus fibrosus or extrudes through tear in annulus, projecting directly into spinal canal (herniated disc). Compresses nerve roots, spinal cord, or both (cord involved only in cervical or thoracic region).

Most commonly affected: C5 to C7 segments in cervical region; L4 to L5 and L5 to S1 in lumbar region (Table 66.1).

Causes of disc herniation: trauma, genetic predisposition. Nerve compression also with spinal stenosis, spondylosis, osteoarthritis.

INCIDENCE

Ruptured intervertebral disc common: peak in fourth to sixth decades; rare before age 25 or after 60. Eighty percent men.

LUMBAR INTERVERTEBRAL DISC RUPTURE

Pain: limited to back or in root distribution; episodic; aggravated by Valsalva maneuvers (sneezing, coughing, straining at stool), heavy lifting, bending or twisting spine; relieved by lying down, worse on standing. Paresthesias in radicular distribution. Typical syndromes in Table 66.1.

Examination: loss of lumbar lordosis, splinting (spine tilted), reduced motion of spine (cannot bend forward to touch toes). Local vertebrae tender. Passive straight-leg raising increases pain.

THORACIC DISC RUPTURE

Rare because mobility limited in thoracic spine; usually with Scheuermann disease or juvenile osteochondritis.

CERVICAL DISC DISEASE

Cervical disc herniation may result in radiculopathy or cord compression. Most frequent sites: C5 to C6, C6 to C7.

TABLE 66.1

COMMON ROOT SYNDROMES OF INTERVERTEBRAL DISC DISEASE

Disc space	L3-4	L4-5	L5-S1	C4-5	C5-6	C6-7	C7-T1
Root affected	L-4	L-5	S-1	C-5	C-6	C-7	C-8
Muscles affected	Quadriceps	Peroneals, anterior tibial, extensor hallucis longus	Gluteus maximus, gastrocnemius, plantar flexors of toes	Deltoid, biceps		Triceps, wrist extensors	Intrinsic hand muscles
Area of pain and sensory loss	Anterior thigh, medial shin	Great toe, dorsum of foot	Lateral foot, small toe	Shoulder, anterior arm, radial forearm		Thumb, middle fingers	Index, fourth, fifth finger
Reflex affected	Knee jerk	Posterior tibial	Ankle jerk	Biceps		Triceps	Triceps
Straight leg raising	May not increase pain	Aggravates root pain	Aggravates root pain	—		—	—

278

Signs and symptoms: stiff neck; discomfort at medial border of scapula. Radicular paresthesias and pain. Worse with movement of neck. Discrete root syndromes (Table 66.1).

EVALUATION

Plain radiographs: abnormal skeletal features (genetic syndromes), degenerative disorders of bone.

MRI: imaging modality of choice. Identifies cord or root compression.

EMG, evoked potential studies: not essential, may help.

DIFFERENTIAL DIAGNOSIS

Tumor (primary or metastatic), infection (e.g., epidural abscess), arachnoiditis.

TREATMENT

Conservative treatment as long as patient improves: analgesics, bed rest for lumbar disc disorders; neck immobilization by collar for cervical disc syndrome. Epidural steroid injections sometimes used but controlled trials needed.

Surgery for Lumbar Disc Disorder

Indications: (a) unable to walk after weeks of activity as tolerated; (b) severe neurologic disorder on examination.

Most common procedure: excision of herniated disc fragment.

Surgery for Cervical Disc Disorder

Acute cord compression may be indication for immediate surgery.

Root syndromes: C5, C8 root involvement a greater indication for surgery than C6, C7.

Chronic Low Back Pain

Among the most common causes pain and lost productivity in adults. Multidisciplinary spine or pain center may be most effective management.

CHAPTER 67 ■ CERVICAL SPONDYLOTIC MYELOPATHY

Cord damage from compression by degenerated intervertebral discs, proliferation of surrounding bone, meninges, supporting tissues of spine.

INCIDENCE

Radiographic evidence of cervical spondylosis increases in each decade: 5% to 10% ages 20 to 30; >50% by age 45; >90% after age 60, but symptomatic myelopathy rare.

PATHOPHYSIOLOGY

Narrow spinal canal from: loss of water from intervertebral disc; degenerative changes in disc; protrusion of annulus fibrosus and osteophytes (spondylotic bars) into spinal canal.

Rare syndrome: ossification of posterior longitudinal ligament.

SYMPTOMS AND SIGNS

Most common: neck pain, spastic gait disorder, hyperreflexia, Babinski sign.
Uncommon: root pain, weakness and wasting of hands, fasciculations, urinary sphincter symptoms; involvement of anterior horn cells rare, if ever.

Slowly progressive, sometimes with stable periods or improvement; natural history not clear.

INVESTIGATIONS

Plain radiographs: narrow disc spaces; osteophytes, especially at C5 to C6, C6 to C7.
MRI: disc degeneration; protruded bars into spinal canal; cord compression, distortion. CT myelography: if MRI not available.

DIFFERENTIAL DIAGNOSIS

(a) Cord compression by other causes: e.g., foramen magnum tumor, Chiari malformation. (b) Myelopathy from MS, ALS, tropical spastic paraparesis, adrenoleukodystrophy, primary lateral sclerosis.

Spondylosis on imaging most often asymptomatic.

TREATMENT

Natural history variable. Indications for surgery and procedure of choice not clearly established.

Decompressive surgery (posterior laminectomy, anterior discectomy, corpectomy) widely used, with improvement reported in 50% to 100%.

Conservative treatment: physical therapy; gait training; neck immobilization by firm collar for mild myelopathy.

Surgery if myelopathy clearly progressive.

CHAPTER 68 ■ LUMBAR SPONDYLOSIS

Age-related degeneration leads to disc bulging and bony spurs, narrowing spinal canal (spinal stenosis); usually confined to one or two lumbar levels, most commonly L4 to L5.

Most patients older than 40; many older than 60. Gradual progression. Back pain often not dominant. Leg pain may be bilateral or unilateral.

Characteristic symptom: unilateral or bilateral discomfort in buttock, thigh, or leg on walking, relieved by rest ("spinal claudication"). Also relieved by flexing forward at waist, or by lying down or sitting. In more common vascular claudication, pain relieved if patient stops walking without flexing spine. Spinal problem also suggested if discomfort brought on by prolonged standing without walking.

Most common findings: weakness of isolated muscles and loss of tendon reflexes. Straight-leg raising often not limited.

Diagnosis: characteristic history, signs, MRI.

Differential diagnosis: (a) peripheral arterial occlusive disease, shows loss of pulses, trophic skin changes, nonradicular pain; (b) osteoarthritis of hip accompanied by pain and limitation of hip rotation, no pain below knee.

Treatment: (a) mild symptoms: nonsteroidal anti-inflammatory drugs, physical therapy; (b) if no medical contraindication, consider surgery for pain and claudication severe enough to impair quality of life without response to conservative therapy.

CHAPTER 69 ■ CRANIAL AND PERIPHERAL NERVE LESIONS

GENERAL PRINCIPLES OF NERVE INJURY

Injury to single nerve (mononeuropathy): most commonly follows trauma. Toxic or metabolic disorders affect many nerves (mononeuropathy multiplex or symmetric polyneuropathy).

PATHOPHYSIOLOGY

Three major types of injury. (1) nerve transection (*neurotmesis*); (2) axonal interruption with distal degeneration but preserved endoneurium (*axonotmesis*); (3) mild ischemic compressive injury resulting in conduction block at site of lesion but without axonal or endoneurial disruption, without degeneration of distal axons (*neurapraxia*).

CLINICAL FEATURES

Motor nerves: flaccid paralysis, wasting of muscles innervated by affected nerve.
Sensory nerves: loss of sensation in distribution of nerve.

Partial injury may cause stabbing pain, pins-and-needles sensation (paresthesias), severe burning pain (causalgia).

Vasomotor disorders, "trophic disturbances" (changes in skin, mucous membranes, bones, nails) more common with injury of sensory or mixed nerves than motor. See also complex regional pain syndrome (reflex sympathetic dystrophy), Chapter 71.

DIAGNOSIS

Distribution of motor and sensory abnormalities (described later in chapter).

Differentiation from spinal root lesions, where weakness, sensory loss segmental, not in nerve distribution.

EMG shows patterns of denervation and reinnervation. Nerve conduction studies ascertain site of injury.

PROGNOSIS

Probability of regeneration lower for injuries near CNS or more severe axonal injury.

TREATMENT

Surgical repair (selected injuries); rehabilitation.

CRANIAL NEUROPATHIES

OLFACTORY NERVE AND TRACT

Lesions of nerve: loss of sense of smell, taste. Injury to CNS connections: often no loss of smell or taste. Temporal lobe lesions, seizures: transient olfactory hallucinations.

Most common cause: head trauma. Usually permanent.

OPTIC NERVE AND TRACT

Manifestations: loss of vision, impaired pupillary light reflexes, abnormal size of pupil (Table 69.1).

Causes: direct trauma, toxins, systemic diseases (e.g., diabetes mellitus, giant cell arteritis), demyelinating; heritable diseases, local conditions (e.g., glaucoma, retinal vein thrombosis), infiltration or compression of nerve, increased intracranial pressure. See also Chapter 7.

Optic neuritis: impaired visual acuity; caused by inflammatory, degenerative, demyelinating, toxic disorders.

Bedside Examination

Visual fields by confrontation. Hemianopia, quadrantanopia: retrochiasmatic lesion.

Visual acuity: optic nerve dysfunction. Also see reduced perception of color saturation (test with small red object).

Blind spot enlargement (test by confrontation): papilledema (e.g., increased intracranial pressure).

Pupil size. Contracted: pontine lesion, sympathetic dysfunction, opiate overdose. Dilated: parasympathetic dysfunction (including lesions in oculomotor nerve).

Pupil reactivity. Failure of one pupil to constrict when light is shone into either eye: parasympathetic dysfunction (e.g., oculomotor nerve compression). Failure of one pupil to constrict when light is shone into the same eye, with intact constriction when light is shown into the other eye (relative afferent pupillary defect): optic nerve (e.g., optic neuritis); see also Chapter 7. Failure to dilate when room is darkened: sympathetic dysfunction (e.g., Horner's syndrome).

Pain on eye movements: optic neuritis.

Convergence, accommodation: abnormal in neurosyphilis, compression of dorsal midbrain (Parinaud syndrome; see Chapter 58).

OCULOMOTOR, TROCHLEAR, ABDUCENS NERVES

Manifestations: diplopia, deviated eye, impaired ocular movement. See also Chapter 7.

Causes: head trauma, tumors or aneurysms at skull base, brainstem stroke, venous sinus thrombosis (e.g., cavernous sinus thrombosis), neurosyphilis, neurosarcoidosis, MS, meningitis, encephalitis, diphtheria, diabetes mellitus, lead poisoning, botulism, Wernicke encephalitis, skull osteomyelitis,

TABLE 69.1

EFFECTS OF LESIONS OF THE OPTIC, OCULOMOTOR, AND SYMPATHETIC PATHWAYS ON THE PUPILS

Site of lesion on right side	Size of pupil		Reaction of ipsilateral pupil to stimulation by light directed into		Consensual reaction of contralateral pupil to stimulation by light directed into		Accommodation-convergence reaction
	Right	Left	Right	Left	Right	Left	
Retina	Normal	Normal	Impaired	Normal	Impaired	Normal	Normal
Optic nerve	Normal	Normal	Lost	Normal	Lost	Normal	Normal
Optic chiasm	Normal	Normal	Normal[a]	Normal[a]	Normal[a]	Normal[a]	Normal
Optic tract	Normal	Normal	Normal[a]	Normal[a]	Normal[a]	Normal[a]	Normal
Optic radiation	Normal	Normal	Normal	Normal	Normal	Normal	Normal
Periaqueductal region[b]	Contracted	Normal	Lost	Normal	Normal	Lost	Normal
Oculomotor nuclear complex or nerve	Dilated	Normal	Lost	Normal	Normal	Lost	Lost on right
Sympathetic pathways	Contracted	Normal	Normal	Normal	Normal	Normal	Normal

[a] No reaction of the pupils if the beam of light is focused sharply on the amblyopic portions of the retina.
[b] Argyll Robertson pupil.

spinal anesthesia, lumbar puncture, increased intracranial pressure.

Third nerve or nucleus: paralysis of medial rectus, superior rectus, inferior rectus, inferior oblique, levator palpebrae superior; paralysis of constrictor ciliary muscles. Ptosis, eye deviated outward; pupil dilated, no reaction to light or accommodation.

Fourth nerve or nucleus: paralysis of superior oblique muscle, impaired ability to turn eye down and in. Diplopia ameliorated by tilting head forward and toward normal eye.

Sixth nerve: paralysis of lateral rectus. Eye deviated inward. Diplopia in all gaze directions.

Sixth nerve nucleus: paralysis of lateral gaze to affected side; neither eye moves beyond midline. Convergence preserved.

Tolosa-Hunt syndrome: painful ophthalmoplegia with MRI evidence of intracavernous inflammation.

FIFTH (TRIGEMINAL) NERVE

Manifestations: paralysis of muscles of mastication with deviation of jaw to side of lesion; loss of sensation for touch, temperature, pain in face; loss of corneal, sneezing reflexes.

Causes: trauma, tumor, aneurysm, meningeal infection, brainstem lesions.

Trigeminal neuralgia ("tic douloureux"): recurrent paroxysms of sharp stabbing pain, distribution of one or more branches of fifth nerve. Rare before age 35. Characteristic feature: trigger zone where stimulation sets off paroxysm of pain. Examination findings normal. Treatment: carbamazepine, baclofen, phenytoin, surgery (microvascular decompression, gangliolysis using stereotactic techniques, rhizotomy).

Atypical facial pain: longer paroxysms of steady dull, aching, crushing, or burning trigeminal pain. Paroxysms always last longer than a few seconds. Often accompanied by depression. Surgical treatment not effective.

SEVENTH (FACIAL) NERVE

Manifestations: paralysis of facial muscles (motor root) with or without loss of taste on anterior two thirds of the tongue or altered secretion of lacrimal and salivary glands (nervus intermedius).

Lesions near origin or near geniculate ganglion: loss of motor, gustatory, autonomic functions. Between geniculate ganglion and origin of chorda tympani: lacrimal secretion not affected. Near stylomastoid foramen: facial paralysis only. Lesions of nucleus: additional associated brainstem findings.

Causes: stab and gunshot wounds, cuts, birth trauma, skull fracture, tumor, aneurysm, meningeal infection, leukemia, osteomyelitis, herpes zoster, Paget disease, bone tumor, sarcoidosis.

Bilateral facial palsy: sarcoidosis, GBS, HIV infection, leprosy, leukemia. Treatment: surgery (anastomosis of 7th cranial nerve with 11th or 12th cranial nerve).

Bell palsy: idiopathic seventh nerve paralysis, followed by partial or full recovery. Frequently treated with steroids and acyclovir, but not formally proven to help.

Blepharospasm: forceful closure of eye in dystonia, hemifacial spasm, parkinsonism. Treatment: botulinum toxin.

Facial myokymia: fine rippling movements of facial muscles. EMG: discharges of rapidly firing motor units in singlets, multiplets, bursts. Seen in MS, brainstem glioma, GBS.

Hemifacial spasm: clonic spasms of facial muscles, usually starting around eye, spreading to other muscles on one side of face. EMG: bursts of muscle action potentials appear regularly or irregularly at 5 to 20 per second. Treatment: carbamazepine, phenytoin, botulinum toxin, surgical decompression of facial nerve.

EIGHTH (ACOUSTIC) NERVE

See Chapter 6.

NINTH (GLOSSOPHARYNGEAL) NERVE

Manifestations: loss of taste on posterior third of tongue; loss of gag reflex on side of lesion. Isolated lesions rare.

Glossopharyngeal neuralgia (tic douloureux of 9th nerve): idiopathic paroxysms of excruciating burning or stabbing pain in region of tonsils, posterior pharynx, back of tongue, middle ear. Often precipitated by swallowing, talking, or touching tonsils or posterior pharynx. Treatment: carbamazepine, alone or with phenytoin; surgical section of nerve.

TENTH (VAGUS) NERVE

Manifestations: *Nucleus ambiguus* lesion: dysarthria, dysphagia. *Dorsal motor nucleus* lesion: asymptomatic (unilateral lesion); severe autonomic dysfunction (bilateral lesion). Pharyngeal branch lesion: dysphagia. Recurrent laryngeal nerve lesion: hoarseness (unilateral lesion); aphonia, inspiratory stridor (bilateral lesion).
Causes: ALS, intramedullary tumor, stroke.
Spasmodic dysphonia: involuntary vocal cord spasm. Cause uncertain. Treatment: botulinum toxin.

ELEVENTH (SPINAL ACCESSORY) NERVE

Spinal portion lesions: weakness, atrophy of trapezius; impaired contralateral head rotation, ipsilateral shoulder shrug; scapular winging (present at rest, worsened by shoulder abduction).

Nerve susceptible to damage during lymph node biopsy, cannulation of internal jugular vein, carotid endarterectomy.

TWELFTH (HYPOGLOSSAL) NERVE

Nucleus or nerve lesion: atrophy, paralysis of muscles of ipsilateral half of tongue, which deviates to paralyzed side when protruded; fibrillations seen in chronic disease of nucleus (ALS, syringobulbia).
Bilateral nucleus or nerve lesion: bilateral tongue atrophy, paralysis of all movement; severe dysarthria, dysphagia.

PERIPHERAL NERVES

Causes of injury: pressure (radial, common peroneal, ulnar, long thoracic nerves), constriction by bands of fascia (median), reaction to injection of serum (axillary), trauma associated with injection of drugs (sciatic); also perforating wounds, bone fractures, stretching of nerves (all nerves).

NERVES OF THE ARM

See Table 69.2.

TABLE 69.2
NERVES OF THE ARM AND PATTERNS OF INJURY

Nerve	Roots	Muscles	Injury	Weak muscles or impaired action	Lost reflexes	Sensory loss
Radial	C5–8	Brachioradialis; supinator; extensors of forearm, wrist, fingers	Mid-arm	Flexion of pronated forearm; extensors of wrist, thumb, proximal fingers; hand adduction; forearm supination (with forearm extended)	Brachioradialis	Posterior radial surface of hand; first and second metacarpals of digits 1–3
			Axilla	As above, plus triceps	As above, plus triceps	
Median	C6–T1	Pronator teres; flexors of wrist, digits 1–3; opponens pollicis	Transverse carpal segment	Forearm pronation; thenar muscles; index flexion; thumb opposition	—	Radial side of palm, volar surface of digits 1–3, radial half of ring finger, distal digits 1–3
Ulnar	C8–T1	Flexor carpi ulnaris, flexor digitorum profundus (digits 4–5), palmaris brevis, abductor digiti minimi, opponens digiti minimi, flexor digiti minimi, all interossei, lumbricals (digits 3–4), flexor pollicis brevis	Elbow	Flexion, adduction of wrist, ring, and little fingers; abduction, opposition of little finger; thumb adduction; adduction, abduction of digits 2–5	—	Palmar, dorsal surfaces of little finger; inner half of ring finger; ulnar side of hand

(continued)

289

TABLE 69.2
NERVES OF THE ARM AND PATTERNS OF INJURY (Continued)

Nerve	Roots	Muscles	Injury	Weak muscles or impaired action	Lost reflexes	Sensory loss
Musculocut-aneous	C5–6	Coracobrachialis, biceps, brachialis	Brachial plexus region	Flexion of supine forearm; forearm supination	Biceps	Anterior outer forearm, posterior outer forearm
Axillary	C5–6	Deltoid	Head of humerus	Outward, backward, forward arm movements	—	Small area on lateral shoulder
Long thoracic	C5–7	Serratus anterior	Shoulder	Arm elevation above horizontal plane; scapular winging with arm fully abducted or anteriorly elevated (vs. cranial nerve XI lesion)	—	
Supra-scapular	C5–6	Shoulder abduction, external rotation	Serum reaction, trauma	Weakness masked by deltoid, teres minor	—	

	Roots/trunk	Muscles	Movements affected	Reflex loss	Sensory loss
Upper BP	C4–6 or upper trunk	Deltoid, biceps, brachialis anticus, brachioradialis, pectoralis major, supraspinatus, infraspinatus, subscapularis, teres major, serratus magnus, rhomboids, levator anguli scapulae	Forearm flexion; arm abduction, internal rotation, external rotation; scapula apposition; backward-inward arm movements	Variable loss of biceps, triceps jerk	Outer surface of arm and forearm
Middle BP	C7 or middle trunk	Radial nerve muscles except brachioradialis	As in radial nerve injury, except for sparing of forearm flexion	Triceps	Dorsal forearm; external dorsal hand
Lower BP	C8–T1 or lower trunk	Flexor carpi ulnaris, flexor digitorum, interossei, thenar and hypothenar muscles	As in combined median and ulnar nerve lesion (flattened hand)	Triceps	Inner arm and forearm; ulnar hand
Lateral cord of BP		Same as musculocutaneous nerve, plus pronator teres, flexor carpi radialis, flexor pollicis, opponens pollicis	Combined musculocutaneous and lateral head of median nerve	Biceps	
Posterior cord of BP		Same as radial and axillary nerves	Combined radial and axillary nerves	Triceps	
Medial cord		Same as ulnar nerve and medial head of median nerve	Combined ulnar and medial head of median nerve (finger flexion)		

BP, brachial plexus.

TABLE 69.3
NERVES OF LEG AND PATTERNS OF INJURY

Nerve	Roots	Muscles	Injury	Weak muscles or impaired action	Lost reflexes	Sensory loss
Obturator	L2–4	Obturator externus, adductor longus, adductor brevis, gracilis, adductor magnus	Tumor, labor	Thigh adduction; external, internal rotation	—	Small area on inner surface of middle side of hip, thigh, knee
Iliohypo-gastric	T12–L1	Internal oblique, transversalis	Inguinal surgery	No significant motor loss	—	Outer and upper part of buttocks, lower part of abdomen
Lateral cuta-neous	L2–3	—		Sensory nerve, loss of sensation in oval area on lateral surface of thigh (meralgia paresthetica)	—	Superior external buttocks (posterior branch), outer surface of thigh (anterior branch)
Femoral	L2–4	Iliopsoas, pectineus, sartorius, quadriceps femoris	Pelvic tumor, diabetic mononeu-ropathy	Extension of leg, flexion of thigh; impossible to walk up stairs	Patellar	Anterior surface of thigh, entire inner surface of leg, anterior internal surface of knee

Sciatic	L4–S2	Semitendinosus, long and short heads of biceps, adductor magnus, semimembranosus	Gunshot, shrapnel, stab wounds	Complete paralysis of all movements of ankle and toes; weakness or paralysis of flexion of leg	Ankle jerk	Outer surface of leg
Common peroneal	L4–S1	Ankle, toe extensors; foot evertor muscles	Pressure during sleep, surgery	Footdrop with burning pains on lateral aspect of leg and in ankle or foot; steppage gait	—	Outer side of leg, front of its lower third, instep, dorsal surface of 4 inner toes over proximal phalanges
Tibial	L5–S2	Muscles on posterior of leg, plantar muscles		Plantar flexion and adduction of foot, flexion and separation of toes	Ankle jerk, plantar reflex	Sole of foot, back and lower part to middle third of leg to outer dorsal surface of foot and to terminal phalanges of toes

Brachial Plexus

Roots: C5 to C8, T1. Trunks: upper (C5 to C6), middle (C7), lower (C8 to T1).

Cords: lateral (musculocutaneous, lateral head of median nerve), posterior (axillary, radial), medial (brachial and antebrachial cutaneous, ulnar, medial head of median).

Note: long thoracic nerve arises from roots (C5 to C7); suprascapular nerve from upper trunk of brachial plexus.

Injury: cuts, gunshot wounds, direct trauma, compression by tumor or aneurysm, stretching in falls, shoulder dislocation, carrying heavy packs on shoulder ("rucksack paralysis"), traction in delivery at birth.

Neuralgic amyotrophy (brachial plexopathy): unilateral or bilateral disorders of brachial plexus, idiopathic or following respiratory infection, surgery, or systemic disease. Local pain, weakness, atrophy. Improves spontaneously but not always completely.

Ischemic Paralysis of Arm

Initial stage: cyanosis, edema of distal limb. Finger and wrist movements limited. Decreased cutaneous sensation. Later: skin smooth, shiny; fibrosis of muscles; anesthesia glove-like.

Distinguishing features: no radial artery pulse; glove-like sensory loss; fibrous feeling on palpation.

NERVES OF LEG

See Table 69.3.

Sciatica: pain in low back and posterior leg from buttock to foot. Most common cause: ruptured intervertebral disc.

CHAPTER 70 ■ THORACIC OUTLET SYNDROME

Syndromes arising from compression of brachial plexus or blood vessels in that area. Compression attributed to anatomic anomalies (cervical rib, fibrous bands) but evidence scarce.

SYMPTOMS AND SIGNS

Pain in shoulder, arm, hand, or all three locations. Hand pain often primarily in fourth, fifth fingers. Pain aggravated by use of arm. Hypesthesia may be present.

"True" neurogenic syndrome: definite clinical and electro-diagnostic abnormalities; rare. Almost always caused by cervical band extending from cervical rib, compressing C8, T1 roots, or lower brachial plexus.

"Disputed" form: no objective signs, no consistent laboratory abnormalities.

DIAGNOSIS AND MANAGEMENT

Consider arteriography to rule out subclavian artery aneurysm.

Surgery indicated when diagnosis unequivocal. Otherwise physical therapy.

CHAPTER 71 ■ NEUROPATHIC PAIN

Estimated to affect 1% of general population, 10% of people with diabetic neuropathy.

DEFINITIONS

Neurogenic pain: resulting from non-inflammatory dysfunction of peripheral or central nervous system, without peripheral nociceptor stimulation or trauma.

Primary nociceptive pain: process injuring tissue stimulates pain receptors.

NEUROGENIC PAIN SYNDROMES

Deafferentation pain: follows interruption of primary afferent nociceptive pathways; term used most often for syndromes that follow CNS injury.

Neuropathic pain: pain associated with peripheral nervous system injury.

Neuralgia: pain in distribution of single peripheral nerve.

Other syndromes: complex regional pain syndrome (CRPS) type I (formerly reflex sympathetic dystrophy), type II (formerly causalgia); thalamic pain syndrome; trigeminal neuralgia; post-herpetic neuralgia.

ETIOLOGY

Most common cause is diabetes mellitus. Others include Sjögren syndrome, alcohol or drug toxicity, AIDS, hyperlipidemia, amyloidosis, Tangier disease, Fabry disease.

CLINICAL FEATURES

Variable pain quality, including burning, aching, electric, stabbing, lancinating.

Pain may be triggered by ordinarily innocuous stimuli (*allodynia*), e.g., contact with bed sheets. Often accompanied by symptoms of small-fiber neuropathy: loss of pain and temperature sensation, numbness, tingling.

DIAGNOSIS

Tendon reflexes often preserved. Electrophysiologic studies may be normal.

Quantitative sensory testing, skin biopsy for counts of small sensory fibers may be helpful.

TREATMENT

General Principles
Response to treatment highly variable. Refractory symptoms best managed by multidisciplinary team including pain specialist and psychiatrist/psychologist to assist with affective component of symptoms.

PHARMACOLOGIC THERAPY

Anti-inflammatory agents, acetaminophen: neuropathic pain often resistant.

Opioids: unlikely to provide chronic relief, though useful as part of multi-modal regimen in refractory patients.

Tramadol: effective for painful neuropathy in placebo-controlled, double-blind, randomized trial. Start at 50 mg per day, gradually increasing weekly to 150 to 200 mg daily or maximal effective dose, whichever is lower. Benefit may be immediate, but increases for 1 to 2 weeks.

Carbamazepine: effective in two placebo-controlled and one comparative study at doses of 300 to 1000 mg/day.

Gabapentin: proven in placebo-controlled trials for several neuropathic pain syndromes. Initial doses of 300 to 600 mg/day in three divided doses are gradually increased to efficacy over several weeks. Daily doses of 1000 to 2000 mg/day are given for adequate pain control in most patients, but some take up to 3600 mg/day. Peak benefit reached after 1 to 2 weeks.

Amitriptyline: effective in numerous double-blind, placebo-controlled trials; equivalent to gabapentin in comparative studies. Anticholinergic effects often limit use. Typical starting doses are 10 to 25 milligrams at bedtime, gradually increasing every two weeks to effect or maximally tolerated dose (not more than 150 mg/day). Benefit may take 4 to 6 weeks to appear.

Lidocaine patch: may reduce regional pain in severely affected areas such as the soles of the feet. However, it transiently worsens numbness and may increase the likelihood of insensate skin injury, especially in diabetics.

Capsaicin cream: effective, but inconvenient to use, because topical application is required three times per day. Also irritates any mucous membranes it may contact (e.g., eye and mouth, after accidental transfer from the hand during application). Neuropathic pain increases during initial one to two weeks of therapy, before producing relief.

OTHER TREATMENTS

Biofeedback, meditation, physical therapy, regular exercise, constructive activity sometimes helpful as adjuvant components of treatment.

Surgery: no established role in treatment of neuropathic pain. Benefit of rhizotomy, thalamotomy usually transient. Sympathectomy for CRPS-I controversial.

CHAPTER 72 ■ RADIATION INJURY

EARLY (ACUTE) EFFECTS (1 TO 6 WEEKS)

Edema, headache, nausea, vomiting, alopecia; hyperpigmentation, desquamation of skin. Complications in 50% for daily dose fractions of 750 cGy; <200 cGy seldom toxic.

MRI: localized swelling of spinal cord or plexus without enhancement. Steroids given prophylactically.

Tissues with fastest turnover rate (skin, bone marrow) affected most often.

EARLY-DELAYED SYNDROMES (WITHIN 6 MONTHS)

Somnolence, headache in children receiving prophylactic whole-brain radiotherapy. Also irritability, anorexia. Focal signs uncommon. Spontaneous recovery.

Ataxia, dysarthria, nystagmus: irradiation to middle ear area for glomus jugulare tumors.

Severe leukoencephalopathy.

Early-delayed radiation myelopathy: Lhermitte sign (sensation of electrical current radiating down back induced by flexing neck).

LATE-DELAYED SYNDROMES (MONTHS TO YEARS)

Radiation Necrosis

About 5% of patients given total doses >5,000 cGy with daily fraction sizes >200 cGy. Median time for symptom onset: 14 months after end of radiotherapy.

Clinical manifestations may simulate those of original tumor.

Imaging: (a) mass lesion at original tumor site or within irradiation path; enhancement mimics original neoplasm, gradually resolving; (b) diffuse white matter changes (hypodensity on CT, increased signal on T2-weighted MRI); usually irreversible.

Distinguishing tumor recurrence from radiation necrosis may be difficult. Radiation necrosis may show hypometabolic areas on PET. Biopsy often needed for diagnosis.

Treatment: steroid therapy or surgical resection. Radiation necrosis rarely progressive, fatal.

Radiation Myelopathy

Delayed injury to spinal cord. One to 3 years after radiotherapy, with one peak at 12 to 14 months and another at 24 to 28 months. Average latency 12 months.

True incidence not known.

Clinical syndrome: painless subacute numbness and paresthesias, spastic gait, sphincter symptoms, limb weakness.

MRI normal or shows cord swelling, atrophy, subarachnoid block, with or without enhancement.

No effective treatment. Steroids may improve symptoms transiently.

Radiation-Induced Vasculopathy

Either intracranial or extracranial circulation affected. Usually follows neck irradiation. Latent period up to 23 years.

Angiography: localized stenosis, occlusion.

Clinical manifestations: TIAs, ischemic stroke.

Radiation-Induced Plexopathy

Either brachial or lumbar plexus; most commonly, arm affected after radiotherapy for breast carcinoma.

Syndromes: (a) transient plexus injury with paresthesias, or less commonly, pain or weakness; median latency 4.5 months; (b) acute ischemic brachial neuropathy following subclavian artery occlusion due to prior irradiation; acute, not progressive, painless; (c) radiation fibrosis with paresthesias or swelling of arm; latency 4 years.

Differentiation from tumor may be difficult. Edema of arm, painless paresis and sensory loss, upper plexus involvement, myokymia (electromyogram) suggest radiation plexopathy. Pain, lack of edema, lower plexus involvement suggest recurrent tumor.

Usually irreversible.

Endocrine Dysfunction

Mostly due to effects on hypothalamus–anterior pituitary axis.

Growth hormone function most vulnerable: growth arrest in children; decreased muscle mass, increased adipose tissue in adults. Treatment includes growth hormone replacement.

Gonadotropin (luteinizing hormone/follicle-stimulating hormone) deficiency: delayed puberty, amenorrhea, infertility, sexual dysfunction, decreased libido. Thyrotropin deficiency: weight gain, lethargy. Hyperprolactinemia: delayed puberty, galactorrhea, amenorrhea, decreased libido, impotence.

Neuropsychological Sequelae

Cognitive impairment common in long-term survivors treated with radiotherapy.

Children under age 5 years, high radiation increase risk. May result in mild delayed IQ decline, learning disability, academic failure. May progress for years.

OTHER COMPLICATIONS OF RADIATION

Peripheral Nerve Damage
Seldom occurs with fractionated doses <6,000 cGy.

Radiation-Induced Tumors
Meningiomas most common. Mean latency 37 years if low-dose irradiation given and 18 months for doses >2,000 cGy. Radiation-induced meningiomas more likely to recur after surgical excision and to undergo malignant degeneration. Radiation-induced sarcomas, CNS gliomas, peripheral nerve tumors also seen.

Radiation Optic Neuropathy
Follows treatment directed to orbit, sinuses, pituitary, intracranial tumors. Painless visual loss, usually monocular, but both eyes may be affected. Symptoms within 3 years. Decreased visual acuity, abnormal visual fields papilledema in most (optic atrophy later), hemorrhagic exudates. About 50% improve, but some become blind. Steroids ineffective.

CHAPTER 73 ■ ELECTRICAL AND LIGHTNING INJURY

High-voltage electric shock or lightning stroke damages CNS, motor neurons, peripheral nerves.

Pathology: lesions in brain or spinal cord. Myelomalacia and other nonspecific lesions seen without change in blood vessels, inflammation, or gliosis.
Pathogenesis: poorly understood.
Epidemiology: electrocution: about 1,000 deaths a year in the United States. Lightning strikes: about 100 deaths a year. M:F ratio 4.5:1.

Immediate symptoms and signs (usually transient): unconsciousness, amnesia, transient limb paralysis or paresthesias. Embolic cerebral infarction may result from cardiac arrhythmia. Cerebral hemorrhage, hypoxic brain damage may occur.

Delayed symptoms and signs: progressive syndrome of parkinsonism, cerebellar disorders, myelopathy, spinal muscular atrophy (with weakness, wasting, fasciculation in affected segments of spinal cord), sensorimotor peripheral neuropathy.

Treatment: acutely, cardiac management. Long-term syndrome: no specific treatment.

CHAPTER 74 ■ DECOMPRESSION SICKNESS

Incidence of decompression sickness in divers: 1% to 30%. Spinal cord most common site of neurologic lesions. Lesions result from bubbles of normally dissolved gases occluding vessels or directly disrupting tissue. Coincident intra-arterial embolism may cause cerebral stroke.

Symptoms and signs: Cord: back pain, leg paresthesias, paresis, urinary retention. Brain: visual impairment, vertigo, hemiparesis, loss of consciousness, seizures.

Treatment: emergency recompression in hyperbaric chamber and concurrent administration of high concentrations of inspired oxygen. For chamber locations and emergency information, physicians should contact: *The Divers Alert Network* at 919-681-4326 (24-hour hotline).

Section VIII

Birth Injuries and Developmental Abnormalities

CHAPTER 75 ■ NEONATAL NEUROLOGY

INTRACRANIAL HEMORRHAGE

Full term: (a) supratentorial subdural (rare; difficult deliveries); (b) primary subarachnoid of venous origin (focal seizures, benign course).

Premature (≤ 32 weeks of gestation): parenchymal, periventricular origin.

PERIVENTRICULAR-INTRAVENTRICULAR HEMORRHAGE (IVH)

Incidence 10–20%, especially in very small premature newborns (<900 g).

Pathophysiology
Arise in vascular germinal plate, near caudate and foramen of Monro (grades I to III), or brain parenchyma (grade IV).

Grade I: blood confined to germinal plate.
Grade II: extension into ventricle.
Grade III: blood filling ventricle, causing distension.
Grade IV: blood in brain parenchyma.
Source of hemorrhage (artery or vein) unclear.

Clinical Features

Grade I: usually asymptomatic.
Grade II: nonspecific irritability or lethargy.
Grade III: usually symptoms of hydrocephalus.
Grade IV: focal signs and mass effect; $\geq 50\%$ mortality. Severe apnea, bradycardia, disconjugate eye movements, pupils fixed, extensor posturing, opisthotonos, clonic limb movements. Death may occur within hours.

Investigations

Hematocrit may drop by 20%.

CSF: many red blood cells; protein 250 to 1,200 mg/dL, but CSF may be normal.

Cranial ultrasound: shows site of blood in parenchyma and ventricles, ventricular size, shifts of major structures.

Treatment and Prognosis

Grades I, II: no treatment. 80% to 90% survival rate without overt neurologic abnormality, but long-term learning and behavior disorders common.

Grade III: no specific treatment if static or reversible ventriculomegaly with normal pressure. If progressive hydrocephalus, consider shunting procedures. Permanent shunts (ventriculoperitoneal) associated with frequent complications in small infants; temporary shunts usually placed in interim (e.g., ventriculo-subgaleal shunt). Overall, 40% incidence of future cerebral palsy and mental retardation.

Grade IV: high mortality; morbidity proportional to size of parenchymal hemorrhage.

PERIVENTRICULAR LEUKOMALACIA (PVL)

Occurs in 10% of surviving infants with birth weight <1500 g; 50% of those with birth weight 500–1000 g.

Imaging: cysts in periventricular white matter (cranial ultrasound); hypomyelination in centrum semiovale, ventricular enlargement due to decreased white matter volume (MRI).

Clinical manifestations: spastic diplegia with damage to corticospinal fibers to the legs.

HYPOXIC-ISCHEMIC ENCEPHALOPATHY (HIE)

Incidence 2 to 4 per 1,000 births. Can occur despite optimal obstetric management.

PATHOLOGY AND PATHOPHYSIOLOGY

Lesion location varies with gestational age. Preterm newborns: periventricular region, centrum semiovale. After 36 weeks of gestation: cerebral gray matter, basal ganglia, brainstem, cerebellar Purkinje cells.

Causes: abruptio placenta, uterine rupture, placental or umbilical cord dysfunction.

CLINICAL FEATURES

At birth: low Apgar score (0–3 for at least 5 minutes); bradycardia, poor respiratory effort, hypotonia, diminished reflexes.

First 72 hours: *mild:* irritability or mild lethargy, hypotonia; *moderate:* above symptoms plus seizures; *severe:* apathy, severe hypotonia, coma, seizures.

First week: variable level of recovery; usually resolution of seizures.

Long-term: microcephaly; signs of static encephalopathy with spasticity or hypotonia, developmental delay, mental retardation. Seizures common. Choreoathetosis may occur.

INVESTIGATIONS

During labor: late deceleration of fetal heart rate relative to uterine contractions, fixed intrauterine heart rate, persistent fetal bradycardia.

Arterial blood gases: metabolic acidosis. Low serum glucose, abnormal liver enzymes. High CSF lactate.

EEG: decreased activity, burst-suppression pattern, or clinically silent seizure activity.

Imaging: areas of diffuse ischemic injury.

TREATMENT AND PROGNOSIS

Support respiration, blood pressure, fluid homeostasis. Brain edema: steroids, osmotic agents ineffective. Seizures: see below. Induced hypothermia being investigated.

Prognosis guarded; better outlook if recovery is rapid. >50% of those with neonatal seizures have significant long-term neurologic deficits.

Prevention: rapid delivery (Cesarean section) when intrauterine fetal distress evident.

NEONATAL INFECTIONS

NEONATAL HERPES ENCEPHALITIS

Neonatal HSV infection: 1 to 3 per 10,000 live births. Acquired in utero or passage through birth canal. Usually herpes simplex virus (HSV) type 2.

CNS manifestations: fever, irritability, seizures.

CSF: lymphocytosis, increased protein. Polymerase chain reaction for HSV establishes diagnosis.

Treatment: 60 mg/kg/day acyclovir intravenously for 21 days if HSV suspected. Mortality ≈33%. Serious neurologic sequelae frequent.

NEONATAL MENINGITIS

Early-onset (first 4 to 5 days of life) usually associated with sepsis; later (first 1 to 2 months) may occur as isolated infection.

Risk factors: prematurity, prolonged ruptured membranes, maternal colonization with group B streptococcus, maternal chorioamnionitis. Predominant organisms in United States: group B streptococcus, gram-negative bacteria.

Symptoms often subtle: lethargy, poor feeding, temperature instability (fever or hypothermia), seizures.

Later: bulging fontanel, opisthotonos.

CSF: as in older children (note: protein levels up to 100 mg/dL are normal in term newborns).

Treatment: appropriate intravenous antibiotics for 3 weeks. High morbidity, mortality.

NEONATAL SEIZURES

Incidence: 0.5% to 1% of all newborns.

CLASSIFICATION

Focal and multifocal clonic: most common form of neonatal seizures; e.g., jerking of one limb, unilateral facial twitching, or rhythmic horizontal deviation of eyes.

Tonic postures: second most common neonatal seizure; e.g., arm extends with or without eye deviation or head turning.

Motor automatisms: e.g., mouthing, pedaling. Often lack clear EEG correlate and may represent subcortical release phenomena.

Generalized tonic-clonic seizures do not occur in newborns due to brain immaturity.

Apnea as sole manifestation of seizure is rare.

ETIOLOGY

Common underlying causes: HIE (term infants), IVH (preterm infants), intracerebral hemorrhage, infarction, CNS infection, cerebral malformations, metabolic disorders, withdrawal (maternal drug use).

Primary epilepsy rare. Recognized syndromes include: benign neonatal convulsions, benign familial neonatal convulsions (autosomal dominant), early infantile epileptogenic encephalopathy (EIEE, Otohara Syndrome), early myoclonic epilepsy (EME).

INVESTIGATIONS

Initial: blood glucose, calcium, magnesium, sodium, acid-base values, blood culture; lumbar puncture (meningitis).

Imaging: Cranial ultrasound (hemorrhage, hydrocephalus); MRI (structural abnormalities, HIE). EEG to characterize abnormal movements, behavioral fluctuations.

Consider also: TORCH titers (toxoplasmosis, rubella, cytomegalovirus, HSV); trials of pyridoxine (50 mg intravenous [IV]) to rule out pyridoxine dependency, folinic acid (1 mg/kg/day for 3 days) to rule out cerebral folate deficiency; blood, urine, CSF for inborn errors of metabolism with neonatal symptoms (phenylketonuria, maple syrup urine disease, lactic or organic acidemias, ammonia cycle abnormalities, nonketotic hyperglycinemia).

TREATMENT

Treat underlying disease when possible (e.g., hypoglycemia: 10% glucose solution IV, initial dose 2 mL/kg).

Phenobarbital: IV loading dose of 20 mg/kg over 5 minutes, followed by maintenance dose of 5 mg/kg/d in two 12-hour doses. Goal: suppression of clinical and electrographic seizures; blood phenobarbital level 20 to 40 g/dL.

If seizures persist despite optimal phenobarbital level: fosphenytoin IV 20 mg/kg over 20 minutes with cardiac monitoring, then maintenance dose 4–7 mg/kg/day.

If seizures remain refractory, consider IV midazolam infusion 0.1–0.4 mg/kg/hour.

PROGNOSIS

Most important determinant of prognosis: underlying cause of seizures (Table 75.1).

TABLE 75.1

RELATIONSHIP OF NEUROLOGIC DISEASE TO PROGNOSIS IN NEONATAL SEIZURES

Disease	Percentage of children who survive with normal development	Comment
Perinatal asphyxia	50%	Most common cause of neonatal encephalopathy
Subarachnoid hemorrhage	90%	Seen in difficult deliveries
Intraventricular hemorrhage	10%	Seizures rare in premature infants
Hypoglycemia	50%	Outcome may be related to early-onset therapy
Late hypocalcemia	90%	Presents day 5 to10
Early hypocalcemia	50%	Presents day 1 to 3 with other encephalopathies
Inborn metabolic errors	10%	Some with phenylketonuria or pyridoxine dependency do well
Bacterial meningitis	30%	Higher mortality in early-onset
Congenital anomalies	0	Includes lissencephaly, polymicrogyria, pachygyria
Drug withdrawal	?	Good follow-up series unavailable; drugs include heroin, methadone
Cause unknown	67%	10% to 20% of neonatal seizures

Normal EEG at time of first seizure usually predicts good outcome. EEG showing burst-suppression, low-voltage background, or continuous multifocal discharges predicts poor outcome in >90%.

Overall, 15% to 30% of infants with neonatal seizures later develop epilepsy.

CHAPTER 76 ■ FLOPPY INFANT SYNDROME

Decreased muscle tone throughout body. Limply hanging limbs when infant held suspended in prone position.

Most common causes (75% of cases): perinatal insult to brain or spinal cord, infantile spinal muscular atrophy, dysgenetic syndromes.

CLUES TO DIAGNOSIS

See Table 76.1.

Age at onset: newborn period or later.

Distinguish *true limb weakness* (decreased movement, reduced or absent tendon reflexes) from low tone with normal strength (often in association with encephalopathy).

Perinatal history: maternal MG, substance abuse; perinatal asphyxia, hemorrhage.

Distribution of abnormality: generalized, symmetric, focal.

FOCAL NEONATAL HYPOTONIA

Trauma (brachial plexus injury, nerve root avulsion) or developmental abnormality.

Hypotonia and weak legs: spinal cord pathology.

TABLE 76.1

FLOPPY INFANT SYNDROMES

	Neuromuscular disorders (weakness prominent)	Central disorders with abnormal neurologic signs or peripheral disorders (little or no weakness)
Neonate	Infantile spinal muscular atrophy	Perinatal asphyxia
	Congenital myotonic dystrophy	Cerebral hemorrhage
	Neonatal myasthenia gravis	Sepsis
	Congenital myopathies[a,b]	Intoxication
	Metabolic myopathies[c]	Spinal cord injury or malformation
	Congenital muscular dystrophies	Failure-to-thrive syndromes
		Congenital hypothyroidism
		Neurotransmitter disorders
		Down syndrome
		Prader-Willi syndrome
		Other dysgenetic syndromes
Age 1–6 months (or later)	Infantile spinal muscular atrophy	Metabolic cerebral degenerations[c]
	Infantile Guillain-Barré syndrome or other neuropathies	Connective tissue disorders[f]
	Congenital myasthenic syndromes[d]	Metabolic and endocrine diseases[g]
	Botulism	Hypotonic cerebral palsy
		Benign congenital hypotonia

[a]Spinal muscular atrophy and congenital myopathies are more likely to become symptomatic *after* the neonatal period.
[b]Congenital myopathies include those characterized by specific histochemical abnormality (nemaline, central cores, myotubules and other structures).
[c]Metabolic myopathies include infantile acid maltase deficiency (Pompe disease), mitochondrial DNA depletion syndrome and benign and fatal infantile cytochrome C oxidase deficiency.
[d]Congenital myasthenic syndromes do not usually cause symptoms, in infants, other than ophthalmoplegia.
[e]Leukodystrophies, lipid storage diseases, peroxisomal diseases, mucopolysaccharidosis, aminoacidurias, Leigh syndrome.
[f]Congenital laxity of ligaments, Ehler-Danlos syndrome, Marfan syndrome.
[g]Organic acidemia, hypocalcemia, hypercalcemia, hypothyroidism, renal tubular acidosis.

DYSGENETIC SYNDROMES

Often associated with distinctive dysmorphic physical features. Include Down syndrome (Chapter 81), Prader-Willi syndrome (Chapter 81), Lowe syndrome (Chapter 82), Zellweger syndrome (Chapter 89), Smith-Lemli-Opitz syndrome, Riley-Day syndrome (familial dysautonomia).

Some disorders of neurotransmitter (serotonin, catecholamine) metabolism may cause neonatal hypotonia.

NEUROMUSCULAR DISORDERS

Clinical features: alert; limb movements decreased; tendon reflexes absent with neural disease, present with myasthenia.

SPINAL MUSCULAR ATROPHY (WERDNIG-HOFFMANN DISEASE)

Most common cause of infantile hypotonia after immediate neonatal period. Autosomal recessive; carrier frequency 1 in 40 in general population. Limb weakness, areflexia, tongue fasciculations. Most affected infants die before age 2 years.

INFANTILE NEUROPATHIES

Uncommon causes of weakness, areflexia, hypotonia (e.g., metachromatic leukodystrophy, neonatal adrenoleukodystrophy, peroneal muscular atrophy). Clues: family history, palpably enlarged peripheral nerves, upper motor neuron signs, elevated CSF protein concentration, slow nerve conduction velocities.

NEUROMUSCULAR JUNCTION DISORDERS

Ophthalmoplegia, difficulty sucking and swallowing; limb weakness; diaphragmatic weakness; tendon reflexes present. (a) *Congenital myasthenic syndromes:* hereditary (autosomal recessive), non-immunologic. (b) *Transient neonatal MG:* autoimmune, due to mother's antibodies. (c) *Juvenile MG:* onset after age 2 years. (d) *Infantile botulism*: ileus, constipation, hypotonia, weakness, pupillary dilation, apneic spells; due to ingestion of *C. botulinum* spores.

See also Chapter 121.

MYOPATHIES

(a) *congenital myopathies with specific structural abnormalities* (e.g., central core disease, multicore disease, nemaline myopathy): muscle weakness, decreased tendon reflexes, dysmorphic physical features, congenital hip dislocation, later scoliosis; (b) *myotonic muscular dystrophy*; (c) *congenital muscular dystrophies* associated with eye and CNS malformations (e.g., Fukuyama muscular dystrophy, muscle-eye-brain disease, Walker-Warburg syndrome); (d) *metabolic myopathies*: e.g., infantile acid maltase deficiency (Pompe disease): weakness, areflexia, cardiomyopathy; cytochrome-*c*-oxidase deficiency, mitochondrial DNA-depletion syndrome.

CHAPTER 77 ■ STATIC DISORDERS OF BRAIN DEVELOPMENT

DEVELOPMENTAL DISORDERS OF MOTOR FUNCTION

MINOR MOTOR DISABILITY

Minor impairments of motor coordination; clumsiness. Neurologic basis rarely known. Often occur in children with other specific learning disabilities or mild mental deficiency.

CEREBRAL PALSY (CP)

Any nonprogressive motor disorder of cerebral or cerebellar origin. Underlying etiology usually not identified; often due to a lesion acquired prenatally or in infancy.

Types of CP

Spastic hemiparesis (hemiplegia): lesion in corticospinal system of one cerebral hemisphere. Often caused by intrauterine cerebral infarct or hemorrhage. Hemiparesis may manifest as early hand preference (less use of weaker side). Seizures frequent when lesion affects cortex.

Spastic diplegia or diparesis: prominent spasticity in both legs, hyperactive reflexes, upgoing toes. Causes: bilateral germinal matrix hemorrhage or periventricular leukomalacia associated with prematurity; perinatal ischemia in watershed parasagittal zone.

Spastic quadriplegia: most severe variant of CP, often with moderate-to-severe mental deficiency. Diffuse malformation or damage to brain, e.g., multicystic leukomalacia following severe ischemia, lissencephaly. Seizures frequent and difficult to control.

Hypotonic CP: child floppy but tendon reflexes hyperactive; usually with severe mental deficiency and diffuse brain involvement.

Dyskinetic CP: athetosis, choreoathetosis, dystonia due to basal ganglia pathology. Causes: neonatal hyperbilirubinemia (kernicterus), severe anoxia. Abnormal movements usually start after age 1 year. Treatment rarely effective.

Ataxic CP: maldevelopment of cerebellum or its pathways; some with cognitive impairment. Does not respond well to physical or drug therapy; may improve with age.

Mixed CP: combination of dyskinetic and spastic CP, or ataxia and athetosis.

Management
Refer to specialized center; neuroimaging; hearing, vision assessment, physical and occupational therapy.

Treatment of spasticity: oral or intrathecal baclofen, diazepam, botulinum toxin, dorsal rhizotomy.

DEVELOPMENTAL DISORDERS OF HIGHER CEREBRAL FUNCTIONS

Global developmental delay: subnormal general intelligence; due to diffuse disorder of neocortical or cortical-subcortical development and function.

Specific developmental disorders: affect certain cognitive abilities selectively; genetic predisposition common.

MENTAL DEFICIENCY (MENTAL RETARDATION)

Global limitation of cognitive function, without loss of previously attained skills (in contrast with dementia). Exclude specific impairment in sensorimotor, visual, auditory, language, other specific cognitive and social skills.

Intelligence test batteries predict success in school or particular vocation.

DEVELOPMENTAL LANGUAGE DISORDERS (DLD; DYSPHASIAS)

Variable manner and age for normal children to acquire aspects of language.

Neurologic basis: unilateral focal lesions in early life do not preclude acquisition of language. Dysphasic children likely have bilateral dysfunction in circuits critical for language.

Predominantly expressive: affects production of sounds and words, grammar, syntax; comprehension and nonverbal aspects of language preserved, e.g., Broca aphasia.

Predominantly receptive: comprehension affected; acquisition of expression also impaired, so "mixed dysphasia."

Semantic-pragmatic: difficulty understanding complex sentences, answering open-ended questions. Basic understanding, fluency, nonverbal aspects preserved. Particularly seen in autistic children.

READING DISABILITY (DYSLEXIA)

Subtypes: inadequate processing of speech sounds, difficulty sequencing words, difficulty learning relationship between letters and sounds, spelling. Never with detectable structural brain lesion. Genetic factors important.

OTHER LEARNING DISABILITIES

Difficulty writing (dysgraphia), calculating (dyscalculia), solving word problems, planning and executing complex tasks.

DISORDERS OF ATTENTION (ATTENTION DEFICIT DISORDER, WITH OR WITHOUT HYPERACTIVITY)

More frequent in boys.

Infancy: difficulty falling asleep, waking too early, nighttime awakenings.

Childhood: restlessness, short attention span, lack of engagement in playing, difficulty sitting through class, impulsivity, distractibility, disorganization, forgetfulness, labile affect.

Management: parental counseling, environmental changes (remove distractions, frequent breaks, opportunities to move about), medication (methylphenidate, dextroamphetamine, atomoxetine). Sedatives avoided.

Prognosis: some symptoms (e.g., motor hyperactivity) tend to abate but some features may persist through life.

AUTISM SPECTRUM DISORDERS (PERVASIVE DEVELOPMENTAL DISORDERS)

Etiology: polygenic inheritance likely cause in most cases. Minority of children with autism have underlying conditions: tuberous sclerosis; hypomelanosis of Ito; fragile X, Rett, or Angelman syndrome; phenylketonuria; congenital rubella; neonatal herpes simplex; hydrocephalus; brain malformation; other static encephalopathy.

Symptoms: variable. Core problems: (a) impaired sociability (lack of interest in others, lack of empathy, difficulty interpreting social cues, occasionally, intrusive behaviors); (b) impaired verbal and nonverbal communication (failure to learn to speak, limited comprehension); (c) restricted range of interests and activities (perseveration, resistance to change, absent imaginative play). Other symptoms: abnormal movements and behaviors (e.g., stereotypic movements, self-injury). Impaired language development in pre-school years is often the presenting complaint.

Course and prognosis: onset in infancy or later. Sociability and language tend to improve. Autistic adults often misdiagnosed as mentally retarded, obsessive-compulsive, schizophrenic, manic-depressive, antisocial personality.

Prognosis also depends on individual's level of cognition: may vary from above-normal intelligence to severe mental retardation.

Management: early individualized education; parental instruction in behavior management; psychotropic drugs for specific behavioral problems.

CHAPTER 78 ■
LAURENCE-MOON-BIEDL SYNDROME

CLINICAL FEATURES

Variable manifestations, primarily combination of obesity and hypogonadism in childhood or adolescence.

Obesity (85% to 95%); mental retardation (70% to 85%); retinitis pigmentosa (92% to 95%); hypogenitalism, hypogonadism (74% to 86% of males and 45% to 53% of females); polydactyly, syndactyly (75% to 80%); renal dysfunction; hypertension; cardiac, hepatic defects.

First decade of life: impaired night vision (retinitis pigmentosa); 73% blind by age 20.

Autosomal recessive inheritance.

DIFFERENTIAL DIAGNOSIS

Alström-Hallgren syndrome: deafness, diabetes mellitus in addition to obesity, hypogonadism; sometimes, retinitis pigmentosa.

Biemond syndrome: as in Laurence-Moon-Biedl, but coloboma of iris rather than retinitis pigmentosa.

Prader-Willi syndrome: obesity, hypogonadism, mental retardation; no visual problems.

CHAPTER 79 ■ STRUCTURAL MALFORMATIONS

MALFORMATIONS OF CEREBRAL HEMISPHERES AND AGENESIS OF CORPUS CALLOSUM

Holoprosencephaly: single-lobed brain, one undivided ventricle. Failure of cleavage of telencephalon and diencephalon. Incomplete variants: semilobar, lobar holoprosencephaly. Associated with defects of skull base, dura, face, eyes, olfactory apparatus.

Polymicrogyria: excessive number of gyri, all smaller than normal. Some familial.

Lissencephaly: ("smooth brain"); absence or primitive appearance of gyri; may occur with chromosome abnormalities or intrauterine insults. Associated with muscle and eye malformations in Walker-Warburg syndrome, Fukuyama muscular dystrophy.

Agenesis of corpus callosum (complete or partial): may occur in isolation or in conjunction with many conditions: holoprosencephaly, septo-optic dysplasia, many syndrome complexes with multiple dysmorphisms, some metabolic diseases (e.g., pyruvate dehydrogenase deficiency).

MACROCEPHALY AND MEGALOENCEPHALY

Macrocephaly: head size >2 standard deviations above mean for age. Causes: hydrocephalus, mass lesions (infant, young child); inherited.

Megaloencephaly: brain weight ≥ 2.5 standard deviations above mean for sex and age or brain weight >1,600 g. May occur alone. Progressive brain enlargement with neurologic deterioration seen with neurocutaneous, neuronal storage, degenerative disorders.

MALFORMATIONS OF OCCIPITAL BONE AND CERVICAL SPINE

BASILAR IMPRESSION (PLATYBASIA)

Base of skull flattened on cervical spine. Compression of pons, medulla, cerebellum, cervical cord; stretching of cranial nerves.

Symptoms and signs: Elongated head; spastic paraparesis, unsteady gait, cerebellar ataxia, nystagmus, lower cranial nerve palsies. Partial or complete subarachnoid block of cerebrospinal flow.
Diagnosis: Skull x-rays, CT, or MRI.
Treatment: Surgical decompression of posterior fossa and upper cervical cord.

MALFORMATIONS OF ATLAS AND AXIS

Neurologic symptoms may result from anterior dislocation of atlas and cord compression between odontoid and posterior rim of foramen magnum: spastic quadriparesis, lower cranial nerve palsies, pain on head movement.

FUSION OF CERVICAL VERTEBRAE (KLIPPEL-FEIL DEFORMITY)

Fusion of upper thoracic vertebrae and cervical spine into one or more separate masses. With short neck, low hairline, limited neck movement. Does not directly cause neurologic symptoms but associated with spinal cord pathology, sometimes syringomyelia or other developmental defects of spinal cord, brainstem, cerebellum. Congenital deafness due to maldevelopment of osseous inner ear in up to 30%.

CRANIOSYNOSTOSIS

Premature closure of cranial sutures. Usually primary congenital disturbance of skull growth without neurologic disorder. Frequency: 1 in 1,900 births; may be inherited. Associated limb or facial anomalies occur in some recognized syndromes (e.g., Apert, Crouzon, Pfeiffer).

Closure of one suture most common, leading to abnormal head shape (e.g., *scaphocephaly*: narrow, elongated skull, with sagittal synostosis). Multiple suture closure often occurs with other craniofacial defects; may lead to increased intracranial pressure, compression of optic or auditory nerves.

Best cosmetic results from surgery before age 3 months.

SPINA BIFIDA AND CRANIUM BIFIDUM

Congenital midline defects due to abnormal closure of neural tube and associated mesodermal and ectodermal elements (*dysraphism*) (Table 79.1).

TABLE 79.1
NEURAL TUBE CLOSURE MALFORMATIONS

Malformation	Characteristics
Anencephaly	Absence of brain plus defects in skull, meninges, scalp; frequency 1:1,000 deliveries
Iniencephaly	Retroflexed head with defects of cervical spine; often with anencephaly or encephalocele
Craniorachischisis	Brain and spinal cord necrosis secondary to exposure to amniotic fluid
Cephalocele	Partial brain protrusion through skull defect (cranium bifidum) with variable covering of meninges and skin; commonly occipital; may be parietal or anterior
Meningocele	Skull or spine defect with meningeal protrusion
Dermal sinus tract	Incomplete separation of neural and epithelial ectoderm; may occur with dermoid; marked externally by skin and hair changes; point of entry for bacteria with subsequent meningitis
Spina bifida	Varying degree of vertebral abnormality
Spina bifida occulta	Vertebral arch defect only; up to 24% of population
Spina bifida cystica	Dura and arachnoid herniation through vertebral defect
Myelomeningocele	Herniation of spinal cord and meninges through defect

Causes: environmental (anticonvulsants), genetic factors.

Associated nervous system abnormalities: tethered cord, diastematomyelia, hydromyelia, hydrocephalus.

Diagnosis: ultrasonography; high maternal alpha-fetoprotein levels in serum, amniotic fluid.

Prevention: Folic acid, taken by mother during periconception period.

Treatment: surgical excision of meningocele or encephalocele. Orthopaedic and urologic approaches to maximize function and prevent skin, bone, renal problems.

Concomitant bone and joint changes: Klippel-Feil syndrome, foot deformities, scoliosis, hip dysplasia; may point to associated cord tethering, hydromyelia, adhesive arachnoiditis, or lipoma.

CHIARI MALFORMATION

Congenital downward elongation of brainstem and cerebellum into cervical spinal canal.

Chiari I malformation: intracranial anomaly alone.

Chiari II malformation: intracranial anomaly with spina bifida occulta, meningocele, or meningomyelocele in lumbosacral region. Hydrocephalus in most.

Symptoms and signs: Onset in first few months of life: usually due to hydrocephalus; prognosis poor. Onset in adult life: ataxia, leg weakness, visual symptoms, downbeat nystagmus, seesaw nystagmus, lower cranial nerve palsies.

Treatment: Infants: excision of sac in spinal region; ventriculoperitoneal shunt. Children, adults: posterior fossa decompression.

CHAPTER 80 ■ MARCUS GUNN AND MÖBIUS SYNDROMES

MARCUS GUNN SYNDROME

Eyelid rises when mouth opens (jaw drops); lid comes down when mouth closes (jaw rises). "Jaw-winking."

Usually accompanied by congenital unilateral ptosis. Comprises 5% of all cases of congenital ptosis. Sometimes autosomal-dominant inheritance. Presumably congenital error of neuronal wiring in brainstem. Trigeminal-oculomotor synkinesis.

Not to be confused with *Marcus Gunn pupil*: afferent-pupillary defect.

MÖBIUS SYNDROME

Congenital facial diplegia, bilateral abducens palsies. Other cranial nerves may be affected (hearing loss, dysarthria, dysphagia). Sometimes with congenital anomalies of limbs or heart, Kallmann syndrome (hypogonadism, anosmia), mental retardation. Rarely, infantile facioscapulohumeral muscular dystrophy.

Typical symptoms: difficulty sucking, lack of facial expression when neonate cries. Incomplete forms seen later: facial weakness often more severe in upper face than lower, in contrast to other supranuclear or lower motor-neuron causes of facial paralysis.

Section IX

Genetic Diseases of the Central Nervous System

CHAPTER 81 ■ CHROMOSOMAL DISEASES

Abnormal total number of chromosomes (aneuploidy) or structural rearrangement (deletion, translocation, duplication).

Clinical manifestations: mental retardation (most common), variable congenital malformations.

TRISOMY 21 (DOWN SYNDROME)

Extra copy of chromosome 21. Incidence 1:800 live births; M:F ratio 3:2. Risk increases with increased maternal age: 1:350 at age 35; 1:110 at age 40.

CLINICAL FEATURES

Round face, short nose, flat nasal bridge. Up-slanting palpebral fissures; epicanthal folds. Small mouth; large protruding tongue. Conductive hearing loss. Short stature; short, broad hands; increased space between first and second toes. Small pelvis.

Atlanto-axial or atlanto-occipital instability in 15% to 20%. Increased incidence of congenital heart defects and intestinal malformations (e.g., duodenal atresia). Infertility in males. Hypothyroidism. Hematologic abnormalities, including increased risk of leukemia.

Neurologic signs: marked hypotonia in infancy; later, mental retardation; after age 35, dementia. Increased incidence of seizures.

NEUROPATHOLOGY

Low neuronal density in diverse cortical areas. Pathology similar to Alzheimer disease (AD), including senile plaques, neurofibrillary tangles.

CYTOGENETICS

Complete extra chromosome 21 in 95%. Mosaic trisomy or translocation in remaining 5%.

DOWN SYNDROME AND FAMILIAL AD

One early-onset familial AD gene linked to chromosome 21: mutations in amyloid precursor protein (APP) gene may be involved in formation of senile plaques. Three copies expressed in patients with Down syndrome; may be responsible for increased APP production and similar histopathology to AD.

MANAGEMENT

Treat associated medical/surgical conditions as required. CT screening for atlantoaxial instability before participating in contact sports.

PRADER-WILLI AND ANGELMAN SYNDROMES

Both syndromes associated with DNA deletion in same region of chromosome 15q.

Genomic imprinting: parent-of-origin–specific gene expression; some autosomal genes are normally inherited in silent state on one parental allele (e.g., paternal), and active state on the other (e.g., maternal).

Disease results when active allele is lost by: (1) mutation (usually deletion), (2) silencing due to imprinting error, (3) duplication of the nonactive allele (*uniparental disomy*).

PRADER-WILLI SYNDROME (PWS)

Due to loss of "PWS critical region" on paternal chromosome 15.

    Incidence 1:25,000 live births. Usually sporadic; hypothalamic dysfunction.

Clinical features: neonatal hypotonia and poor feeding. Then delayed psychomotor development, excessive appetite, childhood obesity, hypogonadism, small external genitalia, short stature, mental retardation.

ANGELMAN SYNDROME (AS)

Due to loss of "AS critical region" on maternal chromosome 15.

Prevalence 1:12,000. Usually sporadic.

Clinical features: feeding difficulty at ages 1 to 2 months; small head circumference, short stature; no speech development; delayed motor development; happy, smiling appearance; wide-based, ataxic gait with tremulous movements. Seizures in infancy.

SUBTELOMERIC CHROMOSOMAL ANOMALIES

Telomeres: complex DNA-protein structures forming 'caps' at ends of chromosomes. Anomalies lead to altered chromosome length and stability.

Fluorescent *in situ* hybridization (FISH) studies with subtelomeric probes may detect subtle chromosomal anomalies in children with idiopathic mental retardation and normal routine karyotype. Positive detection rate up to 25% if criteria include severe mental retardation, positive family history of mental retardation, and at least one physical dysmorphism.

22q11 DELETION SYNDROME

Includes DiGeorge, velocardiofacial, CATCH22 (Cardiac defects, Abnormal facies, Thymic hypoplasia, Cleft palate, Hypocalcemia) syndromes.

Incidence 1:4,000 births.

Clinical features: variable; include cognitive impairment, psychiatric disorders, cardiac malformations, cranial and branchial arch anomalies.

CHAPTER 82 ■ DISORDERS OF AMINO ACID METABOLISM

Incidence: phenylketonuria 1:10,000; defective amino-acid transport 2:10,000; all other aminoacidopathies <8:100,000.

Neurologic damage frequently preventable with early treatment; mass newborn screening important for early diagnosis.

PHENYLKETONURIA (PKU)

Phenylalanine hydroxylase deficiency. Autosomal recessive. Impaired hepatic hydroxylation of phenylalanine to tyrosine. Phenylalanine accumulates in blood and is neurotoxic. If untreated: mental retardation, seizures, imperfect hair pigmentation.

PATHOGENESIS AND PATHOLOGY

Classic PKU: enzyme activity completely or nearly completely absent.
Pathology: defective brain maturation; defective myelination; diminished or absent pigmentation of substantia nigra, locus ceruleus.

CLINICAL FEATURES

Wide range of clinical, biochemical severity. Classic form: normal at birth; vomiting, irritability in first 2 months; delayed intellectual development by 4 to 9 months; seizures (infantile spasms, later grand mal).

Typical features: blond hair, blue eyes, rough and dry skin, eczema, musty odor (phenylacetic acid).
Neurologic features: microcephaly; mental retardation; increased muscle tone; tremor of hands; EEG hypsarrhythmia, foci of spikes or polyspikes; MRI: areas of increased T2 signal in white matter.

DIAGNOSIS AND DIFFERENTIAL DIAGNOSIS

Most identified through newborn screening (blood phenylalanine level).

If positive screen, further testing to 1) confirm persistent hyperphenylalaninemia (HPA), 2) determine cause (2% with HPA have deficiency of cofactor tetrahydrobiopterin (BH_4), with different clinical features and treatment to PKU).

TREATMENT

Lifelong low-phenylalanine diet. Serum phenylalanine level normal in 1 to 2 weeks. Administration of tetrahydrobiopterin or synthetic pterin, and replacement therapy with neurotransmitter precursors, for rare variant with BH_4 deficiency.

PROGNOSIS

Most abnormalities resolve with early treatment, but intellectual development may not be normal.

MAPLE SYRUP URINE DISEASE (MSUD)

Autosomal recessive defect in branched-chain amino-acid metabolism. Urine, sweat have sweet, maple-syrup–like odor. Incidence 1:220,000 to 1:400,000 newborns. Deficiency in mitochondrial branched-chain α-keto acid dehydrogenase leads to accumulation of ketoacid derivatives of three amino acids: leucine, valine, and isoleucine. Manifestations vary from severe MSUD to mild or intermittent forms.

Clinical features (untreated classic form): opisthotonos, increased muscle tone, seizures, rapid deterioration of all cerebral functions, hypoglycemia (in 50%). Imaging: diffuse brain edema, especially severe in white matter of posterior fossa and posterior cerebrum.

Diagnosis: characteristic smell of urine, sweat; quantitation of plasma amino acids.

Treatment: restrict dietary leucine, isoleucine, valine. Nearly normal intellectual development possible with treatment.

DEFECTS IN METABOLISM OF SULFUR AMINO ACIDS

HOMOCYSTINURIA

Second most common metabolic cause of brain damage (after PKU). Incidence 1:45,000 newborns. Autosomal recessive.

Reduced or absent cystathionine synthase. Homocysteine not converted to cystathionine; increased plasma and urine levels of homocystine and its precursor, methionine, lead to endothelial damage and hypercoagulability.

Clinical features: multiple arterial and venous infarcts in various organs; seizures; strokes; developmental delay. Also ectopia of lens; sparse, blond, brittle hair; multiple erythematous blotches on skin; shuffling gait; long limbs and digits; genu valgum.

Diagnosis: increased urinary homocysteine; elevated plasma levels of homocysteine, methionine; reduced cystathionine synthase activity in skin fibroblasts or liver.

Treatment: low-methionine diet supplemented with cysteine, betaine. Pyridoxine helps some. Heterozygotes: increased peripheral vascular disease, premature strokes.

DISORDERS OF AMINO-ACID TRANSPORT

LOWE SYNDROME (OCULOCEREBRORENAL SYNDROME)

Sex-linked recessive. Severe mental retardation, delayed physical development, myopathy, congenital glaucoma or cataract, renal Fanconi (proximal tubule) syndrome, rickets. Generalized aminoaciduria (lysine particularly elevated).

MRI: white matter abnormalities.

HARTNUP DISEASE

Photosensitive dermatitis, intermittent cerebellar ataxia, behavioral abnormality, renal aminoaciduria. Abnormal transport of neutral amino acids.

Other manifestations: red, scaly rash on exposed skin; migraine, photophobia.

Treatment: nicotinic acid, but benefit not proven. Spontaneous improvement occurs over time.

CHAPTER 83 ■ DISORDERS OF PURINE AND PYRIMIDINE METABOLISM

Purines and pyrimidines: heterocyclic compounds with important roles in nucleotide synthesis, generation of energy compounds (ADP, ATP), signaling pathways (cyclic AMP).

Several distinct disorders now recognized; varied clinical phenotypes.

Systemic features: anemia, immunodeficiency, hypo- or hyperuricemia.

Neurologic features: mental retardation, autism, seizures, spasticity, movement disorders, sensorineural hearing loss.

LESCH-NYHAN SYNDROME

X-linked recessive deficiency of hypoxanthine-guanine phosphoribosyltransferase (HPRT); increased rate of purine biosynthesis, high levels of uric acid.

Clinical features: hyperuricemia, mental retardation, choreoathetosis, self-mutilation from biting lips and fingers, gout. Death usually due to renal failure (nephropathy due to urate deposits). Some clinical and biochemical heterogeneity.

Diagnosis: hair root analysis of HPRT; biochemical assay of enzyme in erythrocyte hemolysate or cultured fibroblasts. Prenatal enzymatic diagnosis and DNA analysis possible.

No satisfactory treatment for neurologic symptoms.

CHAPTER 84 ■ LYSOSOMAL AND OTHER STORAGE DISEASES

Storage material (complex lipid, saccharide, or protein) accumulates in lysosomes due to genetically determined deficiency of a catabolic enzyme.

Inheritance recessive, usually autosomal, occasionally X-linked.

Only specific treatment: enzyme replacement therapy for MPS 1, Gaucher, Fabry disease.

See Tables 84.1 through 84.4. Below are notes about selected conditions.

LIPIDOSES

GM2 GANGLIOSIDOSES

Infantile Encephalopathy with Cherry-Red Spots
Classic Tay-Sachs disease: hexosaminidase A absent, hexosaminidase B increased; higher incidence in Ashkenazi Jews.
Infantile Sandhoff disease: hexosaminidase A and B deficient.
AB variant: hexosaminidase A activating protein deficient; hexosaminidase A, B increased.

Myoclonic jerk reaction to sound (hyperacusis); macular cherry-red spot; developmental delay manifesting at age 4 to 6 months, evolving into flaccid weakness with hyperactive reflexes, clonus, Babinski signs. Visual deterioration, seizures, myoclonus, developmental regression. Vegetative state after age 1 year.

Late Infantile, Juvenile, and Adult GM2 Gangliosidoses
Dementia, ataxia; with or without macular cherry-red spot; spasticity, muscle wasting, seizures. Sometimes, signs of motor neuron disease. Rectal biopsy (electron microscopy of autonomic neurons), DNA analysis may aid in diagnosis with variant phenotypes.

TABLE 84.1
SELECTED LIPIDOSES

Disorder	Defective enzyme	Clinical features	Diagnosis
GM2 gangliosidoses	Hexosaminidase	Infantile- to adult-onset phenotypes from infantile encephalopathy with macular cherry-red spots to adult-onset spinal muscular atrophy	Hexosaminidase A, B levels in blood, leukocytes.
GM1 gangliosidoses Infantile form	β-galactosidase	Infantile encephalopathy, organomegaly, skeletal involvement, cherry-red spot (50%), corneal haze (occasionally)	Oligosaccharide pattern in urine; enzyme activity (leukocytes, fibroblasts)
Late infantile form		Onset age 1–3 yr: dementia, seizures, ataxia, dysarthria, spastic quadriplegia. No organomegaly.	Same
Fabry disease	α-galactosidase	X-linked. Purple skin lesions, painful hands and feet, renal disease, leg edema, stroke. ERT effective in reducing symptoms; some still need renal transplant.	Enzyme activity (plasma, leukocytes); mutation analysis
Gaucher disease	β-glucosidase		"Gaucher cells" in bone marrow; enzyme activity (leukocyte, fibroblasts); mutation analysis

(continued)

TABLE 84.1
SELECTED LIPIDOSES (Continued)

Disorder	Defective enzyme	Clinical features	Diagnosis
Infantile neuronopathic		Onset age 3 mo: dementia, organomegaly, poor suck and swallowing, opisthotonos, spasticity, seizures; usually fatal before age 2 years.	
Juvenile neuronopathic		Variable onset of mental defect, splenomegaly, incoordination, seizures, tics	
Adult nonneuronopathic		Splenomegaly (sometimes in infancy) and bony involvement; Ashkenazi Jewish predilection; no neurologic disease. ERT effective.	
Adult neuronopathic		Splenomegaly, bony involvement, seizures, dementia.	
Niemann-Pick disease	Sphingomyelinase		Path: foam ("mulberry") cells in bone marrow Enzyme activity (fibroblasts, leukocytes)
Infantile neuronopathic, type A		Infantile encephalopathy, organomegaly, cherry-red spot (30%), lung infiltrates, especially Ashkenazi Jewish	

Juvenile nonneuronopathic, type B	Sphingomyelinase	Hepatosplenomegaly	Same as type A
Juvenile neuronopathic, type C	Cholesterol esterification induction	Onset at any age: ataxia, dystonia, dementia; seizures in 50%; hepatosplenomegaly variable. Vertical supranuclear gaze palsy characteristic.	Impaired cholesterol esterification in fibroblasts.
Farber disease	Acid-ceramidase	Early infantile painful swollen joints, subcutaneous nodules, organomegaly, enlarged heart, dysphagia, vomiting, normal or impaired mentation	Enzyme activity (fibroblasts, leukocytes)
Wolman disease	Acid lipase	Early infantile organomegaly, vomiting, diarrhea, jaundice, variable CNS involvement	Calcified adrenals; foam cells in bone marrow; enzyme studies (leukocytes)
Refsum disease	Phytanic acid α-hydroxylase	Night blindness, retinitis pigmentosa, ataxia, demyelinating neuropathy, ichthyosis	Serum phytanic acid
Cerebrotendinous xanthomatosis	Mitochondrial enzyme 27-sterol hydroxylase (CYP 27)	Static encephalopathy in first decade; adolescent or adult-onset cataracts, tendon xanthomas, ataxia, spasticity	Mutations in sterol 27-hydroxylase gene

(continued)

TABLE 84.1

SELECTED LIPIDOSES (*Continued*)

Disorder	Defective enzyme	Clinical features	Diagnosis
Neuronal ceroid lipofuscinoses	CLN1, CLN2, CLN3, CLN4, CLN5 gene products		Electron microscopic examination of tissue; (skin, nerve, muscle, or rectal biopsy)
Infantile (Haltia-Santavuori)	Palmitoyl-protein thioesterase enzyme (CLN1 gene)	Infantile onset: progressive visual loss, retinal degeneration, myoclonic jerks, microcephaly. Abnormal electroretinogram	
Late infantile (Jansky-Bielschowsky)	Tripeptidyl peptidase 1 (CLN2 gene)	Onset at age 1–4 yr: seizures, ataxia, dementia, then visual deterioration, retinal degeneration. Abnormal electroretinogram	
Juvenile form (Spielmeyer-Sjögren)	CLN3 gene product	Onset age 5–10 yrs: progressive visual loss, pigmentary retinal degeneration, then seizures, dementia. Abnormal electroretinogram	
Adult (Kufs)		Adult onset: dementia, ataxia, seizures, myoclonus	

ERT, Enzyme replacement therapy.

TABLE 84.2
LEUKODYSTROPHIES

Clinical disorder	Defective enzyme	Clinical features	Diagnosis
Krabbe leukodystrophy			
Infantile form	Galactocerebrosidase	Onset age 3–6 mo: irritability, spasticity, seizures, fevers; developmental slowing then regression; eventual blindness due to optic atrophy, decerebrate posturing, absent tendon reflexes, vegetative state; usually fatal within 2 years	Infantile form: increased CSF protein. All types: slow nerve conduction, enzyme studies (serum, leukocytes, fibroblasts)
Juvenile form	Galactocerebrosidase	Juvenile onset: dementia, optic atrophy, pyramidal tract signs	
Adult form	Galactocerebrosidase	Adult onset: slowly progressive dementia, optic atrophy, pyramidal signs	
Metachromatic leukodystrophy			
Late-infantile form	Sulfatase A	Onset age 1–2 yr: walking difficulty with weakness, ataxia, or spasticity; dementia, optic atrophy, loss of tendon reflexes; eventual quadriplegia, vegetative state	All types: increased CSF protein (except in adult-onset), increased excretion of urine sulfatides, slow nerve conduction; enzyme studies (leukocytes, fibroblasts). Sural nerve biopsy: metachromatic lipids; characteristic "tuffstone" bodies on electron microscopy

TABLE 84.2

LEUKODYSTROPHIES (*Continued*)

Clinical disorder	Defective enzyme	Clinical features	Diagnosis
Juvenile form	Sulfatase A	Onset age 3–10 yr: dementia, gait difficulty, neuopathy, high CSF protein; slower	
Adult form	Sulfatase A	Adult-onset dementia, ataxia, pyramidal signs	
Without sulfatase A deficiency	Sulfatase A activator	Same as late infantile or juvenile form	
Multiple sulfatase deficiency (mucosulfatidosis)	Many sulfatases	Features of both MLD and mucopolysaccharidosis. Onset at age 1–2 yr: developmental delay then regression, seizures, mildly coarse facial features, ichthysis, organomegaly, skeletal changes	Similar to MLD; in addition: increased urine GAG; deficiencies of multiple sulfatases in cultured fibroblasts

GAG, glycosaminoglycans.

TABLE 84.3
MUCOPOLYSACCHARIDOSES

Syndrome	Eponym	Deficient enzyme	Mental defect	Cloudy corneas	Hearing loss	Coarse facial feature	Dwarfing	Dysostosis multiplex	Heart disease	Organomegaly	Other features
MPS I H	Hurler	α-L-iduronidase	3+	3+	2+	3+	3+	3+	3+	3+	Cord compression, pigmentary retinopathy
MPS I H/S	Hurler-Scheie compound	α-L-iduronidase	+−	3+	+−	2+	1+	2+	1+	2+	Severe arachnoid cysts
MPS IS	Scheie	α-L-iduronidase	0	3+	+−	+−	0	1+	1+	+−	Pigmentary retinopathy, carpal tunnel syndrome

(continued)

TABLE 84.3

MUCOPOLYSACCHARIDOSES

Syndrome	Eponym	Deficient enzyme	Mental defect	Cloudy corneas	Hearing loss	Coarse facial feature	Dwarfing	Dysostosis multiplex	Heart disease	Organomegaly	Other features
MPS II A	Hunter (severe)	Iduronate-2-sulfate sulfatase	+	0	3+	2+	2+	2+	+-	1+	Nodular skin lesions
MPS II B	Hunter (mild)	Iduronate-2-sulfate sulfatase	0	0	2+	1+	1+	1+	+-	+-	Pigmentary retinopathy, carpal tunnel syndrome, nodular skin lesions
MPS III A	Sanflippo A	Sulfamidase	3+	0	2+	1+	0	1+	1+	1+	Retinal degeneration; may have seizures

MPS	Eponym	Deficient enzyme									Clinical features
MPS III B	Sanfilippo B	α-N-acetylglucosaminidase	3+	0	2+	1+	0	1+	1+	1+	Retinal degeneration
MPS III C	Sanfilippo C	N-acetyltransferase	3+	0	2+	1+	1+	1+	1+	1+	Odontoid hypoplasia
MPS III D	Sanfilippo D	N-acetylglucosamine-6-sulfate sulfatase	2+	0	1+	0	1+	1+	0	1+	
MPS IV A	Morquio A	Galactose-6-sulfate sulfatase	0	2+	2+	1+	3+	3+	2+	+−	Cord compression, odontoid hypoplasia
MPS IV B	Morquio B	β-galactosidase	0	1+	0	0	0	2+	0	+−	
MPS VI A	Maroteaux-Lamy (severe)	Sulfatase B	0	2+	2+	2+	2+	2+	2+	+−	Cord compression, carpal tunnel syndrome, hydrocephalus
MPS VI B	Maroteaux-Lamy (intermediate)	Sulfatase B	0	2+	+−	+−	1+	2+	2+	0	Carpal tunnel syndrome
MPS VI C	Maroteaux-Lamy (mild)	Sulfatase B	0	1+	+−	+−	1+	1+	1+	0	Cord compression, carpal tunnel syndrome
MPS VII	Sly	β-glucuronidase	2+	+−	1+	1+	2+	2+	1+	1+	Hydrocephalus

MPS, mucopolysaccharidosis; 0, 1+, 2+, 3+ are rough scores of frequency of manifestation.

TABLE 84.4

MUCOLIPIDOSES

Clinical disorder	Defective enzyme	Clinical features	Diagnosis
Sialidoses			
1. Sialidoses with isolated sialidase deficiency	Oligosaccharide sialidase		Abnormal urine sialyloligosaccharides; enzyme studies (fibroblasts)
a. Congenital sialidosis		Premature birth, congenital hydrops fetalis, organomegaly, severe mental and motor defect, death 0–5 mo	
b. Severe infantile sialidosis		Similar to congenital sialidosis, but renal disease; survive to age 2 yr	
c. Nephrosialidosis		Onset age 4–6 mo: organomegaly, facial dysmorphism, psychomotor retardation, renal disease, cherry-red spot, corneal opacities	
d. Mucolipidosis I		Onset age 6 mo: mild Hurler-like facial and skeletal changes, corneal clouding, cherry-red spot, mental defect, myoclonic jerks, cerebellar syndrome, seizures, neuropathy	

Disease	Defect	Clinical features	Diagnostic test
e. Macular cherry-red spot myoclonus syndrome		Onset around age 10 yr: myoclonus, decreasing visual acuity, cherry-red spot; especially in Italians	
2. *Galactosialidoses (Sialidoses with additional β-galactosidase deficiency)*	Stabilizing protein for oligosaccharide sialidase & β-galactosidase		Abnormal urine oligosaccharides; enzyme studies (leukocytes, fibroblasts)
a. Infantile sialidosis (GM1-gangliosidosis phenotype)		Same as GM1-gangliosidosis	
b. Goldberg syndrome		Similar to mucolipidosis I but childhood or adolescent onset, slow; most common among Japanese	
Salla disease (free sialic acid storage disease)	Sialic acid egress from lysosomes	Infantile onset: hypotonia, developmental delay; juvenile ataxia, mental and motor retardation spasticity, athetosis, dysarthria, convulsions; short stature	Free sialic acid markedly increased in urine

(*continued*)

TABLE 84.4

MUCOLIPIDOSES

Clinical disorder	Defective enzyme	Clinical features	Diagnosis
Fucosidosis	a L-fucosidase	Some resemble Hurler phenotype; some have coarse features and neurologic disorder resembling leukodystrophy	Abnormal urine oligosaccharides; enzyme studies (leukocytes, fibroblasts)
α-Mannosidosis	α-Mannosidase	Mild or severe mental defect, organomegaly, coarse features, skeletal involvement, gingival hyperplasia, lenticular opacities, survival into third decade	Abnormal urine oligosaccharides; enzyme studies (leukocytes, fibroblasts)
β-Mannosidosis	β-Mannosidase	Juvenile onset: mental retardation, speech delay, coarse facial features, mild bony changes, angiokeratoma	Abnormal urine oligosaccharides, enzyme studies (leukocytes, fibroblasts)
Aspartylglycosaminuria	Aspartylglucosaminidase	Especially in Finnish people; characteristic facies, thickened skull, scoliosis, diarrhea, respiratory infections, dementia, psychosis, seizures	Abnormal urine oligosaccharides, enzyme studies (leukocytes, fibroblasts)

Mucolipidosis II (I-cell disease)	UDP-N-acetylgalactosamine-1-phosphate: glycoprotein N-acetylgalactosaminyl phosphotransferase	Infantile onset of Hurler-like disorder; but cornea usually clear	Excess sialo-oligosaccharides in urine; enzyme studies (serum, plasma, fibroblasts)
Mucolipidosis III (pseudopolydystrophy)	Same as mucolipidosis II	Onset age 2–4 yr: coarse facies, dwarfism, short neck, claw hands, clear cornea, carpal tunnel syndrome, mental defect, long survival	Same as for mucolipidosis II
Mucolipidosis IV	Mucolipin	Early infantile corneal clouding; juvenile developmental retardation/regression; Ashkenazi Jewish predilection	Elevated serum gastrin; lipid-laden marrow histiocytes (light-microscopy), vacuoles and membranous bodies (electron microscopy: fibroblasts, conjunctiva)

GM1 GANGLIOSIDOSIS

Infantile GM1 Gangliosidosis: Earlier onset, more severe, more rapidly progressive than Tay-Sachs disease. Neonatal onset; hypotonia, poor suck, slow weight gain. Frontal bossing, coarse features, large low-set ears, elongated philtrum. Cherry-red spot in 50%. Hepatosplenomegaly; coarse, thickened skin; bony abnormalities.

LEUKODYSTROPHIES

Genetic metabolic disorders causing dysmyelination.

Krabbe leukodystrophy and **metachromatic leukodystrophy (MLD)**: autosomal recessive conditions that involve both central and peripheral nervous system (Table 84.2).

OTHER LEUKODYSTROPHIES

Adrenoleukodystrophy (ALD): X-linked, adrenal glands affected as well as white matter (see Chapter 89).

Pelizaeus-Merzbacher disease: X-linked, early onset, long course, islands of preserved myelin in demyelinated areas (see Chapter 94).

Childhood ataxia with central hypomyelination (CACH, or vanishing white matter disease).

Unclassified leukodystrophies: orthochromatic or sudanophilic.

MUCOPOLYSACCHARIDOSES (MPS)

Defined by characteristic phenotype, tissue storage, and urinary excretion of acid mucopolysaccharide (Table 84.3). Lack lysosomal hydrolase required for degradation of one or more of three sulfated mucopolysaccharides: dermatan sulfate, heparan sulfate, keratan sulfate.

Screening test: urine glycosaminoglycans (GAG). Confirm diagnosis by enzyme analysis (leukocytes or fibroblasts).

Hurler syndrome (MPS IH): most severe mucopolysaccharidosis. Onset in infancy; fatal before age 10 years.

Hunter syndrome (MPS II): x-linked. Similar to Hurler syndrome; no corneal clouding.

Sanfilippo syndrome (MPS III): prominent dementia, mild somatic involvement. Also spastic quadriparesis, tetraballism, athetosis, incontinence, seizures.

Morquio syndrome (MPS IV): severe skeletal disorder, little neurologic abnormality, urinary excretion of keratan sulfate in type A. Type B: excess urinary oligosaccharides as well.

Maroteaux-Lamy syndrome (MPS VI): prominent skeletal disease, normal intelligence, dermatan sulfate in urine.

MUCOLIPIDOSES

Resemble Hurler phenotype; excess urinary oligosaccharides or glycopeptides (Table 84.4). Screening test: urinary thin-layer chromatography for oligosaccharides (urine).

CHAPTER 85 ■ DISORDERS OF CARBOHYDRATE METABOLISM

GLYCOGEN STORAGE DISEASES

Abnormal metabolism of glycogen, glucose. Due to specific enzyme deficiency (Table 85.1). May present with: fasting hypoglycemia, pathologic glycogen storage (e.g., hepatomegaly), or organ dysfunction (e.g., liver disease, myopathy).

TABLE 85.1

SELECTED GLYCOGEN STORAGE DISEASES

Disease	Affected tissues	Mode of transmission	Clinical presentation
Glucose-6-phosphatase deficiency (Type I, von Gierke)	Liver, kidney	AR	Severe hypoglycemia; hepatomegaly
Infantile acid maltase deficiency (Type II, Pompe)	Generalized	AR	Lethal infantile neuromyopathy: severe cardiomyopathy, hypotonia, respiratory failure, death <1 year.
Acid maltase deficiency, juvenile/adult	Generalized	AR	Slowly progressive myopathy; often with respiratory insufficiency
Debrancher enzyme deficiency (Type III, Cori/Forbes)	Generalized	AR	Hepatomegaly; fasting hypoglycemia; limb weakness
Branching enzyme deficiency (Type IV, Andersen)	Generalized	AR	Hepatosplenomegaly; liver cirrhosis; liver failure
Muscle phosphorylase deficiency (Type V, McArdle)	Skeletal muscle	AR	Exercise-induced myalgia, cramps; myoglobinuria
Phosphoglycerate kinase (PGK) deficiency	Generalized	XR	Variable: hemolytic anemia; seizures; mental retardation; exercise intolerance; myoglobinuria
Glycogen synthetase deficiency	Liver	AR	Severe fasting hypoglycemia with ketosis

AR, autosomal recessive; XR, X-linked recessive.

LAFORA DISEASE AND OTHER POLYGLUCOSAN STORAGE DISEASES

LAFORA DISEASE

Myoclonus epilepsy with Lafora bodies within neurons of cortex, basal ganglia, dentate nucleus. Autosomal recessive.

Clinical features: triad of epilepsy, myoclonus, dementia. Inconstant features: ataxia, dysarthria, spasticity, rigidity. Onset: adolescence; death by age 24 in 90%.

EEG: bilaterally synchronous wave-and-spike formations with myoclonic jerks.

Pathology: Lafora bodies in CNS (round, basophilic, strongly periodic acid-Schiff–positive intracellular inclusions of highly variable size).

Treatment: symptomatic; suppress seizures, reduce myoclonus; benzodiazepines sometimes help.

ADULT POLYGLUCOSAN BODY DISEASE

Progressive upper and lower motor neuron signs plus sensory loss, sphincter problems, neurogenic bladder. Dementia in 50%. No myoclonus or epilepsy. Onset age 40 to 60; duration 3 to 20 years.

Electrophysiologic evidence of axonal neuropathy. Clinically may simulate ALS. Polyglucosan bodies present throughout CNS.

CHAPTER 86 ■ GLUCOSE TRANSPORTER TYPE 1 DEFICIENCY SYNDROME

Clinical features: usual presentation is with seizures in early infancy. Variable features: delayed motor development, microcephaly, ataxia, hypotonia, spasticity. Isolated mental retardation or choreoathetosis may occur. All patients have low CSF glucose (with normal blood glucose) and low-normal to low CSF lactate.

Pathogenesis: insufficiency of glucose-transporter-1 (GLUT1), which facilitates diffusion of glucose across blood-brain barrier.

Treatment: ketogenic diet controls seizures but less effective for cognition, behavior. Antiepileptic drugs ineffective. Thioctic acid may facilitate glucose transport.

CHAPTER 87 ■ DISORDERS OF DNA MAINTENANCE, TRANSCRIPTION, AND TRANSLATION

May be caused by abnormality in: (1) DNA repair following exposure to mutagens (nucleotide excision repair); (2) DNA duplication and transcription, (3) RNA splicing and translation; (4) cell cycle regulation.

Characteristic clinical features: neurodegeneration, impaired growth, premature aging, propensity to develop malignancies.

Specific conditions listed in Table 87.1.

TABLE 87.1

CLINICAL FEATURES OF SELECTED DISORDERS OF DNA SYNTHESIS, MAINTENANCE, TRANSCRIPTION AND TRANSLATION

Disorder	Inheritance	Specific features
DNA Maintenance and Transcription		
Cockayne syndrome, Type 1	AR	Mental retardation, accelerated aging, marked growth retardation, pigmentary retinopathy, optic atrophy, deafness, marble epiphyses, photosensitivity, calcification of basal ganglia, cerebellum.
Cerebro-oculofacioskeletal (COFS) syndrome	AR	Microcephaly, microphthalmia, cataracts, dysmorphism, failure to thrive, recurrent pneumonias, axial hypotonia, limb hypertonia, hyperreflexia, progressive contractures. Calcification in periventricular frontal white matter, basal ganglia.
Progeria	AR	Short stature, failure to thrive; accelerated aging, with loss of scalp hair and subcutaneous fat, joint stiffness, strokes, myocardial infarcts (due to early atherosclerosis), premature death. Cognition spared.
Xeroderma pigmentosum (including de Sanctis-Cacchione syndrome)	AR	Mental retardation, short stature, facial freckles, spasticity, hypogonadism, olivopontocerebellar atrophy.

(*continued*)

TABLE 87.1

CLINICAL FEATURES OF SELECTED DISORDERS OF DNA SYNTHESIS, MAINTENANCE, TRANSCRIPTION AND TRANSLATION (*Continued*)

Disorder	Inheritance	Specific features
Trichothiodystrophy (TTD 1)	AR	Mental retardation, hair shaft abnormalities, ichthyosis, immature sexual development, short stature, facial dysmorphism
Rett syndrome	X-linked	Classic phenotype restricted to females. Normal development for first six months, followed by acquired microcephaly, loss of hand skills and replacement by stereotypies, regression of skills, seizures, spasticity, scoliosis
Spinal muscular atrophy 1, 2, 3	AR	Loss of anterior horn cells; limb weakness, loss of tendon jerks; visible fasciculation may be limited to tongue in infantile type 1.
DNA Translation and Post-translational Modification		
CACH, Cree leukoencephalopathy, ovarioleukodystrophy	AR	Slowly progressive ataxia with diffuse loss of white matter. Episodes of coma with fever, minor trauma
Congenital disorder of glycosylation 1a (CDG 1a)	AR	Mental retardation, short stature, progressive ataxia, peripheral neuropathy, stroke-like episodes, seizures, immune dysfunction, intermittent hepatic failure, coagulopathies

TABLE 87.1

CLINICAL FEATURES OF SELECTED DISORDERS OF DNA SYNTHESIS, MAINTENANCE, TRANSCRIPTION AND TRANSLATION (*Continued*)

Disorder	Inheritance	Specific features
Cell Cycle Regulation		
Angelman syndrome	Multiple mechanisms (see Ch 81)	Psychomotor retardation, ataxia, hypotonia, epilepsy, absence of speech, large mandible, tongue thrusting. Optic atrophy, albinism in some.
Ataxia telangiectasia	AR	Progressive ataxia, choreoathetosis, anterior horn cell loss, immune deficiency, scleral telangiectasia.
Seckel syndrome 1	AR	Short stature, dysmorphism (congenital microcephaly, mental retardation. No immune deficiency or cancers.

CACH, childhood ataxia with CNS hypomyelinization (formerly vanishing white matter disease).

CHAPTER 88 ■
HYPERAMMONEMIA

Causes of high blood ammonia levels: Table 88.1. Differential diagnosis differs according to age of patient.

NEONATAL PERIOD

Transient hyperammonemia of newborn: occurs in some otherwise well premature infants; attributed to metabolic immaturity. Mild, reversible; rarely requires treatment.

In sick neonate with marked hyperammonemia, suspect inborn error of metabolism. Symptoms of hyperammonemia nonspecific: lethargy, vomiting, poor feeding, apneic episodes, seizures. Diagnosis guided by timing of symptom onset (Table 88.1); presence of lactic acidosis (impaired pyruvate metabolism) or ketoacidosis (organic acidurias). Urea cycle defects: respiratory alkalosis with hyperventilation classic finding.

Urea cycle defects (Table 88.2): similar clinical syndromes, except older onset for arginase deficiency. Plasma citrulline and urinary orotic acid levels help rapid determination of site of block (Table 88.2). All autosomal recessive except X-linked ornithine carbamyl transferase deficiency.

MANAGEMENT OF NEONATAL HYPERAMMONEMIA

Outcome worse with higher levels, longer duration hyperammonemia. Acute hyperammonemic coma in newborn a medical emergency.

Treatment: peritoneal dialysis (most effective); exchange transfusion; hemodialysis. Adjuncts: intravenous sodium benzoate; supplemental arginine; temporary elimination of protein from diet.

TABLE 88.1

MAJOR CAUSES OF HYPERAMMONEMIA

Newborn Period
Asymptomatic infant
  Transient hyperammonemia of the newborn
Asymptomatic at birth; symptomatic after 24–72 h protein
  feeding
  Organic acidurias
    Methylmalonicacidemia
    Propionicacidemia
    Isovalericacidemia
    Multiple carboxylase (biotinidase) deficiency
    Others
  Urea cycle defects other than arginase deficiency
Symptomatic at birth or within first day of life
  Asphyxia
  Congenital hepatic disease
  Congenital lactic acidosis
    Pyruvate dehydrogenase deficiency
    Pyruvate carboxylase deficiency (type B)
  Glutaricaciduria, type II
  Short-chain acyl-CoA dehydrogenase deficiency

Older Child and Adult
Primary metabolic disease
  Urea cycle defects
    Incomplete blocks (i.e., ornithine carbamoyltransferase
      deficiency heterozygotes)
    Arginase deficiency
  Dibasic aminoacidurias
    Lysinuric protein intolerance
    Hyperornithinemic states
    Partial defect of ornithine decarboxylase
      (hyperammonemia-hyperornithinemia-
      homocitrullinuria [HHH syndrome])
    Deficiency of ornithine-ketoacid aminotransferase
    Partial
    Severe—associated with gyrate atrophy of the retina
  Primary carnitine deficiency
Liver disease
Drugs
  Valproic acid
  Salicylates
  Others

TABLE 88.2

PLASMA CITRULLINE AND URINARY OROTIC ACID
FINDINGS IN UREA CYCLE DEFECTS

Enzymatic deficiency	Citrulline	Orotic acid
Carbamoyl phosphate synthetase (CPS)	0 to trace	↓
Ornithine carbamoyl transferase (OTC)	0 to trace	↑ ↑
Argininosuccinate synthase (citrullinuria)	↑↑	↑
Argininosuccinase (argininosuccinic aciduria)	↑	Nl
Arginase	Nl	↑
Transient hyperammonemia of newborn	Nl or Sl ↑	Nl

Nl, normal in plasma and urine; ↑, increased in plasma and
urine; ↓, decreased in plasma and urine; sl, slight.
(Modified from Batshaw ML, Brusilow SW, Waber L, et al.
Treatment of inborn errors of urea synthesis: activation of
alternative pathways of waste nitrogen synthesis and excretion.
N Engl J Med 1982;306:1387–1392.)

OLDER CHILDREN AND ADULTS

Most common causes: severe liver disease; drug-induced.

Valproate-associated hyperammonemia: silent, dose-related;
may occur without hepatic dysfunction. If symptomatic,
lethargy, encephalopathy. May prevent by supplementary
L-carnitine.

CHAPTER 89 ■ PEROXISOMAL DISEASES: ADRENOLEUKODYSTROPHY, ZELLWEGER SYNDROME, REFSUM DISEASE

Peroxisomal functions: degrade very long chain fatty acids (VLCFA); initiate synthesis of plasmalogens (myelin sheath lipids).

CLASSIFICATION

Peroxisome biogenesis disorders: abnormalities in more than one metabolic pathway (Table 89.1). Two phenotype groups: (a) Zellweger spectrum (decreased plasmalogens, increased VLCFA); (b) rhizomelic chondrodysplasia punctata (decreased plasmalogens but normal VLCFA degradation).

Single peroxisomal enzyme disorders: single enzyme defects (Table 89.1).

ZELLWEGER SYNDROME (CEREBROHEPATORENAL SYNDROME)

Autosomal recessive. Myelination severely abnormal.

Clinical features: severe neonatal hypotonia; absent Moro, stepping, placing reflexes; poor suck, swallow; absent or decreased tendon reflexes; seizures. Characteristic facial, ophthalmologic, genital, skeletal anomalies. Liver cirrhotic, enlarged or shrunken. Cystic dysplasia of kidneys sometimes. Most succumb within first few months of life.

Laboratory findings: elevated bilirubin levels, abnormal liver function tests, elevated serum iron. VLCFA increased in plasma, fibroblasts, chorionic villus. Increased content of intermediates of bile acid metabolism in plasma, urine. Decreased plasmalogen levels.

TABLE 89.1

HUMAN GENETIC DISEASES CAUSED BY PEROXISOMAL DYSFUNCTION

Peroxisomal biogenesis disorders	Single peroxisomal enzyme disorders
Zellweger spectrum: Zellweger syndrome	X-linked ALD Oxidase deficiency (pseudoneonatal ALD)
Neonatal ALD	Bifunctional enzyme deficiency
Infantile Refsum disease	Thiolase deficiency (pseudo-Zellweger)
Hyperpipecolicacidemia	DHAP acyltransferase deficiency
Rhizomelic chondrodysplasia punctata	Alkyl-DHAP synthase deficiency
	Glutaric aciduria type III (1 case only)
	Refsum disease
	Hyperoxaluria type I
	Acatalasia

ALD, adrenoleukodystrophy.

MRI: poor myelination, brain atrophy, pachygyria, polymicrogyria, neuronal heterotopia.

Pathology: absence of functional peroxisomes in hepatocytes.

ADRENOLEUKODYSTROPHY (ALD)

X-linked, incompletely recessive disorder; variable expressivity.

Childhood cerebral form: most common phenotype. Normal early development, then behavioral change; dementia. Visual loss with optic atrophy, spares outer retina. Progressive gait disturbance, pyramidal tract signs. Seizures common late in disease. Sometimes overt signs of adrenal failure. Death from adrenal crisis or other causes 1 to 10 years after onset.

Adrenomyeloneuropathy: spastic paraparesis, peripheral neuropathy, adrenal insufficiency, begins in second decade. Similar syndrome affects 15% of women heterozygous for ALD mutation.

Adult forms: variable phenotypes; dementia, schizophrenia, focal cerebral syndromes, spastic paraparesis, cerebellar dysfunction, or olivopontocerebellar atrophy. May have adrenal insufficiency without neurologic disorder. Female heterozygotes may become symptomatic with adult ALD. Phenotypic heterogeneity within families common.

Laboratory findings: Plasma: elevated VLCFA levels (confirm diagnosis with elevated VLCFA in cultured skin fibroblasts also). CSF: protein often elevated. CT: characteristic hyperdense and hypodense band-like regions in parietooccipital white matter. MRI: more diffuse abnormalities. Adrenal function tests: adrenal insufficiency even if no clinical signs.

Treatment: steroid replacement for adrenal insufficiency, increased during stressful periods. Bone marrow transplantation cures biochemical defect, but has high morbidity/mortality and does not cause neurologic or radiologic abnormalities to revert; may be considered if diagnosis made early.

REFSUM DISEASE

Autosomal recessive. Stored lipid (phytanic acid) exclusively dietary in origin.

Clinical features: onset: early childhood to fifth decade. Progressive night blindness, then limb weakness, gait ataxia. Abrupt exacerbations and gradual remissions may occur with intercurrent illness or pregnancy. Other findings: pigmentary retinopathy, peripheral neuropathy, ichthyosis, nerve deafness, cataracts, miosis, pupillary asymmetry, pes cavus, bone deformities. Sometimes sudden death from cardiac arrhythmia.

Laboratory findings: CSF protein elevated. Nerve conduction velocities slow. ECG: conduction abnormalities.

Diagnosis: clinical picture; high phytanic acid levels in plasma.

Treatment: limit dietary phytanic acid and precursor, phytol.

CHAPTER 90 ■ ORGANIC ACIDURIAS

Inborn errors of metabolism leading to accumulation of organic acids. As a group, common cause of infantile encephalopathy due to inherited metabolic diseases.

Rapid diagnosis crucial: some curable; in others, metabolic attacks preventable.

Most common organic acidurias involve two principal biochemical pathways: (a) degradation of amino acids; (b) β-oxidation of fatty acids. Lactic acidemia another cause of organic aciduria; usually pyruvate dehydrogenase deficiency or respiratory chain defect (see Chapter 98).

CLINICAL FEATURES

Neonatal acute encephalopathy: signs and symptoms usually nonspecific: vomiting, hypotonia, drowsiness, coma, multisystem failure.

Chronic (infancy/early childhood, through adulthood): (a) intermittent: recurrent episodes of metabolic acidosis, coma, focal neurologic signs; or (b) progressive: poor growth, chronic vomiting, macrocephaly, impaired psychomotor development, hypotonia, dystonia, spastic tetraplegia, intractable seizures.

Early-onset forms tend to be lethal; late-onset forms more benign.

DIAGNOSIS

Hypoglycemia, metabolic acidosis, hyperammonemia suggest organic aciduria. Acute hypoglycemia may be fatal.

Screening tests include urine organic acids, plasma amino acids, plasma carnitine, acylcarnitines. Definite diagnosis: specific metabolites; enzyme assays.

Organic acidurias causing acute encephalopathy include: multiple carboxylase deficiency, maple syrup urine disease (MSUD), methylmalonic aciduria (MMA), propionic aciduria, isovaleric aciduria, fumaric aciduria, glutaric aciduria type I and type II, methylcrotonic aciduria, hydroxymethylglutaric aciduria, dicarboxylic acidurias, 3-hydroxydicarboxylic aciduria.

CLINICAL CLUES IN CHRONIC FORMS

Mental retardation, ataxia, behavioral changes: MSUD, 4-hydroxybutyric aciduria.

Spasticity, ataxia, mental retardation, seizures: L-2–hydroxyglutaric aciduria.

Severe hypotonia, epilepsy, spastic tetraparesis, early death: fumaric aciduria.

Dystonia, spasticity, often normal intellectual development: glutaric aciduria type I.

Choreoathetosis, dystonic posture: 3-hydroxy-3-methylglutaric aciduria.

Mental retardation, movement disorder, osteoporosis, progressive renal failure: MMA.

Seizures, ataxia, alopecia, rash: multiple carboxylase deficiency.

Ataxia, optic atrophy, retinitis pigmentosa: 3-methylglutaconic aciduria.

Infantile spinal muscular atrophy with mental retardation: 3-methylcrotonic aciduria.

Lipid myopathy, cardiomyopathy: carnitine translocase deficiency, mitochondrial trifunctional protein deficiency, very-long-chain acyl-CoA dehydrogenase deficiency, riboflavin-responsive form of glutaric aciduria type II.

THERAPY

Dietary replacement: biotin (multiple carboxylase deficiency), vitamin B12 (methylmalonic aciduria), riboflavin (glutaric aciduria type II).

Dietary restriction: leucine, valine, isoleucine (MSUD); leucine (3-hydroxymethylglutaric aciduria); isoleucine, valine, threonine, methionine (propionic and methylmalonic aciduria); lysine, tryptophan (glutaric aciduria type I).

CHAPTER 91 ■ DISORDERS OF METAL METABOLISM

HEPATOLENTICULAR DEGENERATION (WILSON DISEASE)

Inborn error of copper metabolism; with liver cirrhosis, basal ganglia degeneration. Worldwide prevalence: 30 per 1 million.

PATHOGENESIS AND PATHOLOGY

Autosomal recessive. Gene (chromosome 13) encodes copper transporting protein. Numerous mutations with variable symptom onset, severity.

Fundamental defects: reduced biliary copper transport; impaired formation of plasma ceruloplasmin. Other findings: increased free copper in serum; low to low-normal plasma iron-binding globulin; persistent aminoaciduria (toxic effect of metal on renal tubules).

Copper abnormalities lead to accumulation of copper in liver (cirrhosis), brain (especially basal ganglia), kidney, cornea (Kayser-Fleischer ring).

SYMPTOMS AND SIGNS

Progressive disease, sometimes with temporary clinical arrest or improvement. Symptom onset usually between ages 11 and 25 years.

Ascites, jaundice, esophageal bleeding, other signs of liver damage at any stage.

Neurologic manifestations vary: no characteristic clinical picture. Most common early signs: tremor (often localized to arms; "wing-beating" type), rigidity, psychiatric syndromes. Other findings: dystonia, spasticity of laryngeal or pharyngeal muscles, drooping lower jaw, excess salivation, convulsions, characteristic fixed open-mouth smile.

Tendon reflexes increased; plantar responses almost always flexor. Seizures, usually after starting treatment.

Kayser-Fleischer rings in 75% of patients with hepatic symptoms and 100% those with cerebral symptoms, with or without hepatic symptoms. Never seen before age 7 years.

DIAGNOSIS

Absence of Kayser-Fleischer ring with slit lamp examination in untreated patient with neurologic symptoms rules out diagnosis.

Low serum ceruloplasmin (96% of patients), elevated urinary copper support diagnosis.

Liver biopsy: increased hepatic copper.

MRI: ventricular dilation, diffuse atrophy of cortex, cerebellum, brainstem. Abnormal signal in basal ganglia (putamen, thalamus, head of caudate and globus pallidus).

TREATMENT

Symptomatic and asymptomatic patients require treatment. Homozygotes treated preventively.

Treatment divided into two phases: (1) chelation therapy to control toxic copper levels; (2) maintenance therapy to reduce intestinal copper absorption.

Chelators: ammonium tetrathiomolybdate (60–300 mg/day in 6 divided doses); triethylene tetramine dihydrochloride (trientine).

Zinc acetate: optimum drug for maintenance therapy or treatment of presymptomatic patient.

Neurologic symptoms start to improve 5–6 months after initiation of therapy. Life expectancy normal for patients who complete first few years of treatment.

MENKES DISEASE (KINKY-HAIR DISEASE)

Focal degenerative disorder of gray matter. Incidence: 2 in 100,000 male live births.

PATHOGENESIS AND PATHOLOGY

X-linked. Defect in copper transporter (different from that of Wilson disease), resulting in maldistribution of body copper (low levels in liver and brain, elevated in intestinal mucosa and kidney) and deficient synthesis of several copper-containing enzymes.

CNS pathology: extensive focal degeneration of cortical gray matter in hemispheres and cerebellum.

SYMPTOMS AND SIGNS

Symptoms in neonatal period: hypothermia, poor feeding, impaired weight gain most common. Seizures and progressive deterioration of all neurologic functions follow. Hair colorless, friable. Abnormalities of cerebral and systemic arteries, long bones. Subdural effusions.

DIAGNOSIS

Serum ceruloplasmin and copper levels fail to rise to normal levels at age 1 month.

TREATMENT

Early treatment with copper-histidine beneficial, but does not prevent all complications of disease.

OTHER DISORDERS OF METAL METABOLISM

ACERULOPLASMINEMIA

Autosomal recessive, adult-onset. Complete absence of ceruloplasmin, leading to iron accumulation and neuronal degeneration in basal ganglia, dentate nucleus.

Clinical features: diabetes mellitus, dementia, extrapyramidal symptoms, ataxia, retinal degeneration. Early treatment with desferrioxamine (iron chelator) prevents disease progression.

MOLYBDENUM COFACTOR DEFICIENCY

Autosomal recessive; results in deficiency of molybdenum-containing cofactor essential to function of sulfite oxidase, xanthine dehydrogenase, aldehyde oxidase.

Clinical features: neonatal or infantile seizures, craniofacial dysmorphism, feeding difficulties, dislocation of lens. Diagnosis: increased urinary sulfites, low blood urate. No specific treatment available.

CHAPTER 92 ■ ACUTE INTERMITTENT PORPHYRIA

Neurologic manifestations in two classes: acute intermittent porphyria (AIP) and variegate porphyria. Both autosomal dominant, low penetrance. Prevalence worldwide approximately 1:100,000. More common in women than men. Symptom onset usually in adolescents or young adults.

PATHOGENESIS

Exact nature of abnormality of heme biosynthesis unclear in AIP. Proposed block in porphobilinogen (PBG) deaminase activity in AIP; protoporphyrinogen oxidase in variegate form. Excessive urinary excretion of PBG, δ-aminolevulinic acid (ALA), several porphyrins.

Symptoms caused by interaction of genetic and environmental factors. Porphyric crises result most often from ingestion of drugs that adversely affect porphyrin metabolism (see below), especially barbiturates for sedation or general anesthesia. Attacks also attributed to menses, starvation, emotional stress, intercurrent infections, other drugs.

Pathology: No defining structural change. Electrophysiologic studies show axonal neuropathy.

SYMPTOMS AND SIGNS

Episodic attacks: gastrointestinal (autonomic neuropathy), psychiatric, neurologic. Abdominal pain most common; alone or with neurologic or psychiatric disorder (conversion reaction, acute delirium, mood change, or acute or chronic psychosis). Neuropathic symptoms sometimes purely motor but almost always associated with abdominal pain. Rash may occur in variegate form (approximately 50%) but not in AIP; otherwise clinical features are indistinguishable.

INVESTIGATIONS

Elevated levels of urinary PBG, ALA in individuals with AIP, even between attacks. Variegate form: urinary porphyrins abnormal during acute episodes only. Most reliable test for AIP: assay PBG-deaminase in red blood cell membranes (values 50% of normal diagnostic). DNA mutation analysis available (gene on chromosome 11q).

EMG: denervation pattern; normal or slightly slow nerve conduction.

TABLE 92.1

SELECTED PORPHYROGENIC DRUGS IN
ACUTE PORPHYRIA

Barbiturates
Analgesics
Sulfonamides
Nonbarbiturate hypnotics
Unidentified sedatives
Anticonvulsants
Hormonal

TREATMENT

Autonomic manifestations of attack reversed by propanolol. Neuropathy, abdominal symptoms respond dramatically to intravenous hematin.

Seizures: diazepam or paraldehyde for attacks. Use conventional anticonvulsants cautiously between attacks (may precipitate attack), monitor urinary excretion of ALA, PBG. Gabapentin seems to be safe and effective.

Other drugs for symptomatic relief: codeine, meperidine for pain, chlorpromazine, other psychoactive drugs. Most antibiotics safe.

Major drugs to avoid: barbiturates in any form. Other drugs requiring caution listed in Table 92.1. Patients should wear warning bracelets to identify drug hazards for treatment of trauma, other emergencies.

CHAPTER 93 ■ NEUROLOGIC SYNDROMES WITH ACANTHOCYTES

Acanthocytes ("thorny" erythrocytes) seen in three hereditary neurologic syndromes: abetalipoproteinemia, neuroacanthocytosis, McLeod syndrome.

ABETALIPOPROTEINEMIA (BASSEN-KORNZWEIG SYNDROME)

Autosomal recessive; inability of liver and intestine to secrete apolipoprotein B. Mutations in microsomal transfer triglyceride protein. Lipid malabsorption leads to: (a) demyelination (especially posterior columns, spinocerebellar tracts, corticospinal tracts); (b) abnormalities in cerebellum, peripheral nerve axons; (c) deficiency of fat-soluble vitamins (A, D, E, K).

SYMPTOMS AND SIGNS

Fatty diarrhea with growth retardation from infancy. First neurologic sign: loss of tendon reflexes around age 5 years. Age 10 years: ataxic gait, then limb ataxia; tremor of head, hands; sensorimotor neuropathy; progressive external ophthalmoplegia. Adolescence: retinitis pigmentosa (night-blindness, constricted visual fields, decreased visual acuity). Bleeding diathesis (vitamin K deficiency).

INVESTIGATIONS

Serum: low cholesterol and triglycerides; low ESR.
EMG: axonal neuropathy. Abnormal VER and SSER. ECG abnormal, if cardiomyopathy.

DIAGNOSIS

Clinically resembles Friedreich ataxia (spinocerebellar degeneration, sensorimotor peripheral neuropathy, retinitis pigmentosa), but ophthalmoplegia is distinguishing feature. Diagnosis established by low serum cholesterol, smear for acanthocytes, reduced or absent serum β-lipoprotein and plasma lipids.

TREATMENT

Dietary supplementation with vitamin E (α-tocopherol acetate 100 mg/kg/day); vitamin K (adults). With adequate therapy, arrest progression of neurologic and retinal syndromes.

HYPOBETALIPOPROTEINEMIA

Autosomal dominant; different mutations in gene for apolipoprotein B. Heterozygotes: usually no neurologic symptoms. Homozygotes: syndrome similar to abetalipoproteinemia.

Hypobetalipoproteinemia, acanthocytosis, retinitis pigmentosa, and pallidal degeneration (*HARP syndrome*): caused by mutations in the gene encoding pantothenate kinase 2; clinical features similar to neurodegeneration with brain iron accumulation (Hallervorden-Spatz disease; see Chapter 94).

NEUROACANTHOCYTOSIS (CHOREOACANTHOCYTOSIS)

Multisystem neurodegenerative disorder with acanthocytes; normal plasma lipids, normal lipoproteins; variable neurologic manifestations.

Onset age 30 to 50; rarely juvenile or elderly onset. Usually familial, autosomal recessive.

Due to various mutations on CHAC (choreaacanthocytosis) gene on chromosome 9, encoding chorein.

Clinical features: hyperkinetic movement disorder (chorea, orofacial dyskinesias, dystonia, tics), psychiatric symptoms, progressive dementia, seizures, axonal neuropathy. Characteristic feeding dystonia (tongue pushes food out of mouth), lip and tongue biting.

MRI: caudate atrophy, increased striatal T2 signal.

Treatment limited to symptom control.

McLEOD SYNDROME

X-linked, abnormal expression of Kell blood group antigens, absence of Kx erythrocyte surface antigen.

Clinical features: may be asymptomatic; some have clinical and MRI findings similar to neuroacanthocytosis. Unlike neuroacanthocytosis: chronic hemolysis, myopathy with elevated serum CK typical, some develop progressive cardiomyopathy.

CHAPTER 94 ■ CEREBRAL DEGENERATIONS OF CHILDHOOD

CANAVAN DISEASE (SPONGY DEGENERATION OF THE NERVOUS SYSTEM)

Autosomal recessive megalencephaly and neurologic degeneration. Prevalent among Ashkenazi Jews from eastern Europe and among Saudi Arabians.

Clinical features: macrocephaly, poor head control, lack of psychomotor development, spasticity, optic atrophy, seizures. Symptom onset before age 4 months in >50%. Children eventually become decerebrate, die of intercurrent illness, may survive into third decade.

CT and MRI: increased lucency of white matter, poor demarcation of gray and white matter; later, severe brain atrophy with enlarged CSF spaces.

Pathology: (a) intramyelin vacuolation (spongy degeneration) initially of deep layers of cortex, eventually diffuse; (b) giant abnormal mitochondria in superficial layers of white matter.

Diagnosis: deficiency of aspartoacylase in skin fibroblasts. Gene on chromosome 17p.

Other conditions associated with spongy degeneration of brain: intoxication by triethyltin or hexachlorophene, some neonatal acidurias, some mitochondrial disorders, Aicardi-Goutières syndrome, vanishing white matter disease.

INFANTILE NEUROAXONAL DYSTROPHY

Autosomal recessive, unknown pathophysiology.

Clinical features: symptom onset age 6–18 months with arrest of motor development, then loss of skills. Tone increased or decreased. Ataxia, nystagmus, optic atrophy, dementia common; seizures rare. Death usually by age 10.

Pathology: axonal spheroids (eosinophilic, argyrophilic, ovoid inclusions that distend axons and myelin sheaths) in brain, spinal cord, peripheral nerves. Severe cerebellar atrophy, spongy degeneration of basal ganglia.

Diagnosis: laboratory tests not helpful. Nerve, muscle, rectal, or conjunctival biopsy confirmatory when spheroids found in nerves or NMJ, but false negative results possible. Definite diagnosis at autopsy.

Treatment: symptomatic.

NEURODEGENERATION WITH BRAIN IRON ACCUMULATION (NBIA)

Previously known as Hallervorden-Spatz disease. Includes pantothenate kinase–associated neurodegeneration (PKAN), neuroferritinopathy.

PANTOTHENATE KINASE-ASSOCIATED NEURODEGENERATION (PKAN)

Autosomal recessive, progressive, predominantly motor disorder with onset in childhood or adolescence.

Clinical features: progressive extrapyramidal dysfunction: dystonia, rigidity, dysarthria, choreoathetosis. Sometimes associated spasticity due to corticospinal tract involvement; ataxia, tremor, nystagmus; pigmentary retinopathy (2/3), optic atrophy. Typically presents in first decade, rapidly progressive. Atypical forms present later, course may span decades.

MRI: hypointensity in globus pallidus on T2 images; "eye-of-the-tiger" sign: hypointensity with central region of hyperintensity.

Diagnosis: molecular genetic test: mutations in PANK2 gene found in 50% of patients with clinical features of PKAN, almost all of those with "eye-of-the-tiger" sign on MRI.

Pathology: olive or golden brown discoloration of medial globus pallidus with deposition of iron pigments. Axonal spheroids in affected tissues.

Treatment: limited to symptomatic measures.

PELIZAEUS-MERZBACHER DISEASE

Leukodystrophy; two forms: classic (infantile onset) or connatal (present at birth). Both X-linked recessive, linked to proteolipid protein gene.

Clinical features: prominent, irregular nystagmus and head-tremor in first few months of life (both forms); floppiness, head lag, gray optic discs, stridor, absent development (connatal form). Later: ataxia, spasticity, optic atrophy, seizures, microcephaly, failure to thrive. Most succumb in first years of life; others show protracted course into adolescence.

Laboratory data: nerve conduction velocities normal; CSF protein usually normal (in contrast to MLD, Krabbe disease). Imaging: ventricular dilation, decreased differentiation of gray and white matter, cerebellar atrophy, abnormal white matter signal.

Pathology: absent myelin in brainstem and cerebellar white matter (infantile form), or in brain, cerebellum, brainstem, spinal cord (connatal form). Pathologic hallmark: "tigroid" (striped) appearance of white matter on myelin stains. Peripheral nerves characteristically well myelinated.

ALEXANDER DISEASE

Most cases sporadic; due to mutations in glial fibrillary acidic protein (GFAP) gene. Familial cases autosomal dominant.

Clinical features: Three variants: *Infantile*: megalencephaly, severe motor and developmental delay, seizures, spasticity; rapidly progressive with death in vegetative state in infancy or preschool years. Optic atrophy not usually present (vs. Canavan disease). *Juvenile*: slower, prominent bulbar symptoms, usually without seizures. *Adult*: bulbar palsy, palatal tremor (formerly called palatal myoclonus) and ataxia, with or without intellectual deterioration and spasticity.

Neuroimaging: marked demyelination with frontal predominance; often, enlarged ventricles with zone of increased density in subependymal region. Basal ganglia may appear necrotic.

Pathology: rosenthal fibers (inclusions found exclusively in astrocytic footplates). Characteristically in subpial, subependymal, and perivascular locations. Demyelination in regions rich in Rosenthal fibers. Peripheral nerve myelin spared.

Treatment: symptomatic. Prenatal diagnosis available for families of affected child with identified mutation.

COCKAYNE SYNDROME

See Chapter 87.

RETT SYNDROME

X-linked dominant disorder; affects primarily girls (1:10,000–15,000); due to mutation in the methyl-CpG binding protein 2 (*MECP2*) gene on chromosome Xq28. Most cases sporadic. Rare affected males die soon after birth.

Clinical features: girls with normal birth head circumference and early development; then postnatal deceleration of brain growth occurring anytime between ages 3 months and 4 years, developmental regression, loss of purposeful hand use, continuous stereotypic hand movements, profound cognitive and language impairment, seizures. 25% become nonambulatory during regressive period. Survival into middle age common, but sudden unexplained death may occur.

Neuroimaging: decreased gray matter volume, especially frontal cortex, caudate nucleus.

Diagnosis: established clinical diagnostic criteria; analysis of MECP2 gene detects mutations in 80% of girls with classical Rett syndrome.

Treatment: limited to symptomatic measures.

Other phenotypes associated with *MECP2* mutations: X-linked nonsyndromic mental retardation; X-linked disability with progressive spasticity; Angelman-like syndrome; syndrome characterized by psychosis, pyramidal signs and macro-orchidism.

CHAPTER 95 ■ DIFFUSE SCLEROSIS

Variant of multiple sclerosis; etiology, pathogenesis unknown. Also known as Schilder disease.

Clinical syndrome: leukoencephalopathy (progressive dementia, psychosis, corticospinal signs, loss of vision, brainstem signs); onset usually in childhood.

Pathology: large areas of demyelination in centrum ovale; perivascular infiltration by lymphocytes and giant cells in acute lesions. Lesions similar to those of multiple sclerosis.

Investigations. CT: large areas of ring-enhancing lucency. MRI: gadolinium enhancement. CSF: pleocytosis with evidence of intrathecal synthesis of gamma-globulin, oligoclonal bands.

Differential diagnosis: adrenoleukodystrophy, subacute sclerosing panencephalitis, other leukoencephalopathies.

Treatment: symptomatic.

Prognosis: relentless progression; average survival 6 years.

CHAPTER 96 ■ DIFFERENTIAL DIAGNOSIS

Useful diagnostic resources include two online databases searchable by physical findings: On-Line Mendelian Inheritance in Man (OMIM, http://www.ncbi.nlm.nih.gov/omim); SimulConsult Neurological Syndromes (http://www.simulconsult.com)

Useful clues: inheritance pattern (Table 96.1), ethnic background (Table 96.2), age at onset (Table 96.3), findings on examination (Table 96.4), presence of seizures or myoclonus (Table 96.5), specific motor signs (Table 96.6), specific eye findings (Table 96.7), specific laboratory abnormalities (Table 96.8). Tissue biopsy helpful in some conditions (Table 96.9).

TABLE 96.1
PATTERN OF INHERITANCE OTHER THAN AUTOSOMAL RECESSIVE

Some X-linked recessive diseases
Adrenoleukodystrophy
Pelizaeus-Merzbacher disease
Fabry disease
Hunter syndrome (mucopolysaccharidosis II)
Ornithine transcarbamylase deficiency
Lesch-Nyhan syndrome
Leber optic atrophy
Lowe oculocerebrorenal syndrome
Trichopoliodystrophy (Menkes syndrome)
Duchenne/Becker muscular dystrophy
Norrie disease
Fragile X syndrome
X-linked cortical dysplasias
X-linked mental retardation syndromes

Some X-linked dominant diseases
Incontinentia pigmenti
Pseudo- and pseudopseudohypoparathyroidism
Rett syndrome
Aicardi syndrome
Subcortical band heterotopia

Some autosomal-dominant diseases
Neurofibromatosis

(continued)

TABLE 96.1

PATTERN OF INHERITANCE OTHER THAN AUTOSOMAL RECESSIVE (*Continued*)

Tuberous sclerosis
Von Hippel-Lindau disease
Acute intermittent porphyria
Huntington disease
Some dystonias
Dentatorubralpallidoluysian atrophy
Spinocerebellar ataxias (SCA)

Some mitochondrial cytopathies
MERRF (myoclonic epilepsy with red ragged fibers)
MELAS (mitochondrial encephalomyopathy, lactic acidosis and stroke-like episodes)
LHON (Leber hereditary optic neuropathy)
NARP (neuropathy, ataxia, and retinitis pigmentosa)
Leigh syndrome

TABLE 96.2

PREDOMINANT ETHNIC BACKGROUND IN SOME DISEASES

Ashkenazi Jewish
Classic Tay-Sachs disease
Infantile Niemann-Pick disease
Primary generalized dystonia (DYT1)
Mucolipidosis IV
Canavan disease
Dysautonomia
Juvenile non-neuronopathic Gaucher disease

Saudi Arabia
Canavan disease

Nova Scotia
Type D Niemann-Pick disease

Japan
Sialidosis with chondrodystrophy
Dentatorubralpallidoluysian atrophy

Scandinavia
Finnish ceroid lipofuscinosis (types 1,5)
Juvenile neuronopathic Gaucher disease
Krabbe disease
Aspartylglucosaminuria
Baltic myoclonus (Unverricht-Lundborg disease)

TABLE 96.3

TYPICAL AGE AT ONSET

Neonatal or early infantile onset
Aminoacidurias and organic acidurias
Urea cycle disorders
Galactosemia
Connatal Pelizaeus-Merzbacher disease
Connatal Alexander disease
Congenital sialidosis
Early-onset mitochondrial cytopathies
Canavan disease
Aicardi-Goutières syndrome
Infantile Gaucher disease
Infantile adrenoleukodystrophy
Zellweger syndrome
Neonatal adrenoleukodystrophy
Chondrodysplasia punctata
Infantile Refsum disease
GM_I gangliosidosis (infantile variant)
I-cell disease (mucolipidosis II)
Trichopoliodystrophy (Menkes)
Cerebro-oculo-facial-skeletal syndrome (COFS syndrome)
Neurocutaneous syndromes
Progressive spinal muscular atrophy (Werdnig-Hoffmann disease)
Seckel bird-headed dwarfism

Infantile onset
Aminoacidurias, organic acidurias, urea cycle disorders with partial enzyme deficiency
Many sphingolipidoses, mucopolysaccharidoses, mucolipidoses
Infantile ceroid lipofuscinosis
Leigh syndrome (early types)
Other mitochondrial cytopathies
Lesch-Nyhan syndrome
Sjögren-Larson syndrome
Canavan disease
Wolman disease
Alexander disease
Pelizaeus-Merzbacher disease
Neuroaxonal dystrophy
Alpha-N-acetylgalactosaminidase deficiency
Infantile PKAN (Hallervorden-Spatz disease)
Infantile fucosidosis
Nephrosialidosis
Sialidosis
Pompe disease
Xeroderma pigmentosum neurologic disease
Cockayne disease
Infantile galactosialidosis
Progeria
Rett syndrome

(continued)

TABLE 96.3

TYPICAL AGE AT ONSET (*Continued*)

Onset in preschool years
Aminoacidurias, organic acidurias, urea cycle disorders with
partial enzyme deficiency
Aspartylglucosaminuria
Marinesco-Sjögren syndrome
Alexander disease
Ataxia telangiectasia
Xeroderma pigmentosum neurologic disease
Chédiak-Higashi disease
Metachromatic leukodystrophy
Late infantile gangliosidoses
Niemann-Pick disease, Nova Scotia variant
Late infantile ceroid lipofuscinoses
Sanfilippo syndromes
Maroteaux-Lamy disease
Mild Hunter disease
Leigh syndrome and other mitochondrial cytopathies
Kearns-Sayre syndrome
Disintegrative psychosis
Other autistic regression
Leukodystrophy with vanishing white matter

Onset in school age or adolescence
Wilson disease
Acute intermittent porphyria
Juvenile ceroid lipofuscinosis
Adrenoleukodystrophy
Late variants of the gangliosidoses
Niemann-Pick type C disease
Sialidosis with cherry-red spot myoclonus (variants with and
without chondrodystrophy)
Fabry disease
Cerebrotendinous xanthomatosis
Leigh syndrome (some variants)
Other mitochondrial cytopathies (e.g., MERRF and MELAS
syndromes)
Refsum disease
Friedreich ataxia
Bassen-Kornzweig disease
Other spinocerebellar degenerations
Primary generalized dystonia (DYT1)
Juvenile Huntington disease
Juvenile parkinsonism
Classic Hallervorden-Spatz disease (PKAN)
Lafora disease
Baltic myoclonus
Subacute sclerosing panencephalitis (SSPE)
Cockayne disease (late variants)
Xeroderma pigmentosum neurologic disease (late variants)

TABLE 96.4

HELPFUL CLUES IN THE PHYSICAL EXAMINATION

Big head
Tay-Sachs disease
Alexander disease
Canavan disease
Hurler disease
Glutaric aciduria type 1
Other mucopolysaccharidoses with hydrocephalus
Leukodystrophy with subcortical cysts

Small head
Krabbe disease
Infantile ceroid lipofuscinosis
Some infantile mitochondrial cytopathies
Neuroaxonal dystrophy
Incontinentia pigmenti
Cockayne disease
Rett syndrome
Seckel bird-headed dwarfism
Chromosomal abnormalities

Hair abnormalities
Stiff, wiry
    Trichopoliodystrophy (Menkes)
Frizzy
    Giant axonal neuropathy
Hirsutism
    Infantile GM_1 gangliosidosis
    Hurler, Hunter, Sanfilippo syndromes
    I-cell disease
Gray
    Ataxia telangiectasia
    Cockayne disease
    Chédiak-Higashi disease
    Progeria

Skin abnormalities
Telangiectasia
    Ataxia telangiectasia
Angiokeratoma
    Fabry disease
    Juvenile fucosidosis
    Galactosialidosis
    Adult-onset Alpha-N-acetylgalactosaminidase deficiency
Ichthyosis
    Refsum disease
    Sjögren-Larsson syndrome
Hypopigmentation
    Trichopoliodystrophy (Menkes)
    Chédiak-Higashi syndrome
    Tuberous sclerosis (ash-leaf spots)
    Hypomelanosis of Ito

(*continued*)

TABLE 96.4

HELPFUL CLUES IN THE PHYSICAL EXAMINATION
(*Continued*)

Prader-Willi syndrome
Phenylketonuria
Hyperpigmentation
   Niemann-Pick disease
   Adrenoleukodystrophy
   Farber disease
   Neurofibromatosis (café-au-lait spots)
   Xeroderma pigmentosum neurologic disease
   Incontinentia pigmenti
Thin atrophic skin
   Ataxia telangiectasia
   Cockayne disease
   Xeroderma pigmentosum neurologic disease
   Progeria
Thick skin
   I-cell disease
   Mucopolysaccharidoses I, II, III
   Infantile fucosidosis
Subcutaneous nodules
   Farber disease
   Neurofibromatosis
   Cerebrotendinous xanthomatosis
Xanthomas
   Niemann-Pick disease
Blotching
   Dysautonomia

Enlarged nodes
Farber disease
Niemann-Pick disease
Juvenile Gaucher disease
Chédiak-Higashi disease
Ataxia telangiectasia (lymphoma)

Stridor, hoarseness
Infantile-onset peroxisomal disorders
Farber disease
Infantile Gaucher disease
Connatal Pelizaeus-Merzbacher disease

Enlarged orange tonsils
Tangier disease

Severe swallowing problems
(Present late in the course of all patients with severe bulbar, pseudobulbar, cerebellar, or basal ganglia pathology)
Infantile Gaucher disease
Dysautonomia
Hallervorden-Spatz disease (PKAN)
Primary generalized dystonia (DYT1)
Zellweger syndrome

(*continued*)

TABLE 96.4

HELPFUL CLUES IN THE PHYSICAL EXAMINATION
(*Continued*)

Heart abnormalities
Pompe disease
Hurler disease and other mucopolysaccharidoses
Fabry disease
Infantile fucosidosis
Refsum disease
Friedreich ataxia
Abetalipoproteinemia (Bassen-Kornzweig disease)
Tuberous sclerosis
Progeria
Zellweger syndrome
Disorders of carnitine metabolism
Duchenne muscular dystrophy
Kearns-Sayre syndrome

Strokes
Fabry disease
Trichopoliodystrophy (Menkes)
Progeria
MELAS syndrome
Homocystinuria
Sickle-cell diseases

Organomegaly
Mucopolysaccharidoses (most types)
Infantile GM_1 gangliosidosis
Niemann-Pick disease
Gaucher disease
Generalized peroxisomal disorders
Galactosemia
Pompe disease
Mannosidosis

Gastrointestinal problems
Malabsorption
    Wolman disease
    Bassen-Kornzweig disease
Nonfunctioning gallbladder
    Metachromatic leukodystrophy
    Infantile fucosidosis
Jaundice
    Zellweger disease
    Galactosemia
    Niemann-Pick disease
Vomiting
    Dysautonomia
    Urea cycle defects
Diarrhea
    Hunter syndrome

(*continued*)

TABLE 96.4

HELPFUL CLUES IN THE PHYSICAL EXAMINATION
(*Continued*)

Dysmotility
   Mitochondrial neurogastrointestinal
     encephalomyopathy (MNGIE)

Kidney problems
Renal failure
   Fabry disease
   Nephrosialidosis
   Some mitochondrial cytopathies
Cysts
   Zellweger syndrome
   Von Hippel-Lindau disease
   Tuberous sclerosis
   Neonatal olivopontocerebellar atrophy (OPCA)
   Joubert syndrome
Stones
   Lesch-Nyhan disease
   Aminoacidurias
   Lowe syndrome
   Wilson disease

Bone and joint abnormalities
Stiff joints
   Mucopolysaccharidoses (all but type I–S)
   Mucolipidoses (most types)
   Fucosidosis
   Farber disease
   Sialidoses (some forms)
   Zellweger syndrome
   Rhizomelic chondrodysplasia punctata
   Cockayne disease
Scoliosis
   Friedreich ataxia
   Ataxia telangiectasia
   Primary generalized dystonia (DYT1)
   All chronic diseases with muscle weakness
   Rett syndrome
Kyphosis
   Mucopolysaccharidoses

Endocrine dysfunction
Adrenals
   Adrenoleukodystrophy
   Wolman disease
Hypogonadism
   Xeroderma pigmentosum neurologic disease
   Ataxia telangiectasia
   Some spinocerebellar degenerations
Diabetes
   Ataxia telangiectasia

(continued)

TABLE 96.4

HELPFUL CLUES IN THE PHYSICAL EXAMINATION
(*Continued*)

Dwarfing
  Morquio disease
  Other mucopolysaccharidoses
  Cockayne syndrome
  Progeria
  Diseases with severe malnutrition
Hypothalamic dysfunction
  De Sanctis-Cacchione syndrome

Neoplasms
Ataxia telangiectasia
Xeroderma pigmentosum neurologic disease
Neurofibromatosis
Von Hippel-Lindau disease
Tuberous sclerosis

Hearing loss
Hunter disease
Other mucopolysaccharidoses
Generalized peroxisomal disorders
Refsum disease
Cockayne disease
Kearns-Sayre and Leigh syndromes
Other mitochondrial cytopathies
Some spinocerebellar degenerations
Usher syndrome
Olivopontocerebellar atrophy

TABLE 96.5

DISEASES WITH PROMINENT SEIZURES OR MYOCLONUS

Pyridoxine dependency
Acute intermittent porphyria
Gangliosidoses (infantile especially)
Ceroid lipofuscinoses (late infantile variant especially)
MERRF and MELAS syndromes
Glucose transporter protein deficiency syndrome (GLUT1)
Trichopoliodystrophy (Menkes)
Zellweger syndrome
Generalized peroxisomal disorders
Infantile Alexander disease
Krabbe disease
Lafora disease
Baltic myoclonus
Sanfilippo disease
Juvenile Huntington disease
Tuberous sclerosis
Juvenile neuronopathic Gaucher disease
Subacute sclerosing panencephalitis

TABLE 96.6
MOTOR SIGNS HELPFUL TO DIAGNOSIS

Floppiness in infancy
Progressive spinal muscular atrophy
Congenital myopathies
Zellweger syndrome
Pompe disease
Trichopoliodystrophy
Neuroaxonal dystrophy
Gangliosidoses (early variants)
Fucosidosis (infantile variant)
Infantile ceroid lipofuscinosis
Canavan disease
Leigh syndrome (early variant)
Neonatal OPCA

Peripheral neuropathy
Acute intermittent porphyria
Metachromatic leukodystrophy
Fabry disease
Krabbe disease
Neuroaxonal dystrophy
Refsum disease
Tangier disease
Bassen-Kornzweig disease
Sialidosis (some variants)
Mucolipidosis III
Cerebrotendinous xanthomatosis
Ataxia telangiectasia
Adrenomyeloneuropathy
Mucopolysaccharidoses I, II, VI, VII (entrapment)
Cockayne syndrome (demyelinating)
Xeroderma pigmentosum neurologic disease (axonal)
Some mitochondrial cytopathies
Giant axonal neuropathy

Prominent cerebellar signs
Wilson disease
Late infantile ceroid lipofuscinosis
Pelizaeus-Merzbacher disease
Neuroaxonal dystrophy
Metachromatic leukodystrophy
Ataxia telangiectasia
Leigh syndrome
Niemann-Pick disease type C
Some late-onset gangliosidoses
Some sialidoses
Friedreich ataxia
Bassen-Kornzweig disease
Cerebrotendinous xanthomatosis
Spinocerebellar ataxias (SCAs)

(*continued*)

TABLE 96.6

MOTOR SIGNS HELPFUL TO DIAGNOSIS *(Continued)*

Lafora disease
Baltic myoclonus
Chédiak-Higashi disease
Usher syndrome
Neonatal OPCA
De Sanctis-Cacchione syndrome
Phosphomannomutase deficiency (CDG-Ia)

Abnormal posture or movements
Wilson disease
Lesch-Nyhan disease
Hallervorden-Spatz syndrome
Familial striatal necrosis
Primary generalized dystonia (DYT1)
Niemann-Pick disease type C
Chronic GM_1 and GM_2 gangliosidoses
Pelizaeus-Merzbacher syndrome
Crigler-Najjar disease
Ataxia telangiectasia
Juvenile ceroid lipofuscinosis
Juvenile Huntington disease
Juvenile parkinsonism
Gilles de la Tourette syndrome
De Sanctis-Cacchione syndrome (xeroderma pigmentosum
    with endocrine dysfunction)
Dentatorubralpallidoluysian atrophy
Glutaric aciduria type 1

Spasticity
Too common to be discriminating.

TABLE 96.7

EYE FINDINGS

Conjunctival telangiectasia
Ataxia telangiectasia
Fabry disease

Corneal opacity
Wilson disease (Kayser-Fleischer ring)
Mucopolysaccharidoses I, III, IV, VI
Mucolipidoses III, IV
Fabry disease
Galactosialidosis
Cockayne disease
Xeroderma pigmentosum neurologic disease
Zellweger syndrome (inconstant)

(continued)

TABLE 96.7

EYE FINDINGS (*Continued*)

Lens opacity
Wilson disease
Galactosemia
Marinesco-Sjögren syndrome
Lowe disease
Cerebrocutaneous xanthomatosis
Sialidosis (rarely significant clinically)
Mannosidosis
Zellweger syndrome
Cockayne disease

Glaucoma
Mucopolysaccharidosis I (Hurler-Scheie syndrome)
Zellweger syndrome (infrequent)

Cherry-red Spot
Tay-Sachs disease
Sialidosis (usually)
Infantile Niemann-Pick disease (50% of cases)
Infantile GM_1 gangliosidosis (50% of cases)
Farber disease (inconstant)
Multiple sulfatase deficiency (metachromatic
  leukodystrophy variant)

Macular and retinal pigmentary degeneration
Ceroid lipofuscinosis (most types)
Mucopolysaccharidoses I-H and I-S, II, III
Mucolipidosis IV
Bassen-Kornzweig syndrome (abetalipoproteinemia)
Peroxisomal disorders
OPCA variant
Refsum disease (all types)
Kearns-Sayre syndrome
Leber congenital amaurosis
Other mitochondrial cytopathies
Hallervorden-Spatz syndrome (some types)
Cockayne disease
Sjögren-Larsson syndrome (not always)
Usher syndrome
Some other spinocerebellar syndromes
Neurocutaneous syndromes

Optic atrophy
Krabbe disease
Metachromatic leukodystrophy
Most sphingolipidoses late in their course
Adrenoleukodystrophy
Alexander disease
Canavan disease
Pelizaeus-Merzbacher disease
Neuroaxonal dystrophy

(continued)

TABLE 96.7

EYE FINDINGS (Continued)

Neonatal mitochondrial cytopathies
Leber congenital amaurosis
Leber hereditary optic neuropathy
Joubert syndrome
Some spinocerebellar degenerations
Diseases with retinal pigmentary degeneration

Nystagmus
Diseases with poor vision (searching nystagmus)
Pelizaeus-Merzbacher syndrome
Metachromatic leukodystrophy
Friedreich ataxia
Other spinocerebellar degenerations and cerebellar atrophies
Neuroaxonal dystrophy
Ataxia telangiectasia
Joubert syndrome
Leigh syndrome (inconstant)
Marinesco-Sjögren syndrome
Opsoclonus-myoclonus syndrome
Chédiak-Higashi syndrome

Ophthalmoplegia
Leigh syndrome
Kearns-Sayre syndrome
Niemann-Pick disease type C
Bassen-Kornzweig syndrome
Ataxia telangiectasia
Infantile Gaucher disease
Tangier disease

TABLE 96.8

USEFUL LABORATORY TESTS

Urine
Amino acids, organic acids
Galactose, other sugars
Mucopolysaccharides, sialidated oligosaccharides
N-Acetylaspartic acid
Copper excretion
Porphyrins
Metachromatic granules
Oxalate, cysteine crystals, uric acid

Blood chemistry
Ammonia (urea cycle disorders, some mitochondrial
  encephalopathies, organic acidemias)
Lactate-pyruvate ratio (Leigh syndrome, other
  mitochondrial cytopathies)

(*continued*)

TABLE 96.8

USEFUL LABORATORY TESTS (*Continued*)

Amino acids and other special metabolites
C26/C22 very-long-chain fatty acid ratio
 (adrenoleukodystrophy, Zellweger disease, other
 peroxisomal diseases)
Phytanic acid
Pipecolic acid
Isoelectrofocusing of serum sialotransferrins
 (congenital disorders of glycosylation)
Long-, medium-, and short-chain fatty acids

White blood cells
Lysosomal enzymes and other enzymatic assays
DNA tests for genetic mutations
Lipid and other inclusions (ceroid lipofuscinoses,
 gangliosidoses)

Red blood cells
Enzymatic assays for galactosemia, porphyria

Cultured skin fibroblasts
Enzymatic assays for most diseases with known deficits
Lipid and other inclusions (in mucolipidosis IV, I-cell
 disease, mucopolysaccharidoses, Chédiak-Higashi
 syndrome)
DNA repair after ultraviolet or radiation exposure
 (ataxia telangiectasia, Cockayne disease, xeroderma
 pigmentosum)
DNA tests for genetic mutations

Cerebrospinal fluid
CSF glucose decreased with normal blood glucose
 (GLUT 1 deficiency)
CSF protein increased in metachromatic
 leukodystrophy, Krabbe disease, infantile
 adrenoleukodystrophy (not always in classic
 variant), Friedreich ataxia, and other spinocerebellar
 degenerations (inconstant), Zellweger disease
 (sometimes), Refsum disease, Cockayne disease
CSF lactate/pyruvate (Mitochondrial cytopathies)
CSF neurotransmitter metabolites

Amniotic cells
Enzymatic assays for disease of known enzymatic defect
Abnormal inclusion in mucolipidosis IV
Karyotype in X-linked disease
C26/C22 very-long-chain fatty acid ratio
DNA tests for genetic mutations

Intradermal histamine test
Dysautonomia

TABLE 96.9

DISEASES IN WHICH BIOPSIES FOR HISTOLOGY ARE LIKELY TO HELP

Skin
Ceroid lipofuscinosis
Mucopolysaccharidoses
Mucolipidosis IV
Neuroaxonal dystrophy
Lafora disease

Conjunctiva
Mucopolysaccharidoses
Mucolipidoses
Neuroaxonal dystrophy

Bone marrow
Niemann-Pick disease
Gaucher disease
Mucopolysaccharidoses

Muscle
Glycogenoses
Mitochondrial myopathies (Kearns-Sayre and Leigh
　syndromes)
Other myopathies
Neuroaxonal dystrophy
Lafora disease

Nerve
Neuroaxonal dystrophy
Metachromatic leukodystrophy
Other diseases with neuropathies

Brain
(Rarely needed except possibly for the following)
Neuroaxonal dystrophy
Undiagnosed disease with probable cortical
　involvement

Section X
Mitochondrial Disorders

CHAPTER 97 ■
MITOCHONDRIAL ENCEPHALOMYOPATHIES: DISEASES OF MITOCHONDRIAL DNA

Two genomes control mitochondria: mitochondrial DNA (mtDNA) and nuclear DNA (nDNA). Diseases caused by nDNA mutations: Mendelian inheritance (see Chapter 99). Diseases caused by mutations in mtDNA: maternal inheritance or sporadic; *mitochondrial encephalomyopathies.*

GENERAL PRINCIPLES

Mitochondrial Genetics
Human mtDNA encodes proteins in respiratory chain, translational proteins.

Each cell contains multiple copies of mtDNA (*polyplasmy*). Both mutant and wild-type mtDNA may coexist in individual (*heteroplasmy*). Manifestations of mtDNA mutation depend on amount of heteroplasmy (*threshold effect*). Distribution of mitochondria in tissue continues to change after birth (*mitotic segregation*); phenotype changes over time. Inheritance *maternal* (mitochondria contributed by oocyte, not sperm); distinguished from autosomal dominant disorders by absence of paternal transmission.

Multiple deletions in mtDNA may result from mutation in nDNA; inheritance is autosomal (dominant or recessive).

CLINICAL FEATURES

Common neurologic findings: ophthalmoplegia, myopathy, peripheral neuropathy, sensorineural deafness, pigmentary retinopathy.

Prevalent systemic abnormalities: short stature, cardiomyopathy, cardiac conduction defects, diabetes mellitus, other endocrine disorders, lipomatosis.

Laboratory data: lactic acidosis in blood and CSF.

Pathology: ragged red fibers (RRFs) in muscle fibers (proliferation of mitochondria; not present in all conditions).

Diagnosis: (a) recognize appropriate clinical syndrome; (b) lactic acidosis; (c) RRFs; (d) document impaired respiration in biochemical assay of muscle extracts or isolated mitochondria; (e) identify mutation in mtDNA in blood or muscle. Not all criteria present in each syndrome.

No effective treatment proven to date.

DISEASES DUE TO mtDNA MUTATIONS

DELETIONS AND DUPLICATIONS

Usually sporadic.

Progressive External Ophthalmoplegia (PEO)

Symptom onset usually in childhood, occasionally in adolescence or adulthood: ptosis, then bilateral, symmetric ophthalmoparesis. May have pharyngeal and proximal limb weakness. Relatively benign condition, lifespan normal.

Kearns-Sayre Syndrome (KSS)

Invariant triad: onset before age 20, PEO, pigmentary retinopathy. One of following three: heart block, cerebellar syndrome, CSF protein >100 mg/dL. Endocrine disorders (e.g., hypoparathyoidism, diabetes mellitus) frequent. Survival beyond age 20 years rare.

Treatment: pacemaker for heart block.

POINT MUTATIONS

Usually maternally inherited.

MELAS

Mitochondrial *e*ncephalomyopathy, *l*actic *a*cidosis, and *s*troke. Stroke before age 40, often in childhood. Also: seizures, migraine, vomiting, dementia.

MRI: encephalomalacic foci, usually occipital; does not conform to distribution of major vessels.

Muscle biopsy: cytochrome c oxidase (COX)-positive RRFs.

Point mutation in transfer RNA (tRNA)^{Leu} gene of mtDNA in 80% of patients.

MERRF
*M*yoclonus with *e*pilepsy and *r*agged *r*ed *f*ibers. Myoclonus, generalized seizures, cerebellar ataxia, myopathy; sometimes multiple symmetric lipomas.

Onset: childhood or adult.
Muscle biopsy: COX-negative RRFs.

Point mutation in tRNA^{Lys} gene of mtDNA in most patients.

NARP
Various combinations of sensory *n*europathy, *a*taxia, seizures, dementia, *r*etinitis *p*igmentosa. Onset in early adult years.

Investigations: lactic acidosis may be lacking. No RRFs in muscle.

Point mutation in gene encoding adenosine triphosphatase (ATPase) 6.

Leber Hereditary Optic Neuropathy
See Chapter 98.

DEFECTS OF INTERGENOMIC SIGNALLING

Multiple Deletions of mtDNA
Several syndromes with PEO and variable multisystem involvement. Mutations in nuclear DNA lead to multiple mitochondrial deletions (nDNA control of mtDNA). Inheritance may be autosomal dominant or recessive.

MNGIE
*M*itochondrial *n*eurogastro*i*ntestinal *e*ncephalomyopathy.
Autosomal recessive. Mutation in gene on chromosome 6 encoding thymidine phosphorylase. Onset in childhood or adolescence with: chronic diarrhea, PEO, proximal limb weakness, sensory neuropathy, leukodystrophy.

Depletion of mtDNA
Markedly decreased levels of mtDNA in one or more tissues. Three syndromes, all autosomal recessive: (a) congenital myopathy; (b) infantile myopathy; (c) hepatopathy.

Acquired mtDNA depletion: reversible mitochondrial myopathy after treatment of HIV infection with zidovudine (AZT).

CHAPTER 98 ■ LEBER HEREDITARY OPTIC NEUROPATHY

Loss of central vision. Maternal inheritance; point mutation in mtDNA. 60% to 90% of patients are men.

CLINICAL FEATURES

Onset: adolescence or early adult years; progressive painless clouding of central vision: usually begins in one eye, affects both within weeks to months. Visual loss often severe, permanent.

Other features (less common): cardiac conduction abnormalities, mild neurologic abnormalities.

Fundus: blurred or normal disc early; optic atrophy later.

Leber-plus syndromes: (a) optic neuropathy and dystonia; (b) optic neuropathy and spastic dystonia; (c) optic neuropathy and Leigh-like syndrome; (d) optic neuropathy and MELAS, (e) optic neuropathy, athetosis, tremor, corticospinal tract signs, posterior column dysfunction, psychiatric disorder, acute encephalopathy.

GENETICS

Different mtDNA point mutations in different patients; usually homoplasmic (all mutant mtDNA). Clinical manifestations similar regardless of genotype. Pedigree: father never affected.

DIFFERENTIAL DIAGNOSIS

Demyelinating, toxic-nutritional optic neuropathy (including tobacco-alcohol amblyopia), other types of hereditary optic atrophy, occasionally glaucoma or ischemic optic neuropathy, compressive lesions.

Leber congenital amaurosis: severe congenital visual loss due to degeneration of retina, not optic nerve. Autosomal recessive. Electroretinogram abnormal.

THERAPY

Products to enhance respiratory enzymes (coenzyme Q10, idebenone, thiamine), antioxidants: commonly used though not of proven value. Tobacco, alcohol avoided in family members at risk.

CHAPTER 99 ◼
MITOCHONDRIAL DISEASES WITH MUTATIONS OF NUCLEAR DNA

Most autosomal recessive, lack ragged red fibers (RRFs). Onset: infancy or childhood. Can be classified biochemically (Table 99.1). Selected disorders described below.

LEIGH SYNDROME (SUBACUTE NECROTIZING ENCEPHALOMYOPATHY)

Clinical features: onset from infancy to adulthood. Infancy: poor feeding, feeble cry, respiratory difficulty, impaired vision and hearing, ataxia, limb weakness, intellectual deterioration, seizures, nystagmus. Later onset: progressive external ophthalmoplegia, dystonia, ataxia.

Investigations: elevated CSF lactate, pyruvate; MRI: characteristic symmetrical, necrotizing lesions in the midbrain, pons, medulla, thalamus, basal ganglia.

Genetics: inheritance autosomal recessive, X-linked, or maternal. Many different mutations in mitochondrial DNA (mtDNA) or nuclear DNA (nDNA), impaired cerebral oxidative metabolism: pyruvate dehydrogenase; biotinidase;

TABLE 99.1

CLASSIFICATION OF MITOCHONDRIAL DISEASES
ASSOCIATED WITH MUTATIONS OF NUCLEAR DNA

Biochemical abnormality	Clinical examples
Substrate transport	Carnitine deficiency
Substrate use	Pyruvate dehydrogenase deficiency
Citric acid cycle	Fumarase deficiency
Respiratory chain	Cytochrome-*c*-oxidase deficiency
Oxidation-phosphorylation	Luft disease (molecular basis not known)
Protein importation	Mohr-Tranebjaerg (deafness-dystonia) syndrome
Intergenomic signaling	Depletion of mtDNA
Membrane lipid milieu	Barth syndrome, Coenzyme Q deficiency
Mitochondrial motility	Spastic paraplegia 4
Metal metabolism	Friedreich ataxia

mtDNA, mitochondrial DNA.

complex I, II, IV deficiency. Most common: complex IV (cytochrome *c* oxidase [COX]) deficiency. No RRFs.

PYRUVATE DEHYDROGENASE COMPLEX DEFICIENCY

Most common cause of congenital lactic acidosis. Male predominance (most mutations: E1 α subunit, encoded on X chromosome). Onset usually neonatal.

Clinical features: see those for Leigh Syndrome (above). Female carriers may have mental retardation, ataxia.

PYRUVATE CARBOXYLASE DEFICIENCY

Congenital hypotonia, psychomotor retardation, failure to thrive, seizures, metabolic acidosis (ketoacidosis).

COENZYME Q10 DEFICIENCY

Clinical features: myopathy with variable associated findings: mild: recurrent myoglobinuria, RRF; severe: ataxia, seizures, mental retardation. Responds to coenzyme Q10 replacement therapy. Presumed autosomal recessive inheritance.

Section XI

Neurocutaneous Disorders

CHAPTER 100 ■
NEUROFIBROMATOSIS

Cardinal features: multiple pigmented birthmarks on skin ("café-au-lait" spots), multiple neurofibromas.

Two forms: neurofibromatosis type 1 (NF-1; von Recklinghausen disease, peripheral neurofibromatosis), neurofibromatosis type 2 (NF-2; central neurofibromatosis, bilateral acoustic neuromas).

Both autosomal dominant. NF-1 prevalence 1:3,000.

MOLECULAR GENETICS AND PATHOGENESIS

NF-1: chromosome 17; neurofibromin gene.
NF-2: chromosome 22; merlin gene. Both tumor-suppressor genes; mutations lead to tumors.

SYMPTOMS AND SIGNS

NF-1: variable, progressive manifestations (see below).
NF-2: bilateral acoustic neuromas at about age 20. In contrast to NF-1, few café-au-lait spots, neurofibromas.
Segmental neurofibromatosis: café-au-lait spots, neurofibromas limited, usually affect upper body segment.
Cutaneous neurofibromatosis: pigmentary changes only.

Cutaneous Symptoms
Café-au-lait macules: pathognomonic lesion, present in almost all patients. Axillary or inguinal freckling.

Ocular Symptoms
Pigmented iris hamartomas (Lisch nodules) pathognomonic; almost all patients over age 20; only in NF-1.

Neurologic Symptoms

Neurofibromas: evident at age 10 to 15. Always involve skin. Found on deep peripheral nerves, nerve roots, autonomic nerves. Symptoms usually limited to pain from pressure on nerves, nerve roots, cauda equina, spinal cord.

Other lesions: optic glioma, astrocytoma, acoustic neuroma, neurilemmoma, meningioma. Optic glioma slowly progressive.

NF-1: learning disabilities, attention-deficit disorder common. Intellectual retardation, seizures, occlusive cerebrovascular disease (moyamoya type) rare.

NF-2: hearing loss, tinnitus, imbalance, headache around age 20. Few café-au-lait spots and neurofibromas. Intracranial and intraspinal meningioma, schwannoma, gliomas.

Symptoms of the Skull, Spine, and Limbs

(a) Unilateral defects in posterior superior wall of orbit; pulsating exophthalmos; (b) underdevelopment of mastoid; (c) large spinal canal, scalloped vertebral bodies; (d) kyphoscoliosis; (e) pseudoarthrosis; (f) "twisted ribbon" rib deformities; (g) enlargement of long bones.

TABLE 100.1

DIAGNOSTIC CRITERIA FOR NEUROFIBROMATOSIS

Neurofibromatosis 1 (any two or more)
Six or more café-au-lait macules
   Before puberty >5 mm diameter
   After puberty >15 mm diameter
Freckling in the axillary or inguinal areas
Two or more neurofibromas or one plexiform neurofibroma
Optic glioma
Two or more Lisch nodules (iris hamartomas)
Bone lesion, e.g,:
   sphenoid dysplasia
   thinning of cortex of long bones with or without
      pseudoarthrosis
A first-degree relative with NF-1

Neurofibromatosis 2
Bilateral eighth nerve tumor (MRI, CT, or histologic
   confirmation)
A first-degree relative with NF-2 and a unilateral eighth nerve
   tumor
A first-degree relative with NF-2 and any two of the following:
   Neurofibroma, meningioma, schwannoma, glioma, or
      juvenile posterior subcapsular lenticular opacity

NF-1, neurofibromatosis type 1; NF-2, neurofibromatosis type 2. Modified from Conference statement, National Institutes of Health consensus development conference: neurofibromatosis. *Arch Neurol* 1988;45:575–578.

Miscellaneous Complications

Hypertension due to pheochromocytoma (never in children), renal artery neurofibroma. Malignant tumors: leukemia, Wilms tumor, ganglioglioma, neuroblastoma. Precocious puberty (hypothalamic glioma or hamartoma). Pulmonary: cystic pulmonary lesions, malignancy, interstitial pneumonia.

DIAGNOSIS

See Table 100.1.

TREATMENT

Treat complications. Genetic counseling.

CHAPTER 101 ■ ENCEPHALOTRIGEMINAL ANGIOMATOSIS

Also called Sturge-Weber-Dimitri Syndrome.

SYMPTOMS AND SIGNS

Characteristic syndrome: cutaneous vascular port-wine nevus of the face, contralateral hemiparesis and hemiatrophy, glaucoma, seizures, mental retardation.

Neurologic: epilepsy most common neurologic manifestation, usually starting before age 1 year with focal motor, generalized major motor, or partial complex seizures. Onset of seizures before age 2 years, refractory epilepsy associated

with increased risk of intellectual impairment. Homonymous hemianopia due to occipital lobe atrophy. Behavioral
problems include attention-deficit disorder.

Ophthalmologic: raised intraocular pressure with glaucoma
and buphthalmos in approximately 30% of patients.
Coloboma of iris; deformity of lens.

INVESTIGATIONS

CT: curvilinear ("trolley-track") calcifications following cerebral convolutions (usually after age 2 years); unilateral cerebral
atrophy, affecting occipital lobe most often (ipsilateral to facial nevus). MRI: leptomeningeal disease (angiomatosis). EEG:
wide area of low potentials over affected areas.

GENETICS

Most cases sporadic; autosomal recessive, dominant inheritance also seen. Incomplete penetrance with marked variability
of clinical manifestations.

TREATMENT

Facial nevus: laser therapy available when cosmetics inadequate. Seizures often refractory to anticonvulsants; lobectomy,
hemispherectomy may be effective. Physical, occupational therapy for hemiparesis. Yearly monitoring for glaucoma recommended for all patients.

CHAPTER 102 ■ INCONTINENTIA PIGMENTI

INCONTINENTIA PIGMENTI

CLINICAL FEATURES

Cutaneous: linear vesicobullous lesions at birth, rarely as late as 1 year. Lesions change to linear verrucous and dyskeratotic growth. Pigmentary changes follow: slate-gray blue or brown, irregular marbled or wavy lines; later fade to depigmented, atrophic skin. Skin lesions in lines of Blaschko.
Neurologic (20%): slow motor development, spastic hemiparesis, quadriparesis, or diplegia; mental retardation; seizures.
Ocular (20%): strabismus, cataracts, visual loss.
Other manifestations: partial or total anodontia, peg-shaped teeth.

INVESTIGATIONS

Eosinophilia, leukocytosis.

GENETICS

X-linked dominant, lethal in males. Sometimes sporadic.

INCONTINENTIA PIGMENTI ACHROMIANS

Also called hypomelanosis of Ito.

CLINICAL FEATURES

Cutaneous lesions hypopigmented, in contrast to incontinentia pigmenti. Other features: hypotonia, pyramidal tract dysfunction, mental retardation (80%), seizures; strabismus, optic atrophy, micro-opthalmia, heterochromia iridis, ptosis.

GENETICS

Most cases sporadic; genetic abnormality identified in most cases: somatic mosaicism for chromosomal trisomies.

CHAPTER 103 ■ TUBEROUS SCLEROSIS COMPLEX

GENETICS AND INCIDENCE

Autosomal dominant; often sporadic.

2 recognized genes: chromosomes 9 (TSC1: *hamartin*), 16 (TSC2: *tuberin*); both tumor suppressor genes.

Incidence 1:10,000. Prevalence 1:10,000 to 1:170,000.

SYMPTOMS AND SIGNS

Cardinal features: skin lesions, seizures, mental retardation.

Cutaneous: (a) depigmented or hypomelanotic macules (ash-leaf spots), sometimes need examination with Wood lamp; congenital; (b) facial adenoma sebaceum (facial angiofibroma) in butterfly distribution on nose, cheeks, by age 4 in most children; (c) shagreen patch (rough, elevated plaque) after age 10; usually lumbosacral; (d) fingernail or toenail (ungual) fibromas, (e) café-au-lait spots.

Neurologic: (a) seizures: myoclonic spasms, hypsarrhythmia in infants; generalized tonic-clonic or partial complex seizures later; (b) mental retardation (in correlation with refractory seizures), (c) autism.

Ophthalmic: hamartomas of retina or optic nerve (50% of patients); multinodular near disc (mulberry appearance); flat, circular at periphery.

Visceral: (a) renal hamartoma (angiomyolipomas), cysts, rare carcinoma; (b) cardiac rhabdomyoma; (c) pulmonary hamartoma.

INVESTIGATIONS

EEG: may show hypsarrhythmia, focal or multifocal spike or sharp-wave discharges, generalized spike-and-wave discharges.

CT, MRI: calcified subependymal nodules encroach on lateral ventricle; calcified cortical or cerebellar nodules (cortical tubers).

DIAGNOSIS

Clinical. Infancy: depigmented cutaneous lesions, infantile spasms strongly suggestive; cardiac rhabdomyoma sometimes detected on prenatal ultrasound. Older child or adult: see Table 103.1.

TABLE 103.1

DIAGNOSTIC CRITERIA–TUBEROUS SCLEROSIS COMPLEX CONSENSUS CONFERENCE (1998)

Major features	Minor features
Facial angiofibromas or forehead plaques	Multiple randomly distributed pits in dental enamel
Nontraumatic ungual or periungual fibroma	Hamartomatous rectal polyps
Hypomelanotic macules (three or more)	Bone cysts
Shagreen patch (connective tissue nevus)	Cerebral white matter radial migration lines
Multiple retinal nodular hamartomas	Gingival fibromas
Cortical tuber	Nonrenal hamartoma
Subependymal nodule	Retinal achromic patch
Subependymal giant cell astrocytoma	"Confetti" skin lesions
Cardiac rhabdomyoma, single or multiple	Multiple renal cysts
Angiomyolipoma	

Diagnosis of tuberous sclerosis complex is established when two major features or one major plus two minor features can be demonstrated.

Section XII
Peripheral Neuropathies

CHAPTER 104 ■ GENERAL CONSIDERATIONS

DEFINITIONS

Peripheral neuropathy, polyneuropathy: diffuse lesions of peripheral nerves, manifest by weakness, sensory loss, autonomic dysfunction.

Mononeuropathy: single nerve affected (trauma, entrapment).

Mononeuropathy multiplex: two or more nerves affected individually; can identify nerves by clinical pattern or nerve conduction studies.

Neuronopathy: motor or sensory neuron affected.

CLASSIFICATION BY SYMPTOMS AND SIGNS

Predominantly motor: lead toxicity, dapsone or hexane intoxication, tick paralysis, porphyria, some cases of GBS, multifocal conduction block, anti-GM_1 antibodies.

Predominantly sensory: thallium poisoning, acute idiopathic sensory neuronopathy or ganglioneuritis, pyridoxine (vitamin B_6) deficiency, inherited sensory neuropathies, primary biliary cirrhosis, diabetes mellitus, amyloidosis, carcinoma, lepromatous leprosy.

Predominantly autonomic: acute or chronic autonomic neuropathy, amyloidosis.

Mononeuropathy multiplex: diabetes mellitus, periarteritis nodosa, HIV-1 infection, rheumatoid arthritis, brachial neuropathy, leprosy, nerve trauma, sarcoid compression. Asymmetric motor neuropathy in multifocal neuropathy.

Hypertrophic nerves: Charcot-Marie-Tooth (CMT) disease type 1, Dejerine-Sottas syndrome, Refsum disease, neurofibromatosis type 1, leprosy, amyloidosis, chronic demyelinating polyneuropathy, sarcoid, acromegaly (hyperpituitarism).

Fasciculations: spontaneous contractions of individual motor units; visible twitch of limb muscle under skin; also identified in EMG. Anterior horn cell diseases, multifocal motor neuropathy.

ETIOLOGY AND DIAGNOSIS

See Table 104.1.

TREATMENT

Specific: see Chapters 105, 106.

Symptomatic: specific therapy if indicated, physical therapy, foot orthosis (lightweight splint to support paretic foot), prevention of pressure sores, general care.

TABLE 104.1

CLASSIFICATION AND EVALUATION OF MOST COMMON POLYNEUROPATHIES

Cause or diagnosis	Presentations	Laboratory tests
Vitamin Deficiencies	S, SM, SYM	Vitamins B_{12}, B_6, B_1
Infectious		
Lyme disease	S, SM, SYM, MF, CN	Serology, PCR
HIV-1	S, SM, SYM, MF, CN	Serology, PCR
Hepatitis C	S, SM, SYM, MF, CN	Serology, PCR
Herpes Zoster	S, radicular	Serology, PCR
Cytomegalovirus	SM, M, SYM, MF	Serology, PCR, culture
Immune Mediated		
Guillain-Barré and variants	SM, S, M, SYM, CN	IgG anti-ganglioside antibodies (GM1,GD1a,GQ1b, GD1b), urine porphyrins
IgM antibody associated	M, MF	IgM anti-GM1, GD1a
	S, SM, SYM	IgM anti-MAG, sulfatides, GD1b, GQ1b
Monoclonal gammopathy	M, S, SM, SYM, MF	Serum immunofixation electrophoresis, quantitative immunoglobulins

(continued)

TABLE 104.1

CLASSIFICATION AND EVALUATION OF MOST COMMON POLYNEUROPATHIES (*Continued*)

Cause or diagnosis	Presentations	Laboratory tests
Autonomic neuropathy	Autonomic dysfunction	Anti-nicotinic acetylcholine receptor antibodies
Vasculitis	SM, S, MF, SYM	ESR, cryoglobulins, hepatitis C serology or PCR
Sarcoid	SM, S, MF, SYM	ACE, chest X-ray
Celiac disease	S, SM, MF, SYM	Anti-gliadin, endomysial, transglutaminase antibodies
CIDP	Chronic motor or sensorimotor, demyelinating	EMG, CSF
Rheumatologic diseases (Sjögren syndrome, lupus erythematosus, Wegener granulomatosis, rheumatoid arthritis)	SM, S, MF, SYM	SSA-Ro, SSB-La antibodies, ANA, ANCA (PR3, myeloperoxidase), dsDNA Ab, RNP, rheumatoid factor
Paraneoplastic		
Lung cancer	S, SYM	Anti-HU Ab, chest X-ray
Waldenström macroglobulinemia	SM, S, M, SYM, MF	Serum immunofixation electrophoresis
Myeloma	SM, M, SYM, MF	Serum and urine immunofixation electrophoresis, skeletal survey

Hereditary		
CMT1-1	Demyelinating, SM, SYM, MF	DNA tests for PMP-22, MPZ, EGR2, Cx32
CMT-2	Axonal, SM, SYM	DNA tests for NF-L, Cx32, MPZ
Mitochondrial	NARP, SM, MF, MNGIE	Serum lactate, thymidine phosphorylase (MNGIE), DNA testing
Other	Axonal S, SM, amyloid, porphyria	DNA test for transthyretin, periaxin; urine porphyrins; porphobilinogen, delta aminolevulinic acid; muscle nerve biopsy for amyloid.
Nutritional		
Alcoholism	SM, autonomic	
Vitamin B$_1$ deficiency	SM, autonomic	Serum B$_1$
Vitamin B$_{12}$ deficiency	S, SM	CBC count serum B$_{12}$
Vitamin B$_6$ deficiency	S	Serum B$_6$
Vitamin E deficiency	S	Serum vitamin E

(continued)

TABLE 104.1

CLASSIFICATION AND EVALUATION OF MOST COMMON POLYNEUROPATHIES (*Continued*)

Cause or diagnosis	Presentations	Laboratory tests
Metabolic/Toxic		
Diabetes	S, SM, SYM, MF, CN	Chem 7, HgbA1c, glucose tolerance test
Renal failure	S, SM, SYM	Chem 7
Thyroid disease	S, SM, SYM, MF	TSH, T4
Heavy metal toxicity	S, SM, SYM	Urine lead, mercury, arsenic

CN, cranial nerves; Cx32, connexin; EGR, early growth response protein; GM_1, GD_{1a}, ganglioside component of myelin; MPZ, myelin protein zero; NF-L, neurofilament light chain; M, motor; MF, multifocal; MNGIE, Myopathy with ophthalmoplegia, Neuropathy, and Gastro-Intestinal disease with Encephalopathy; NARP, neuropathy, ataxia, retinitis pigmentosa; PMP, peripheral myelin protein; PCR, polymerase chain reaction; RNP, ribonucleoprotein; S, sensory; SM, sensorimotor; SSA, SSB, antigens for Sjögren syndrome severe antibodies; SYM, symmetric.

CHAPTER 105 ■ HEREDITARY NEUROPATHIES

Selected inherited neuropathies and their features listed in Table 105.1. Clinical classification in Table 105.2.

CHARCOT-MARIE-TOOTH DISEASES (CMT)

Also known as *hereditary motor and sensory neuropathies* (HMSN). Most common inherited neuropathies.

CLASSIFICATION AND MOLECULAR GENETICS

CMT type 1 (CMT-1): most common; demyelinating; slow conduction velocity; autosomal dominant. Histology = demyelination and remyelination ("onion bulb" formations lead to nerve hypertrophy).

CMT-2: clinically similar to CMT1 but no demyelination; normal nerve conduction; autosomal dominant or recessive.

CMT-3 (Déjerine-Sottas syndrome): most severe form. Onset in early childhood, ultimately extreme disability. Hypertrophic demyelinating; extremely slow conduction. Most autosomal recessive. Same syndrome from mutation in any of three genes.

CMT-4: Refsum disease (see Chapter 89).

CMT-5: spastic paraplegia with amyotrophy.

CMT-6: CMT with optic atrophy.

CMT-7: with retinitis pigmentosa.

CMT-X: x-linked (dominant or recessive); demyelinating.

Hereditary neuropathy with liability to pressure palsies (HNPP): intermittent clinical manifestations. Transient paralysis of muscles innervated by specific peripheral nerves (especially median and ulnar) or brachial plexus. Nerve conduction often slow between attacks, sometimes with conduction block. Autosomal dominant. Maps to 17p11; gene product PMP22 (peripheral myelin protein) as in CMT1A.

TABLE 105.1
INHERITED NEUROPATHIES

Disorder	Locus/gene	Inheritance	Protein	Testing method
CMT1A	17p11.2/PMP22	AD	Peripheral myelin protein 22	Pulse-field gel electrophoresis, FISH, Southern blot
HNPP	17p11.2/PMP22	AD	Peripheral myelin protein 22	Mutation analysis, FISH, Long PCR-RFLP, Southern blot
CMT1B	1q22/MPZ	AD	Myelin protein zero	Sequencing, mutation scanning, mutation analysis
CMT1C	16p13.1-p12.3/LITAF	AD	SIMPLE	
CMT1D	10q21.1-q22.1/EGR2	AD	Early growth response protein 2	Sequencing, mutation scanning, mutation analysis
CMT2A	1p36.2/KIF1B	AD	Kinesin-like protein KIF1B	Direct DNA, linkage analysis
CMT2B	3q21/RAB7	AD	*Ras*-related protein Rab-7	Direct DNA, linkage analysis
CMT2C	12q23–24/unknown	AD	Unknown	Direct DNA, linkage analysis
CMT2D	7p15/GARS	AD	Glycyl-tRNA synthetase	Direct DNA, linkage analysis
CMT2E	8p21/NEFL	AD	Neurofilament triplet L protein	Sequencing
CMT2F	7q11–21/unknown	AD	Unknown	Linkage
CMT4A	8q13-q21.1/GDAP1	AR	Ganglioside-induced differentiation protein-1	Sequencing
CMT4B1	11q22/MTMR2	AR	Myotubularin-related protein 2	
CMT4BB2	11p15/CMT4B2	AR	SET binding factor 2	
CMT4C	5q32/KIAA1985	AR	Unknown	

CMT4D	8q24.3/NDRG1	AR	NDRG1 protein	Mutation analysis, sequencing
CMT4E	10q21.1-q22.1/EGR2	AR	Early growth response protein 2	Mutation analysis, sequencing
CMT4F	19q13.1-q13.2/PRX	AR	Periaxin	Sequencing, mutation scanning, mutation analysis
CMTX	Xq13.1/GJB1	X-linked	Gap junction beta-1 protein (Connexin 32)	
dHMN I	Unknown	AD	Unknown	
dHMN II	12q24.3/Unknown	AD	Unknown	
dHMN III	1q21-23/Unknown	AR	Unknown	
dHMN V	7p15/GARS	AD	Glycyl-tRNA synthetase	
dHMN VI	Unknown	AR	Unknown	
dHMN VII	2q14/Unknown	AD	Unknown	
dHMN Jerash	9p21.1-p12/Unknown	AR	Unknown	
ALS4	9q34/Unknown	AD	Unknown	
HMN Dynactin	2p13/DCTN1	AD	Dynactin	
HSAN I	9q22.1-q22.3/SPTLC1	AD	Serine palmitoyltransferase light chain 1	Sequencing
HSAN II	Unknown	AR	Unknown	
HSAN III (Riley Day)	9q31/IKBKAP	AR	I-kappa-B kinase complex-associated protein	Mutation analysis, quantitative PCR
HSAN IV	1q21-q22/NTRK1	AR	Tyrosine kinase for nerve growth factor	

CMT, Charcot-Marie-Tooth disease; HNPP, hereditary neuropathy with liability to pressure palsies; DHMN, distal hereditary motor neuropathy; HSAN, hereditary sensory and autonomic neuropathy.

TABLE 105.2

DYCK AND LAMBERT CLASSIFICATION OF HEREDITARY MOTOR AND SENSORY NEUROPATHIES

Type	Features
HMSN Type I A and B (dominantly inherited hypertrophic neuropathy)	Slow nerve conduction velocities Distal weakness, mild sensory loss Palpable nerves Decreased reflexes Pathology demonstrating segmental demyelination, remyelination, onion bulb formation, and axonal loss Autosomal dominant
HMSN Type II (neuronal type of peroneal muscular atrophy)	Normal nerve conduction velocities Distal weakness, mild sensory loss Nonpalpable nerves Pathology demonstrating degeneration of motor and sensory nerves Autosomal dominant
HMSN Type III (hypertrophic neuropathy of infancy; Dejerine and Sottas)	Delayed motor development Severe motor-sensory loss Slow nerve conduction velocities Autosomal recessive
HMSN Type IV Hypertrophic neuropathy (Refsum; associated with phytanic acid excess)	Refsum disease
HMSN Type V (associated with spastic paraplegia)	Spastic paraplegia present
HMSN Type VI (with optic atrophy)	Optic atrophy present
HMSN Type VII	Retinitis pigmentosa present

CLINICAL FEATURES

Onset in childhood or adolescence. Initial symptoms: foot deformity (*pes cavus*), scoliosis, foot drop, steppage gait. Later: hand weakness. Slow progression. Motor involvement greater than sensory. Variable severity.

HNPP may be asymptomatic between attacks.

LABORATORY STUDIES

Nerve conduction studies for classification. DNA analysis diagnostic.

TREATMENT

Limited to mechanical assistance for leg weakness, surgical correction of joint deformities and scoliosis, physical therapy.

HEREDITARY SENSORY AND AUTONOMIC NEUROPATHY (HSAN)

"Sensory neurogenic arthropathy": mutilating painless injuries of skin and bone cause deformities of hands and feet.

HSAN1: autosomal dominant. Types 2, 3, 4 all autosomal-recessive forms of congenital indifference to pain.

FAMILIAL AMYLOIDOTIC POLYNEUROPATHY

Autosomal dominant.

CLINICAL FEATURES

Onset age 20 to 35. Distal sensory loss, chronic diarrhea, impotence. Severe sensory symptoms disabling; neurogenic arthropathy common. Weakness years later. Cardiomyopathy with heart block. Fatal in 7 to 15 years.

PATHOLOGY AND PATHOGENESIS

Amyloid deposits in extracellular spaces of many organs, including autonomic and peripheral nerves. Both demyelinating and axonal. Abnormal protein: transthyretin.

TREATMENT

Plasmapheresis used with limited success. Liver transplantation may arrest progression.

OTHER INHERITED NEUROPATHIES

See Table 105.1.

CHAPTER 106 ■ ACQUIRED NEUROPATHIES

GUILLAIN-BARRÉ SYNDROME (GBS) AND VARIANTS

Also "acute inflammatory demyelinating polyneuropathy." Acute onset of peripheral and cranial nerve dysfunction. Frequently preceded by respiratory or gastrointestinal infection immunization, or surgery.

Incidence: 0.6 to 1.9/100,000 persons/year. Most frequent acquired demyelinating neuropathy.

Symptoms and signs: rapidly progressive (days); symmetric limb weakness, loss of tendon reflexes, facial diplegia, oropharyngeal and respiratory weakness, paresthesias and impaired sensation in hands and feet. About 20% require mechanical ventilation.

Variants: *acute motor axonal neuropathy (AMAN)*: motor axonal degeneration; little or no demyelination or inflammation. Many follow *Campylobacter jejuni* infection. *Miller-Fisher syndrome*: triad of gait ataxia, areflexia, ophthalmoparesis; sometimes pupillary abnormalities. Nerve conduction normal. CSF changes as in GBS.

Laboratory data: elevated CSF protein, normal cell count. Nerve conduction slow; often normal at first. AMAN: anti-GM_1 or GD_{1a} ganglioside antibodies. Miller-Fisher: anti-GQ_{1b} antibodies.

Pathology: focal segmental demyelination with perivascular and endoneurial infiltrates of lymphocytes and monocytes or macrophages.

Differential diagnosis: acute West Nile viral infection (can present as acute paralytic syndrome), HIV neuropathy, porphyric neuropathy, toxic neuropathy (n-hexane, thallium, arsenic), botulism, tick paralysis.

Course: worsens for days to 3 weeks; then plateaus, followed by gradual improvement to normal or nearly normal function. Autonomic instability (blood pressure instability, arrhythmia) may seriously complicate course.

Treatment: early plasmapheresis or IVIG accelerates recovery, reduces long-term neurologic disability. Intensive care unit observation, mechanical ventilation, aspiration precautions. Mortality 5%.

CHRONIC INFLAMMATORY DEMYELINATING POLYNEUROPATHY (CIDP)

Clinical features: insidious or acute onset limb weakness, depressed tendon reflexes, impaired sensation. Often follows viral infection.

Laboratory data: CSF protein usually increased. Slow nerve conduction.

Pathology: segmental demyelination, lymphocytic infiltrates in peripheral nerves. Nerves may be enlarged.

Course: chronic progressive or relapsing.

Treatment: glucocorticoids, plasmapheresis, IVIG, immunosuppressive drugs often beneficial.

MULTIFOCAL MOTOR NEUROPATHY

Weakness, wasting, fasciculation with active or absent tendon reflexes. Can mimic ALS (lower motor neuron syndrome). Often asymmetric. Nerve conduction studies define multifocal motor conduction block. Anti-GM_1, anti-GD_{1a} antibodies sometimes found. Reversible with IVIG or immunosuppressive drug therapy.

SENSORY NEURONOPATHY AND NEUROPATHY

Numbness, paresthesias, pain; distal, radicular, or whole body; tendon reflexes present or absent; normal strength. EMG: reduced or absent sensory potentials. CSF protein normal or slightly elevated. Variable response to glucocorticoids or immunosuppressive therapy.

Etiology: autoimmune disease, HIV-1 infection, vitamin B_6 deficiency, paraneoplastic neuropathy, amyloidosis, toxic neuropathy.

IDIOPATHIC AUTONOMIC NEUROPATHY

Acute or subacute onset of postural syncope, diminished tearing, sweating; impaired bladder function; marked intestinal dysmotility; diminished sexual potency in men. May follow viral infection. Self-limited, with partial or complete recovery.

VASCULITIC AND CRYOGLOBULINEMIC NEUROPATHIES

Mononeuritis multiplex or distal symmetric polyneuropathy. Nerve and muscle biopsies: inflammatory cell infiltrates, necrosis of blood vessel walls.

Vasculitis confined to peripheral nerves or associated with systemic disease: periarteritis nodosa, cryoglobulinemia, Churg-Strauss syndrome, Sjögren syndrome, Wegener granulomatosis, rheumatoid arthritis, systemic lupus erythematosus, systemic sclerosis.

May respond to prednisone, cyclophosphamide. Plasmapheresis for cryoglobulinemia.

NEUROPATHIES WITH MYELOMA OR NONMALIGNANT IgG OR IgA MONOCLONAL GAMMOPATHY

Peripheral neuropathy in 50% of patients with osteosclerotic myeloma and immunoglobulin G (IgG) or IgA monoclonal gammopathy. Also with primary amyloidosis, cryoglobulinemia. Demyelination, axonal degeneration both present.

NEUROPATHIES WITH IgM MONOCLONAL ANTIBODIES THAT REACT WITH PERIPHERAL NERVE GLYCOCONJUGATE ANTIGENS

Anti-MAG (myelin-associated glycoprotein) autoantibodies: chronic demyelinating sensorimotor neuropathy. Treatment: plasmapheresis, chemotherapy, IVIG.

Anti-GM_1 ganglioside antibodies: syndrome of motor neuropathy or lower motor neuron. EMG: denervation, conduction block. Treatment: immunosuppressive chemotherapy, IVIG.

AMYLOID NEUROPATHY

Principal forms of amyloid protein that cause neuropathy: immunoglobulin light chains (primary amyloidosis, plasma cell dyscrasias), transthyretin (hereditary amyloidosis).

Variable combination of painful, autonomic dysfunction, symmetric loss of pain and temperature sensations with spared position and vibration senses, carpal tunnel syndrome. Prognosis poor.

NEUROPATHY ASSOCIATED WITH CARCINOMA (PARANEOPLASTIC NEUROPATHY)

Most characteristic syndrome: sensory neuropathy; subacute onset, small cell carcinoma of lung. Anti-Hu antineuronal antibodies often present. Other neuropathy syndromes also sometimes with cancer.

HYPOTHYROID NEUROPATHY

Usually entrapment neuropathy. Painful paresthesias in hands and feet, without weakness. "Hung-up" tendon reflexes. Reversible with thyroid replacement.

HYPERTHYROID NEUROPATHY

(a) ALS-like syndrome: diffuse weakness, fasciculations, preserved or hyperactive tendon reflexes; reverses with treatment of hyperthyroidism; (b) GBS.

ACROMEGALIC NEUROPATHY

Usually entrapment neuropathies. Weakness may be severe.

CELIAC NEUROPATHY

Most common complication of celiac disease. Gastrointestinal symptoms absent in half of patients with neuropathy. Most commonly small fiber sensory neuropathy, often multifocal. Anti-gliadin antibodies often present. Gluten-free diet only sometimes results in improvement of neuropathy.

UREMIC NEUROPATHY

Sensorimotor neuropathy; axonal; painful paresthesias feet, glove-stocking loss of sensation, distal weakness. Dialysis may stabilize symptoms; renal transplantation may reverse neuropathy.

Mononeuropathy, usually carpal tunnel syndrome distal to implanted arteriovenous fistula.

NEUROPATHIES ASSOCIATED WITH INFECTION

LEPROSY

Most common treatable neuropathy in the world. Tuberculoid leprosy: mononeuritis or mononeuritis multiplex. Lepromatous leprosy: patchy loss of cutaneous sensation; tendon reflexes preserved. Treatment: dapsone.

DIPHTHERIA

Impaired accommodation and paresis of eye muscles; also oropharyngeal; then quadriparesis. Demyelinating.

HIV-RELATED NEUROPATHIES

Early (before seroconversion): GBS.

Before evidence of immunodeficiency: subacute demyelinating neuropathy like idiopathic CIDP but with CSF pleocytosis.

AIDS: distal sensorimotor polyneuropathy, axonal; severe painful paresthesias in feet first. Carbamazepine, amitriptyline may help.

Any stage of HIV infection: mononeuropathy multiplex. Consider cytomegalovirus when CD4 count <50; treatment may be life-saving.

Medication-induced neuropathy: dideoxynucleotide antiretroviral medications may cause painful sensory neuropathy indistinguishable from AIDS-related neuropathy.

HERPES ZOSTER

(a) Painful sensory radiculopathy (shingles) before or after characteristic skin lesions. Weakness rare. Most common in elderly, malignancy, immunosuppression. Facial nerve zoster: vesicular herpetic eruption in external auditory meatus, vertigo, deafness, and facial weakness (Ramsay Hunt syndrome). (b) GBS with CSF pleocytosis.

LYME NEUROPATHY

Painful sensory radiculitis 3 weeks after erythema migrans. Cranial neuropathy, limb weakness may follow. Facial nerves affected most frequently.

SARCOID NEUROPATHY

Most common forms: single or multiple cranial nerve palsies; fluctuating; especially facial nerve. Symmetric limb polyneuropathy later. Mixed axonal and demyelinating. Steroids may help.

POLYNEUROPATHY ASSOCIATED WITH DIETARY STATES

Vitamin B$_1$(thiamine) deficiency: severe burning dysesthesias, feet more than hands; weakness and wasting distal more than proximal; trophic changes (shiny skin, hair loss), sensory loss, worse distally. Axonal.

Niacin (nicotinic acid) deficiency neuropathy: does not improve with niacin supplements; improves only when thiamine and pyridoxine added to diet.

Vitamin B_{12} deficiency: subacute combined degeneration of spinal cord plus sensorimotor peripheral neuropathy. May occur without hematologic abnormalities.

Vitamin B_6 (pyridoxine) deficiency: axonal, sensory more than motor. Most common cause: treatment with isoniazid; increases pyridoxine excretion.

Vitamin B_6 (pyridoxine) excess: severe sensory neuropathy.

Vitamin E deficiency: resembles spinocerebellar degeneration with ataxia, severe loss joint position and vibration, hyporeflexia. Sensory evoked responses: low amplitude or absent; delay in central conduction. Occurs in fat malabsorption syndromes, including abetalipoproteinemia, congenital biliary atresia, pancreatic dysfunction, surgical removal of large portions of small intestine.

Strachan syndrome: visual loss, oral ulcers, skin changes, painful neuropathy. Originally described in Jamaican sugar workers. Likely due to diet deficient in B vitamins.

Gastric bypass surgery associated sometimes followed by subacute axonal neuropathy. Vitamin deficiency presumed responsible.

CRITICAL ILLNESS POLYNEUROPATHY

Often suspected if difficulty weaning from ventilator. Sensorimotor axonal. Acute quadriplegic myopathy may follow use of neuromuscular blocking agents for intubation in patient also receiving steroid therapy.

Mononeuritis or mononeuritis multiplex in 2% of patients with bacterial endocarditis.

NEUROPATHIES CAUSED BY HEAVY METALS

ARSENIC

Most common heavy metal–induced neuropathy but rare. Painful paresthesias in legs, then distal weakness with loss of tendon reflexes. Hair loss. Axonal. May show fingernail "Mees lines."

LEAD

Atypical because of motor predominance and arm involvement. Focal weakness of extensor muscles of fingers and wrist, then other arm. Basophilic stippling of red cells. History of exposure needed for diagnosis; now rare.

MERCURY

Organic mercury: distal paresthesias attributed to dorsal root ganglion degeneration. Inorganic mercury: primarily weakness and wasting.

THALLIUM

Neuropathy in adults exposed to rat poison. Primarily sensory and autonomic. Acute-onset severe dysesthesias; diffuse alopecia. Axonal.

OTHER CHEMICALS

Include acrylamide monomer (not polyacrylamide); triorthocresyl phosphate; dimethylaminopropionitrile; methylbromide; pyriminil; n-hexane; methyl-N-butyl ketone; fish neurotoxins (ciguatera, saxitoxin, brevitoxin, tetrodotoxin).

NEUROPATHIES CAUSED BY THERAPEUTIC DRUGS

Vincristine: symmetric progressive sensorimotor distal neuropathy in legs; areflexia.

Cisplatinum: pure sensory distal neuropathy with paresthesias, impaired vibration sense, loss of ankle jerks.

Paclitaxel (Taxol): predominantly sensory neuropathy.

Dapsone, disulfiram: predominantly motor neuropathy.

Isoniazid: vasculitic mononeuropathy multiplex (rare).

ALCOHOLIC NEUROPATHY

Most commonly small fiber sensory neuropathy. Vibratory sensation, position sense usually affected later. Abstinence may lead to recovery.

DIABETIC NEUROPATHY

Transient: acute painful neuropathy, mononeuropathy (third, sixth cranial nerve; femoral nerve radiculopathy). Spontaneous remission common.

Progressive: sensorimotor polyneuropathy; sometimes with autonomic neuropathy. Predominantly sensory. Usually irreversible.

Diabetic amyotrophy: pain, severe asymmetric muscle weakness, weakness of iliopsoas, quadriceps, adductor muscles. Onset may be abrupt. Prominent weight loss ("neurogenic diabetic cachexia"). Little or no sensory loss. Usually resolves spontaneously but may last 1 to 3 years.

Treatment of pain: amitriptyline, desipramine.

BRACHIAL NEURITIS

Also known as neuralgic amyotrophy (Parsonage-Turner syndrome). Acute pain localized to shoulder region, followed by weakness of ipsilateral shoulder girdle or arm muscles; sometimes bilateral and asymmetric. Patterns: mononeuropathy multiplex, mononeuropathy, plexopathy. Predominantly axonal.

RADIATION NEUROPATHY

Radiotherapy for breast cancer: brachial plexopathy; or lumbosacral plexus after radiotherapy for testicular cancer. In

Hodgkin disease: caudal roots affected. Severe pain followed by paresthesias, sensory loss. Latent period of years. Fasciculation, myokymia may be prominent. Axonal.

IDIOPATHIC NEUROPATHY

Sometimes identified later as immune-mediated or hereditary neuropathy.

Section XIII
Dementias

CHAPTER 107 ■ ALZHEIMER DISEASE AND OTHER DEMENTIAS

Definition of dementia (according to DSM-IV): "Multiple cognitive deficits that are sufficiently severe to cause impairment in occupational or social functioning." Must involve memory plus other cognitive domains; must show decline from premorbid function; exclude delirium. See also Chapter 1.

DEGENERATIVE DISEASES

ALZHEIMER DISEASE (AD)

Clinical Syndrome

First symptom: memory impaired for newly acquired information; memory for remote events less impaired. Later: impaired language, abstract reasoning, executive functions; delusions, other psychotic behavior; major depression; agitation, hallucinations.

Rigidity, bradykinesia, shuffling gait, postural instability common.

Progressive, terminates in complete incapacity, then death in 4 to 16 years.

EEG: generalized slowing. MRI: diffuse atrophy, particularly frontotemporal. PET: temporoparietal hypometabolism.

Epidemiology

Prevalence: <1% before age 65; 5% to 10% at age 65; 30% to 40% after 85.

Lifetime risk double in siblings of patients. The ε4 polymorphism of apolipoprotein E gene (chromosome 19) increases risk. Autosomal inheritance in 5% with mutation in one of three genes (synuclein, presenilins).

Other risk factors: traumatic head injury, lower educational achievement, parental age at time of birth, smoking, Down syndrome in first-degree relative.

Pathology and Biochemistry

(a) Diffuse atrophy of cerebral cortex, especially frontal, parietal, temporal.

(b) Senile neuritic plaques: core of extracellular amyloid surrounded by enlarged axonal endings.

(c) Neurofibrillary tangles: fibrillary intracytoplasmic structures within neurons, containing paired helical filaments, tau protein.

(d) 50% to 90% reduction of activity of choline acetyltransferase (CAT); decreased synthesis of acetylcholine, in cerebral cortex and hippocampus. Loss of CAT correlates with severity cognitive loss.

Diagnosis

Mental status examination, neuropsychologic testing most helpful. Brain imaging (CT or MRI) to exclude other causes of dementia.

Treatment

Anticholinesterases: tacrine (use limited by hepatotoxicity), donepezil, rivastigmine, galantamine. Small benefit on cognitive performance; unclear effect on functional capacity.

Psychotropic drugs for agitation, delusions, psychosis, depression in AD.

FRONTOTEMPORAL DEMENTIA

Pick disease: progressive dementia, personality change, speech disturbance, inattentiveness; sometimes parkinsonian signs. Rare; some familial. Frontotemporal atrophy; round intraneuronal inclusions (Pick bodies) contain tau protein; ubiquitinated inclusions (Table 107.1).

Frontotemporal dementias other than Pick disease: personality change, deterioration of memory and executive functions,

TABLE 107.1

DEGENERATIVE DISEASES ASSOCIATED WITH DEMENTIA AND WITH SPECIFIC TAU GENE MUTATIONS

Familial frontotemporal dementia and parkinsonism
Progressive supranuclear palsy
Familial progressive subcortical gliosis
Corticobasal ganglionic degeneration
Familial multiple system tauopathy with presenile dementia

stereotypical behavior; parkinsonism prominent. Rare; mutations in tau gene, chromosome 17. Neurofibrillary tangles present. Atrophy of frontal and temporal cortex, basal ganglia, substantia nigra. May be associated with motor neuron disease (ALS).

DEMENTIA WITH PARKINSON DISEASE (PD)

Third most common dementia. Affects up to 40% patients with Parkinson disease. Risk increases with age of onset of PD symptoms, presence depression, advanced motor disease. Often with mild PD-type cognitive loss (impaired mental speed, visuospatial abilities).

DEMENTIA WITH LEWY BODIES

Also known as diffuse Lewy body disease (DLBD). Cognitive decline, visual hallucinations, parkinsonism, repeated falls, sensitivity to neuroleptics. Fluctuating cognitive function; episodic confusion, delusions, hallucinations may differ from AD.

HUNTINGTON DISEASE

See also Chapter 109. Memory loss, difficulty performing complex or sequential mental activities prominent early in disease. Frank dementia follows.

VASCULAR DISEASES

CEREBROVASCULAR DISEASE AND DEMENTIA

Stroke: second most frequent cause of dementia. 15% to 20% of patients with acute ischemic stroke over age 60 have dementia at stroke onset. Risk 5% per year thereafter.

Risk factors: advancing age, diabetes, history of prior stroke, size, location of stroke.

Definition of vascular dementia unsettled. Etiology may be multifactorial. Diagnosis difficult due to high prevalence of stroke and AD.

Mechanisms: critically located single infarcts; multiple large infarcts; extensive small vessel disease; hemorrhagic stroke.

Cortical syndrome: repeated atherothrombotic or cardioembolic strokes, focal sensorimotor signs, aphasia, abrupt onset cognitive failure.

Subcortical syndrome (deep white matter lesions): pseudobulbar signs, pyramidal signs, depression, emotional lability, "frontal" behavior, mildly impaired memory, disorientation, poor response to novelty, restricted interests, difficulty passing from one idea to another, inattention, perseveration.

CADASIL: cerebral autosomal dominant inherited arteriopathy with subcortical infarcts and leukoencephalopathy.

TABLE 107.2

LABORATORY INVESTIGATIONS OF INHERITED METABOLIC DEMENTIAS

Disease	Laboratory tests
Wilson disease	Serum ceruloplasmin, urinary copper
Adrenoleukodystrophy and adrenomyeloneuropathy	Very-long-chain fatty acids
Cerebrotendinous xanthomatosis	Serum cholestanol
Kufs disease	Urinary dolichols, skin or brain biopsy
Membranous lipodystrophy	Hand x-rays, bone biopsy
MERRF, MELAS	Lactic acid, muscle biopsy
Metachromatic leukodystrophy	Leukocyte arylsufatase A
Mucopolysaccaridosis III	α-N-acetylglucosaminidase
Gaucher disease	Glucocerebrosidase
Niemann-Pick type C	Sphingomyelinase
Krabbe disease	Leukocyte galactocerebroside β-galactosidase
GM_2-gangliosidosis	Leukocyte hexosaminidase A
GM_1-gangliosidosis	Leukocyte β-galactosidase
Adult polyglucosan body disease	Sural nerve biopsy
Lafora disease	Muscle biopsy; DNA for laforin at EMP2 locus at 6p22.

MELAS, mitochondrial encephalomyopathy with lactic acidosis and stroke; MERRF, myoclonic epilepsy with ragged red fibers.

Autosomal dominant. Onset age 20 to 40. Mutations of notch3 gene, chromosome 19. See Chapter 41.

TRANSMISSIBLE DISEASES

PRION-RELATED DISEASES

See Chapter 34.

HIV-1–ASSOCIATED DEMENTIA COMPLEX

See Chapter 25.

INHERITED METABOLIC DISEASES

Rarely cause dementia in adults, but may be treatable. Clues: young-onset dementia; involve other areas of CNS, viscera. See Table 107.2.

Section XIV
Ataxias

CHAPTER 108 ■ HEREDITARY ATAXIAS

See Table 108.1 for list of disorders; Tables 108.2, 108.3 for clinical features and inheritance. Notes about selected conditions follow.

Note: syndrome of myoclonus, progressive ataxia, previously called Ramsay Hunt syndrome, is now recognized as including several diseases, including mitochondrial encephalomyopathy with ragged red fibers (MERRF; Chapter 97, Unverricht-Lundborg disease (progressive myoclonus epilepsy type 1 [EPM1]), Lafora body disease (EPM2), neuronal ceroid lipofuscinosis.

AUTOSOMAL RECESSIVE ATAXIAS

Most have early onset. Clinically heterogeneous; ataxia-plus; inherited; pathology involves cerebellum or connections.

Friedreich ataxia (FRDA): most common early-onset ataxia. Prevalence 2:100,000; carrier frequency 1:120. Expansion GAA triplet repeat in frataxin gene (chromosome 9). Hypertrophic cardiomyopathy in 25%; diabetes mellitus in 10%. Most cannot walk 15 years after onset; mean age at death 40 to 60. Late-onset (after age 25) forms exist, with milder severity, slower progression.

Ataxia telangiectasia: defective DNA repair. Cutaneous telangiectasias characteristic but not invariable. Median age at death 20 years.

Ataxia with vitamin E deficiency: normal lipid absorption. Usually mimics FRDA. Vitamin E replacement prevents or reverses ataxia.

X-LINKED ATAXIAS

Fragile X-tremor ataxia syndrome: associated with premutation expansions (55–200 CCG repeats) in fragile X mental

TABLE 108.1

HEREDITARY ATAXIAS BY MODE OF INHERITANCE

Autosomal Recessive Ataxias
(onset usually before age 20, although some have
  late-onset forms)
Friedreich ataxia (FRDA)
Ataxia telangiectasia (AT)
Ataxia with vitamin E deficiency (AVED)
Abeta and hypobetalipoproteinemia
AOA1 (ataxia with oculomotor apraxia 1)
AOA2 (ataxia with oculomotor apraxia 2)
ARSACS (autosomal recessive spastic ataxia of
  Charlevoix Saguenay)
IOSCA (infantile onset cerebellar ataxia)
Ataxia-telangiectasia variant (ATV1)/Nijmegen
  Breakage Syndrome
Spinocerebellar ataxia with neuropathy

Other Recessive Ataxias
  With hypogonadism
  With myoclonus
  With optic atrophy and mental retardation
  With deafness
  With cataracts and mental retardation
  (Marinesco-Sjögren)
Childhood ataxia with CNS
  hypomyelination/vanishing white matter (CACH)
Carboxylase deficiencies
Urea cycle defects
Aminoacidurias
Biotinidase deficiency
Wilson disease
Hypoceruloplasminemia with ataxia and dysarthria
  (onset in 40s)
Sialidosis
Refsum
Ceroid lipofuscinosis (Batten disease)
Leukodystrophies
Cerebrotendinous xanthomatosis
Hexosaminidase deficiency
Xeroderma pigmentosum
Cockayne syndrome
Leigh (also mitochondrial inheritance)

X-Linked
Fragile X-Tremor Ataxia
X-linked sideroblastic anemia with ataxia
Uncomplicated ataxia
Ataxia with spasticity
  With mental retardation
  With deafness

(continued)

TABLE 108.1

HEREDITARY ATAXIAS BY MODE OF INHERITANCE
(*Continued*)

Autosomal Dominant Ataxias
Spinocerebellar ataxias:
SCA type 1, 2, 3 (Machado-Joseph disease), 4, 5, 6, 7,
8, 10, 11, 12, 13, 14, 15, 16, 17, 18, 20, 21, 25
Dentatorubral pallidoluysian atrophy (DRPLA)
Episodic ataxia type 1 (EA1)
Episodic ataxia type 2 (EA2)

Mitochondrial Inheritance
Coenzyme Q10 (Co-Q10) deficiency
Mitochondrial encephalomyopathies (MERRF, NARP,
KSS)
Leigh Syndrome

KSS, Kearns-Sayre syndrome; MERRF, mitochondrial
encephalomyopathy with ragged red fibers; NARP, neuropathy,
ataxia, retinitis pigmentosa.

retardation gene (FMR1). Ataxia, intention tremor, with possible dementia, parkinsonism, neuropathy, proximal leg weakness, autonomic dysfunction. Penetrance increases with age.

AUTOSOMAL DOMINANT ATAXIAS

Also known as autosomal dominant cerebellar ataxias
(ADCA). Genetic classification: spinocerebellar ataxias (SCA),
types 1 to 25 (some numbers skipped). See Table 108.3.

Distinct clinical features present in some SCAs but most
SCAs share clinical features. Early: gait, limb ataxia, possible
hyperreflexia. Later: loss of tendon reflexes, often along with
vibration, position sense. Eye signs include nystagmus, slow
saccades, abnormal pursuit. Additional features may include
dementia, dystonia, parkinsonism, tremor, neuropathy, distal
wasting. Severe disability 10 to 20 years after onset in most
SCAs.

Mutation: unstable expansion of CAG triplet repeat in protein-
coding region of respective gene in all except SCA8, 10,
12, 14. Inverse relation between repeat length and age at
onset. Anticipation (earlier onset), potentiation (increasing
severity of symptoms) in successive generations observed
in most SCAs (most dramatic in SCA7, DRPLA; absent in
SCA6).

TABLE 108.2
CLINICAL FEATURES IN SELECTED AUTOSOMAL RECESSIVE ATAXIAS

Disorder	Typical age of onset (range in years)	Clinical features (all have ataxia)
Friedrich ataxia (FRDA)	Childhood–teens (infant–40)	Hyporeflexia, position sense loss, sensory loss, dysarthria, Babinski sign, cardiomyopathy, scoliosis; may be manifest by late-onset spastic paraparesis without much or any ataxia
Ataxia-telangiectasia (AT)	Early childhood (infant to 27)	Oculocutaneous telangiectasia, immunodeficiency, elevated alpha-fetoprotein, malignancy
Ataxia with oculomotor apraxia type 1 (AOA 1)	7 (2–16)	Dysarthria, dysmetria, axonal neuropathy with areflexia, chorea, dystonia, decreased serum albumin and total cholesterol
Ataxia with oculomotor apraxia type 2 (AOA2)	15 (10–25)	Sensorimotor neuropathy, oculomotor apraxia, chorea, dystonia, increased alpha-fetoprotein
Autosomal recessive spastic ataxia of Charlevoix Saguenay (ARSACS)	Childhood	Retinal striations, spasticity, peripheral neuropathy
Infantile onset spinocerebellar ataxia (IOSCA)	Infancy	Peripheral neuropathy, chorea, optic atrophy, hearing loss
Marinesco- Sjögren	Infancy	Cataracts, mental retardation, hypotonia, myopathy
Ataxia with Vitamin E Deficiency (AVED)	Child to teen (2–52)	FRDA-like, titubation

TABLE 108.3

CLINICAL FEATURES IN SELECTED AUTOSOMAL DOMINANT ATAXIAS

Disorder	Mean age of onset (range)	Distinguishing clinical features (ataxia including dysarthria is common for all)
SCA1[a]	30s (childhood to >60)	Pyramidal signs, dysphagia, ophthalmoparesis, neuropathy
SCA2[a]	20s–30s (infant to 67)	Slow saccades, neuropathy, hyporeflexia, dementia
SCA3[a]	30s (6–70)	Ophthalmoparesis, pyramidal and extrapyramidal signs, amyotrophy, sensory loss
SCA4	30s (19–59)	Sensory neuropathy, pyramidal signs
SCA5	30s (10–68)	Slowly progressive
SCA6[a]	48 (19–75)	Slowly progressive, sometimes episodic, downbeat nystagmus
SCA7[a]	30s (infant–60s)	Visual loss with optic atrophy and pigmentary retinopathy, ophthalmoparesis, pyramidal signs, extreme anticipation
SCA8[a]	39 (18–65)	Hyperreflexia, decreased vibratory sense, maternal bias for transmission
SCA10[a]	36	Seizures, polyneuropathy
SCA11	30 (15–70)	Slowly progressive, hyperreflexia, vertical nystagmus
SCA12	33 (8–55)	Early tremor, bradykinesia, dystonia, dementia, dysautonomia, hyperreflexia
SCA13	child	Mental retardation, short stature
SCA14[a]	28 (12–42)	Early axial myoclonus
SCA15	Childhood to teens	Dysarthria (pure ataxia)
SCA16	39 (20–66)	Head tremor, nystagmus, dysarthria
SCA17[a]	6–34	Dementia, parkinsonism, dystonia, chorea, seizures, cerebral and cerebellar atrophy on MRI

(continued)

TABLE 108.3

CLINICAL FEATURES IN SELECTED AUTOSOMAL
DOMINANT ATAXIAS (*Continued*)

Disorder	Mean age of onset (range)	Distinguishing clinical features (ataxia including dysarthria is common for all)
SCA18	teens	Motor > sensory neuropathy
SCA19		Tremor, myoclonus cognitive impairment
SCA20	46 (19–64)	Palatal tremor/myoclonus, dysarthria, hypermetric saccades, pyramidal signs, dentate calcification on CT
SCA21	6–30	Akinesia, rigidity, tremor, cognitive impairment
SCA22	10–46	Slowly progressive
SCA25	1–39	Sensory neuropathy
DRPLA[a]	30s (child–70)	Early onset myoclonus and epilepsy, late-onset chorea. Dementia in both
EA1	Child (2–15)	Exercise- or startle-induced ataxia, myokymia (attack duration: seconds-minutes), no vertigo
EA2	Child (3–52)	Stress- or fatigue-induced episodic ataxia (attack duration: minutes–hours), later permanent ataxia, acetazolamide responsive

[a]Genetic test commercially available.

SCA3: Machado-Joseph disease (MJD); common cause of ADCA in diverse populations.

DRPLA: dentatorubral-pallidoluysian atrophy. Most common in Japan (20% of ADCA families). Expansion of CAG repeat in DRPLA gene; anticipation. Variable phenotype. Early-onset: severe, rapid progression, myoclonus, epilepsy, cognitive decline. Late-onset: ataxia, chorea, dementia. Haw River syndrome: variant in African American family in North Carolina.

MRI: atrophy of cerebral cortex, cerebellum, pontomesencephalic tegmentum; increased signal in white matter of cerebrum and brainstem.

Unmapped ADCAs: other loci for ADCA remain to be identified.

Treatment of SCAs: levodopa for rigidity, other parkinsonian features (especially MJD/SCA3).

EPISODIC OR PAROXYSMAL ATAXIAS

Episodic ataxia with myokymia (EA type 1): attacks of ataxia, dysarthria, tremor. Attacks last a few minutes; provoked by startle, sudden movement, change in posture, exercise. Onset: childhood, adolescence. Not progressive. Myokymia persists between attacks around eyes and in hands. Acetazolamide may reduce frequency of attacks; phenytoin, other anticonvulsants may reduce myokymia. Mutations in voltage-gated potassium channel gene.

Episodic ataxia with nystagmus (EA type 2): attacks of ataxia, nystagmus, headache, sweating, nausea, vertigo, ataxia, dysarthria, ptosis, ocular palsy. Attacks last hours to days. Provoked by stress, exercise, fatigue, alcohol. Onset from infancy to 40 years. Cerebellar syndrome (dysarthria, ataxia) may progress. Interictal nystagmus. Acetazolamide almost always reduces attack frequency. Mutation in voltage-gated calcium channel gene; allelic to mutation associated with familial hemiplegic migraine.

SPORADIC CEREBELLAR ATAXIA OF LATE ONSET

Small minority due to SCA mutations. Onset in sixth decade; rapid course; parkinsonism, upper motor neuron signs, autonomic dysfunction sometimes present (multiple system atrophy of olivopontocerebellar type).

MANAGEMENT OF HEREDITARY ATAXIAS

No treatments influence the course of most hereditary ataxias. Symptomatic treatments mentioned above.

Section XV
Movement Disorders

CHAPTER 109 ■ HUNTINGTON DISEASE

Progressive; autosomal dominant; usually adult onset; with movement disorder (usually chorea), personality disorder, dementia.

Pathology: generalized brain atrophy; striatum (caudate nucleus, putamen) most affected.

Biochemistry: loss of striatal and nigral neurons synthesizing γ-aminobutyric acid (GABA); possible excitotoxicity.

Prevalence: 4 to 8/100,000 in United States, Europe; 10 times less prevalent in Japan.

GENETICS

Expansion of CAG trinucleotide repeat in HD gene (chromosome 4). Number of repeats inversely correlated with age at symptom onset. Expansion unstable in sperm only: paternal transmission associated with increased number of repeats, younger onset age in offspring. Neuronal accumulation of gene product (huntingtin).

SIGNS AND SYMPTOMS

Symptom onset usually age 35 to 40 (range: 5 to 70). Movement disorder, personality disorder, mental deterioration together or in any order.

Typical course: clumsiness, drop objects, fidgetiness, irritability, slovenliness, neglect duties, then frank chorea, dementia. Duration variables, around 15 to 20 years; more rapid with earlier age onset.

Chorea
Defined in Chapter 9. All muscles randomly involved. Arm and leg movements result in dancing, prancing, stuttering gait.

Other motor signs: motor impersistence (inhibitory pauses during voluntary contraction), slow saccades, irregular smooth pursuit; dysarthria, dysphagia.

In advanced stages, chorea may be replaced by rigidity, dystonia, immobility.

Cognitive and Psychiatric Signs

Early: irritability, impulsive behavior, bouts of depression, fits of violence.

Later: progressive impairment of memory, loss of intellectual capacity, apathy, inattention to personal hygiene.

Other Neurologic Manifestations
Seizures in late stages.

Westphal variant: akinetic-rigid syndrome, in childhood or adolescent onset (10% of all HD cases); dementia, convulsive seizures. Fatal in <10 years.

LABORATORY DATA

CT or MRI: enlarged ventricles; butterfly appearance of lateral ventricles, small caudate nucleus. Akinetic-rigid form: striatal hyperintensity on T2-weighted MRI. 18-FDG-PET: hypometabolism in striatum.

DIFFERENTIAL DIAGNOSIS

HD-like syndromes (HDL1, 2, 3); other causes of chorea: see Chapter 110. Also consider: other inheritable disorders (leukodystrophies, gangliosidosis).

TREATMENT

Symptomatic. Antipsychotics with lower risk of motor side effects (quetiapine, clozapine) preferred for psychosis. Dopamine depleting agents (reserpine, tetrabenazine) useful for chorea.

Counseling crucial before and after genetic testing.

CHAPTER 110 ■ SYDENHAM AND OTHER FORMS OF CHOREA

Most common causes of chorea: Tables 110.1, 110.2.

SYDENHAM CHOREA

Etiology: manifestation of rheumatic fever. Autoimmune; follows infection with group A β-hemolytic streptococcus (GAS). Chorea may be delayed for months. Presumed cross-reaction of streptococcal antibodies with neurons in caudate, subthalamic nuclei.

PANDAS (pediatric autoimmune neuropsychiatric disorders associated with streptococcal infection): term for possible relationship between infection with GAS and tic disorders, obsessive-compulsive disorder; controversial.

Epidemiology: 80% ages 5 to 15. M:F ratio 1:2. Rare in developed countries.

Clinical features: rapid, irregular, aimless, involuntary movements of limbs, face, trunk. Behavioral, mental.

Laboratory data: tests for rheumatoid factor, antinuclear antibodies, antistreptolysin titers, CSF oligoclonal bands. EEG: diffuse slowing. 18-FDG-PET scan: striatal hypermetabolism.

Course: complete recovery of almost all patients in 3 to 6 weeks. Recurrence in 35%.

Complications: cardiac, usually endocarditis, in 20%. Mental, behavioral abnormalities may persist.

Treatment: bed rest, sedation, dopamine-depleting agents (reserpine, tetrabenazine) for chorea. Prophylactic penicillin for at least 10 years recommended to prevent rheumatic fever.

OTHER IMMUNE CHOREAS

Chorea in systemic lupus erythematosus: intermittent; with antiphospholipid antibodies (lupus anticoagulant).

TABLE 110.1

COMMON CAUSES OF CHOREA

Hereditary
Huntington disease
Huntington disease-like syndromes (HDL1, HDL2, HDL3)
Hereditary nonprogressive chorea
Neuroacanthocytosis
Dentatorubral pallidoluysian atrophy
Spinocerebellar atrophy 17 (SCA17)
Wilson disease
Ataxia-telangiectasia
Lesch-Nyhan syndrome

Secondary
Infections/immunologic
  Sydenham chorea
  Encephalitis
  Systemic lupus erythematosus
  Antiphospholipid syndrome
Drug-induced
  Levodopa
  Anticonvulsants
  Anticholinergics
  Antipsychotics
Metabolic and endocrine
  Chorea gravidarum
  Hyperthyroidism
  Birth control pills
  Hyperosmolar nonketotic hyperglycemic encephalopathy
Vascular
  Hemichorea/hemiballismus with subthalamic nucleus lesion
  Post-pump choreoathetosis after cardiac surgery
  Periarteritis nodosa

Unknown etiology
Senile chorea
Essential chorea

Chorea gravidarum: isolated, transient chorea during pregnancy. May be mediated by anti-basal ganglia antibodies.

Chorea in primary antiphospholipid antibody syndrome: young women; spontaneous abortions, venous and arterial thrombosis, thickened cardiac valves, livedo reticularis, Raynaud phenomenon, strokes, multi-infarct dementia.

TABLE 110.2

OTHER CAUSES OF SYMPTOMATIC CHOREA
IN CHILDHOOD

Adrenal insufficiency
Anoxic encephalopathy
Antiphospholipid antibody
Benign hereditary chorea
Cardiopulmonary bypass, complication of encephalitis, e.g.,
   ECHO virus type 25, mononucleosis, HIV infection,
   bacterial endocarditis, typhoid fever, Lyme disease
GM_1 gangliosidosis
Human immunodeficiency virus (HIV)
Huntington disease, Juvenile
Hypocalcemia, hypercalcemia
Hypothermia, deep
Lesch-Nyhan syndrome
Moyamoya disease
Systemic lupus erythematosus
Wilson disease
Withdrawal emergent syndrome (a form of tardive dyskinesia)

VASCULAR CHOREA AND BALLISM

Stroke (occlusive, hemorrhagic): hemichorea, hemiballism.
Usual lesion in contralateral subthalamic nucleus. Also seen
with nonvascular lesions of same nucleus.

Hyperosmolar hyperglycemic nonketotic syndrome: diffuse
chorea, ballism, probably striatal hypoperfusion.

Post-pump chorea: after surgery for congenital heart disease
with prolonged time on cardiac pump, deep hypothermia,
circulatory arrest. Usually persists; difficult to treat.

NEUROACANTHOCYTOSIS

See Chapter 93.

DENTATORUBRAL-PALLIDOLUYSIAN ATROPHY

See Chapter 108.

HUNTINGTON DISEASE-LIKE SYNDROMES

Huntington Disease-Like Syndromes 1, 2 (HDL1, HDL2): both autosomal dominant. Phenotype like Huntington disease (HD). HDL2 affects exclusively or predominantly people of African origin.

HDL3: autosomal recessive neurodegenerative disease beginning at 3 to 4 years of age. Chorea, dystonia, ataxia, gait disorder, spasticity, seizures, mutism, intellectual impairment. MRI: bilateral frontal, caudate atrophy.

DNA: mutation at HDL1, HDL2, or HDL3 locus, not at HD locus.

SPINOCEREBELLAR ATROPHY 17

Although labelled a spinocerebellar degeneration, SCA17 can present with chorea, other features of HD.

HEREDITARY NONPROGRESSIVE CHOREA

Childhood onset; nonprogressive; no other neurologic abnormalities. Autosomal dominant; if no other cases in family called "essential chorea" but could be new mutation.

SENILE CHOREA

Late-onset generalized chorea; no other cases in family; no dementia. Most cases have defined etiology (e.g., HD, antiphospholipid syndrome).

CHAPTER 111 ■ MYOCLONUS

Brief, "lightning-like" muscle jerks with typically brief EMG bursts (20 to 100 msec). "Negative" myoclonus: sudden, brief lapse of contraction (e.g., asterixis).

Prevalence 8.6/100,000.

Differential diagnosis: no other movement associated with similarly rapid EMG bursts. In addition, tics often more complex; chorea slower, often random in location.

Classification: clinical, anatomic, etiologic (Table 111.1).

Localization principles: rhythmicity almost always denotes segmental origin (brainstem or spinal cord). Generalized appearance suggests brainstem origin. Focal myoclonus cortical or subcortical.

Cortical myoclonus: usually focal, reflex-induced. Cortical origin established by back-averaging EMG jerks with EEG spikes. Often with large somatosensory evoked potentials. May be idiopathic (rhythmic form, also called familial cortical tremor) or associated with other diseases (e.g., corticobasal degeneration). *Epilepsia partialis continua:*

TABLE 111.1

CLASSIFICATION OF MYOCLONUS

Clinical	Anatomic	Etiology
1. At rest action, reflex	1. Cortical focal multifocal generalized Epilepsia partialis continua	1. Physiologic
2. Focal axial, multifocal generalized		2. Essential
		3. Epileptic
		4. Symptomatic
		Storage diseases
3. Irregular, oscillatory rhythmic	2. Thalamic	Cerebellar degenerations
	3. Brain stem reticular startle palatal	Basal ganglia degenerations
		Dementias
		Infectious encephalopathy
	4. Spinal segmental propriospinal	Metabolic encephalopathy
	5. Peripheral	Toxic encephalopathy
		Hypoxia
		Focal damage

rhythmic focal jerking; within the cortical myoclonus family.

Palatal myoclonus: also classified as palatal tremor. Rhythmic (approximately 2 Hz) contractions of soft palate muscles.

(a) **Primary:** cause unknown; often with constant clicking sounds in ear; disappears in sleep.

(b) **Secondary:** lesion in medullary Guillain-Mollaret triangle; persists in sleep; often with vertical ocular myoclonus.

Essential myoclonus: familial or sporadic; no other neurologic abnormality; no progression.

Serotonin syndrome: sometimes accompanies treatment serotonergic agents (e.g., fluoxetine, paroxetine); myoclonus, diaphoresis, flushing, rigidity, hyperreflexia, shivering, confusion, agitation, restlessness, coma, autonomic instability.

Polyminimyoclonus: small amplitude, resembles continuous generalized irregular tremor. Eyes often involved (opsoclonus-myoclonus syndrome). With neuroblastoma in infants; paraneoplastic or postviral in adults.

Exaggerated startle syndromes (hyperekplexia): brainstem origin; sudden response (range from small movement to complex motor or verbal acts) to unexpected stimulus.

Encephalomyelitis with rigidity: severe sudden-onset variant of stiff-person syndrome. Stiffness, excessive startle, stimulus-triggered myoclonic jerks. Often responds to steroid therapy.

Treatment of myoclonus: often requires polypharmacy. Valproic acid, clonazepam, primidone, levetiracetam. Clobazam reported effective for hyperekplexia.

CHAPTER 112 ■ GILLES DE LA TOURETTE SYNDROME

Most common cause of tics. Diagnostic criteria: multiple motor and phonic tics; change in character over time; onset before age 21 years; symptoms wax and wane; last more than 1 year. Tics defined in Chapter 9.

Other causes of tics: neuroacanthocytosis, encephalitis, neuroleptics, head trauma.

Tics usually begin in face and neck; may spread to limbs; often with vocal or other sounds (words, sniffing, throat clearing, barking); obscene utterances (coprolalia) characteristic but uncommon (10%).

Obsessive-compulsive disorder, attention-deficit/hyperactivity disorder, impulse control problems frequently present.

Inheritance pattern complex. Linkage to specific chromosomes in some families. Possible immune etiology not substantiated.

Prevalence in adolescents: highly variable estimates; about 5:10,000 in males, 3:10,000 in females.

Treatment: Clonidine, clonazepam; dopamine antagonists (e.g., newer antipsychotics), dopamine depleters (e.g., tetrabenazine) more effective but more adverse effects.

CHAPTER 113 ■ DYSTONIA

Sustained muscle contractions, frequently cause twisting repetitive movements or abnormal postures (see also Chapter 9). Also called "torsion dystonia." Movements sometimes rhythmic (dystonic tremor).

EMG in dystonia: simultaneous contraction of agonist and antagonist muscles with prolonged bursts and overflow to extraneous muscles.

DEFINITIONS

Task-specific dystonia: movements and postures elicited by specific actions. *Action dystonia*: Evoked by any action of involved body part. *Overflow dystonia*: evoked by action of other body parts. *Sensory trick*: simple touch diminishes dystonic movement (touching chin or side of face reduces torticollis).

Focal dystonia: single area affected. *Segmental*: two or more contiguous body parts. *Generalized*: involves leg plus some other area. *Multifocal*: two or more noncontiguous parts. *Hemidystonia*: half-body.

CLASSIFICATION OF DYSTONIA

See Table 113.1. Age at onset: most important prognostic factor for primary dystonia; younger onset, more likely dystonia later becomes severe and spreads to other body parts.

Onset of dystonia in leg second predictor of more rapid progression course. Adult-onset dystonia more often focal than generalized.

TABLE 113.1

CLASSIFICATIONS OF TORSION DYSTONIA

By Age at Onset
Childhood onset, 0–12 yr
Adolescent onset, 13–20 yr
Adult onset, >20 yr

By Distribution
Focal
Segmental
Multifocal
Generalized
Hemidystonia

By Etiology
Primary (also known as idiopathic) dystonia
Dystonia plus
Secondary dystonia
Heredodegenerative diseases (usually presents as dystonia-plus)

TABLE 113.2
GENE NOMENCLATURE FOR THE DYSTONIAS

Name	Inheritance pattern	Phenotype
DYT1	AD	Young, limb-onset (Oppenheim)
DYT2	AR	Early-onset
DYT3	XR	Filipino, dystonia/parkinsonism ("lubag")
DYT4	AD	Whispering dysphonia
DYT5	AD	DRD/ parkinsonism (Segawa)
DYT6	AD	Mixed type, Mennonite/Amish
DYT7	AD	Adult cervical
DYT8	AD	PNKD (FDP1) (Mount-Rebak)
DYT9	AD	CSE, episodic choreoathetosis with spasticity
DYT10	AD	PKD (EKD1 &2)
DYT11	AD	Myoclonus-dystonia
DYT12	AD	Rapid-onset dystonia-parkinsonism
DYT13	AD	Cervical/cranial/brachial
DYT14	AD	DRD
DYT15	AD	Myoclonus-dystonia

Genetic nomenclature is presented in the chronologic order named. AD, autosomal dominant; AR, autosomal recessive; CSE, choreoathetosis/spasticity episodic; DRD, dopa-responsive dystonia; FPD1, familial paroxysmal dyskinesia type 1; PKD, paroxysmal kinesigenic dyskinesia; PNKD, paroxysmal non-kinesigenic dyskinesia; RDP, rapid-onset dystonia parkinsonism; XR, X-linked recessive.

PRIMARY TORSION DYSTONIAS

Restricted to dystonic postures and movements; sometimes tremor. Include familial and sporadic conditions. See Table 113.2.

OPPENHEIM (DYT1) DYSTONIA

Onset in childhood or adolescence in leg (most patients) or arm, then neck or larynx. Mean onset age 13 years; rarely after 26.

Progresses to generalized or multifocal dystonia in 65% of all patients. Probability of progression higher with onset in childhood and in leg. Rate of progression varies; mostly in first 5 to 10 years.

Mutation in DYT1 gene; chromosome 9. Autosomal dominant, but penetrance 30% to 40%, highly variable. Phenotype expression also highly variable. Gene product: torsin-A, a heat-shock protein.

Affects most ethnic groups. Accounts for great majority of childhood and adolescent-onset primary dystonia in Ashkenazi Jews, about 30% to 50% in non-Jews. Higher frequency in Ashkenazi Jews due to founder effect.

Genetic testing for DYT1 mutation: indicated for any primary dystonia starting before age 26. Counseling especially important given highly variable penetrance, phenotype.

OTHER EARLY-ONSET NON-DYT1 PRIMARY DYSTONIAS

DYT6 dystonia: autosomal dominant; onset in childhood or adulthood. Disabling dysphonia, dysarthria. Especially in Amish/Mennonite population.

DYT13 dystonia: described in one Italian family. Autosomal dominant. Jerking movements of neck, shoulder; variable spread to cranial and brachial muscles. Mild disability in most.

ADULT ONSET PRIMARY DYSTONIA

DYT7 dystonia: predominantly cervical; northwest Germany.

Cervical dystonia (spasmodic torticollis): most common focal dystonia. Onset age 20 to 60. Sustained turning, tilting, flexing, or extending neck. Neck pain in 66%.

Blepharospasm: contractions of orbicularis oculi; onset after age 50; increased frequency of blinking, then closure of eyelids intermittent at first, then more firm and prolonged. More common in men. Worsened by walking, bright light. Meige syndrome: blepharospasm plus facial or other cranial dystonia.

Writer's cramp: dystonic movements and postures of hand elicited by writing; spreads to other arm in 15%.

Dystonia of vocal cords: (a) spastic (spasmodic) dysphonia more common; vocal muscles contract; voice high pitched, strangled, coarse, broken with pauses; (b) breathy (whispering) dysphonia caused by contractions of vocal cord abductor; patient cannot talk in loud voice, tends to run out of air trying to speak.

DYSTONIA-PLUS SYNDROMES

Dystonia coexistent with parkinsonism or myoclonus.

DOPA-RESPONSIVE DYSTONIA (DRD)

Also known as Segawa disease, DYT5.

About 10% of patients with childhood-onset dystonia. Autosomal dominant. Responds well to treatment.

Features besides dystonia: (a) parkinsonism; (b) diurnal fluctuations, improve after sleep, worse as day wears on; (c) spastic-like straight-legged gait, tend to walk on toes; (d) hyperreflexia, particularly in legs, sometimes with Babinski signs; (e) excellent response to low doses levodopa, dopamine agonists, or anticholinergic drugs.

Onset any age, usually 6 to 16. Usually with mutations of gene for GTP cyclohydrolase I.

RAPID-ONSET DYSTONIA-PARKINSONISM

Autosomal dominant. Onset both symptoms ages 14 to 45. Maximum involvement in hours to days.

MYOCLONUS-DYSTONIA

Onset: childhood or adolescence. Autosomal dominant with reduced penetrance; most affected people inherit disorder through father. Neck, arms most commonly involved. Jerks respond dramatically to alcohol. Psychiatric symptoms, including obsessive compulsive disorder, may be present, even if motor signs are absent.

Most cases due to mutation in epsilon sarcoglycan gene on chromosome 7 (DYT11). Other cases: sporadic; mutation on second locus (DYT15); other unknown mutations.

SECONDARY DYSTONIA

Dystonia attributed to environmental factors (Table 113.3). Clinical clues may suggest secondary dystonia (Table 113.4) or psychogenic dystonia (Table 113.5).

TABLE 113.3

CAUSES OF SECONDARY DYSTONIA

Perinatal cerebral injury
  Athetoid cerebral palsy
  Delayed onset dystonia
  Pachygyria
Encephalitis, infections, post-infectious sequelae
  Subacute sclerosing panencephalitis
  Wasp sting
  CJD
  HIV infection
Head trauma
Thalamotomy
Primary antiphospholipid syndrome
Focal cerebral vascular injury
Arteriovenous malformation
Hypoxia
Brain tumor
Multiple sclerosis
Brainstem lesion, including pontine myelinolysis
Posterior fossa tumors
Cervical cord injury or lesion
Peripheral injury
Electrical injury
Drug induced
  Levodopa
  Dopamine D2 receptor blocking agents
    Acute dystonic reaction
    Tardive dystonia
  Ergotism
  Anticonvulsants
Toxins
  Manganese, carbon monoxide, carbon disulfide, cyanide,
  methanol, disulfiram, 3-nitroproprionic acid
Metabolic (hypoparathyroidism)
Psychogenic

TABLE 113.4
CLUES SUGGESTIVE OF SYMPTOMATIC DYSTONIA

1. History of possible etiologic factor, e.g., head trauma, peripheral trauma, encephalitis, toxin exposure, drug exposure, perinatal anoxia
2. Presence of neurologic abnormality, e.g., dementia, seizures, ocular, ataxia, weakness, spasticity, amyotrophy, parkinsonism
3. Onset of rest, instead of action, dystonia
4. Early onset of speech involvement
5. Leg involvement in an adult
6. Hemidystonia
7. Abnormal brain imaging
8. Abnormal laboratory workup
9. Presence of "give-way" weakness on sensory examination, or other clues of psychogenic etiology (see Table 113.5)

TABLE 113.5
CLUES SUGGESTING PSYCHOGENIC DYSTONIA

Clues relating to movements
1. Abrupt onset
2. Inconsistent movements (changing characteristics)
3. Incongruous movements and postures (movements do not fit recognized patterns or normal physiologic patterns)
4. Presence of additional types of abnormal movements not consistent with basic abnormal movement pattern or not congruous with known movement disorder, particularly rhythmic shaking, bizarre gait, deliberate slowness carrying out requested voluntary movement, bursts of verbal gibberish, and excessive startle (bizarre movements induced by sudden unexpected noise or threatening movement)
5. Spontaneous remissions
6. Movements disappear with distraction
7. Response to placebo, suggestion, or psychotherapy
8. May be paroxysmal
9. Dystonia begins as fixed posture
10. Twisting facial movements move mouth to one side or other (note: organic dystonia of facial muscles does not usually move mouth sideways)

Clues relating to other medical observations
1. "Give-way" weakness (absence of resistance due to lack of effort)
2. Sensory complaints changing with time or inconsistent with neuroanatomy
3. Multiple somatization or undiagnosed conditions

(continued)

TABLE 113.5

CLUES SUGGESTING PSYCHOGENIC DYSTONIA
(*Continued*)

4. Self-inflicted injuries
5. Evident psychiatric symptoms
6. Employed in health profession or insurance claims field
7. Presence of secondary gain, including continuing care by "devoted" spouse
8. Litigation or compensation pending

HEREDODEGENERATIVE DYSTONIA

Other neurologic features, especially parkinsonism, also present (Table 113.6).

DIFFERENTIAL DIAGNOSIS

See Tables 113.7, 113.8.

TREATMENT

Oral drugs: anticholinergics (e.g., trihexyphenidyl); baclofen; benzodiazepines (clonazepam, diazepam); antidopaminergics (reserpine, dopamine receptor blockers). Test levodopa therapy first in all patients with possible dopa-responsive dystonia.

Botulinum toxin: injections frequently effective in focal dystonia. Effect usually lasts 3 months.

Intrathecal baclofen: especially helpful for spasticity and dystonia.

Surgery: bilateral globus pallidum deep brain stimulation used for generalized primary dystonia unresponsive to other therapies; sometimes considered for severe tardive dystonia (Chapter 117).

TABLE 113.6

HEREDODEGENERATIVE DISEASES (TYPICALLY NOT PURE DYSTONIA)

X-Linked Recessive
Lubag (X-linked dystonia-parkinsonism) (DYT3)
Pelizaeus-Merzbacher disease
Deafness, dystonia, retardation, blindness syndrome

Autosomal Dominant
Juvenile parkinsonism (presenting with dystonia) (can be autosomal dominant or recessive)
Huntington disease (usually presents as chorea)
Machado-Joseph disease (SCA-3)
Dentatorubral pallidoluysian atrophy
Other spinocerebellar degenerations
Familial basal ganglia calcification

Autosomal Recessive
Wilson disease
Juvenile neuronal ceroid lipofuscinosis (sea-blue histiocytosis, dystonic lipidosis; Batten disease)
Gangliosidosis
Metachromatic leukodystrophy
Lesch-Nyhan syndrome
Homocystinuria
Glutaric acidemia
Triosephosphate isomerase deficiency
Methylmalonic aciduria
Hartnup disease
Ataxia telangiectasia
Neurodegeneration with brain iron accumulation (Hallervorden-Spatz disease)
Neuroacanthocytosis
Neuronal intranuclear hyaline inclusion disease
Hereditary spastic paraplegia with dystonia

Probable Autosomal Recessive
Progressive pallidal degeneration
Rett syndrome

Mitochondrial
Leigh syndrome
Leber hereditary optic neuropathy
Other mitochondrial encephalopathy

Associated with Parkinsonian Syndromes
Parkinson disease
Progressive supranuclear palsy
Multiple system atrophy
Corticobasal ganglionic degeneration
SCA, spinocerebellar ataxia

Adapted from Fahn S, Marsden CD, DeLong MR, eds. Dystonia 3. *Adv Neurol* 1998;78.

TABLE 113.7

OTHER MOVEMENT DISORDERS IN WHICH DYSTONIA MAY BE PRESENT

Tic disorders with dystonic tics
Paroxysmal dyskinesias with dystonia
   Paroxysmal kinesigenic dyskinesia
   Paroxysmal nonkinesigenic dyskinesia
   Paroxysmal exertional dyskinesia
   Benign infantile paroxysmal dyskinesias
Hypnogenic dystonia (sometimes these are seizures)

TABLE 113.8

PSEUDODYSTONIAS (NOT CLASSIFIED AS DYSTONIA BUT CAN BE MISTAKEN FOR DYSTONIA BECAUSE OF SUSTAINED POSTURES)

Sandifer syndrome (gastroesophageal reflux disease)
Stiff-person syndrome
Isaacs syndrome
Satoyoshi syndrome
Rotational atlantoaxial subluxation
Soft tissue nuchal mass
Bone disease
Ligamentous absence, laxity or damage
Congenital muscular torticollis
Congenital postural torticollis
Juvenile rheumatoid arthritis
Ocular postural torticollis
Congenital Klippel-Feil syndrome
Posterior fossa tumor
Syringomyelia
Arnold-Chiari malformation
Trochlear nerve palsy
Vestibular torticollis
Seizures manifesting as sustained twisting postures
Inflammatory myopathy

CHAPTER 114 ■ ESSENTIAL TREMOR

Chronic, progressive neurologic condition; 4 to 12 Hz tremor may involve arms, neck, voice, chin.

Tremor primarily with movement (kinetic) or sustained posture. Rarely present at rest, in contrast Parkinson tremor (see also Chapter 9).

Other possible manifestations: gait ataxia, eye movement abnormalities, mild cognitive impairment, impaired smell.

Prevalence 0.4% to 3.9%. One of most common adult-onset movement disorders. May be inherited (autosomal dominant) or sporadic.

Onset at any age; incidence increases with advancing age; may become progressively worse; often ameliorated temporarily by drinking alcoholic beverages.

Treatment: most effective drugs β-blockers (propranolol), primidone, or both. Also: clonazepam, methazolamide, glutethimide, clozapine, gabapentin. For severe problems: thalamotomy, deep brain thalamic stimulation.

CHAPTER 115 ■ PARKINSONISM

Characterized by any combination of: tremor at rest, rigidity, bradykinesia (slowing of movements), hypokinesia (less frequent spontaneous movements), flexed posture, loss of postural reflexes, "freezing" (motor block).

Categories: idiopathic, symptomatic, Parkinson-plus syndromes, heredodegenerative diseases with parkinsonism (Table 115.1).

Core biochemical pathology: decreased dopaminergic neurotransmission in basal ganglia, leading to disinhibition of subthalamic nucleus and medial globus pallidus.

TABLE 115.1

CLASSIFICATION OF MAJOR PARKINSONIAN SYNDROMES

Idiopathic Parkinsonism
Parkinson disease

Symptomatic Parkinsonism
Drug-induced: dopamine antagonists and depleters
Hemiatrophy-hemiparkinsonism
Hydrocephalus; normal pressure hydrocephalus
Hypoxia
Infectious; postencephalitic
Metabolic; parathyroid dysfunction
Toxins: manganese, carbon monoxide, MPTP, cyanide
Trauma
Tumor
Vascular; multi-infarct state

Parkinson-plus Syndromes
Cortical-basal ganglionic degeneration
Dementia syndromes
  Alzheimer disease
  Diffuse Lewy body disease (dementia with Lewy bodies)
Lytico–Bodig (Guamanian parkinsonism–dementia–ALS complex)
Multiple system atrophy syndromes
  Striatonigral degeneration
  Shy-Drager syndrome
  Sporadic olivopontocerebellar degeneration
  Motor neuron disease-parkinsonism
Progressive pallidal atrophy
Progressive supranuclear palsy

Heredodegenerative Diseases
Neurodegeneration with brain iron accumulation (NBIA; Hallervorden-Spatz disease)
Huntington disease
Lubag (X-linked dystonia-parkinsonism)
Mitochondrial cytopathies with striatal necrosis
Neuroacanthocytosis
Wilson disease

ALS, amyotrophic lateral sclerosis; MPTP, methyl-4-phenyl-1,2,3,6-tetrahydropyridine

Rest tremor: 4 to 5 Hz; usually involves limbs, especially distally; also lips, chin, tongue. Disappears with action, but reemerges with maintained posture. Worsened by stress, walking.

Rigidity: increased resistance to passive movement; equal in all directions; often with palpable "cogwheeling."

Flexed posture: commonly begins in arms, spreads to body.

Bradykinesia: slow movements, difficulty starting movement, loss of automatic movements (arm-swing).

Hypokinesia: reduced amplitude of movement, particularly repetitive movements ("decrementing" finger or toe-tapping).

Akinesia: reduced frequency of movements.

Examples of bradykinesia, hypokinesia, akinesia: hypomimia (decreased facial expression), decreased blinking, loss of gestures, setting motionless, hypophonia, dysarthria, tachyphemia (rapid speech), aprosody (monotonous speech; loss of rhythm of speech), drooling (impaired swallowing), micrographia, impaired fine motor skills, short stride (festinating gait), difficulty rising from seat. Advanced bradykinesia—major impediment in activities of daily living. If feet involved, should stop driving.

Freezing phenomenon (motor block): transient inability to perform active movements. Manifest in legs (gait freezing), eyelids (apraxia of lid opening), speech (palilalia), writing. Lasts several seconds. Triggers: starting to walk, turning, approaching a destination, revolving doors, elevator doors, crossing heavily trafficked streets. Often overcome by visual clues.

PARKINSON DISEASE (PD)

Also known as idiopathic Parkinson disease or primary parkinsonism.

PATHOLOGY

Degeneration of neuromelanin-containing neurons in pars compacta of substantia nigra, locus ceruleus; Lewy bodies in surviving neurons.

EPIDEMIOLOGY

About 80% of cases of parkinsonism outlined in Table 115.2. Mean onset age 55, range 20 to 80. M:F ratio 3:2. Prevalence 160:100,000; incidence 20:100,000/year.

TABLE 115.2

CLUES INDICATING THE LIKELY TYPE OF PARKINSONISM

Clinical	Most likely form of parkinsonism
Never responded to levodopa	Other than PD
Predominantly unilateral	PD; HP-HA syndrome; CBGD
Symmetric onset	PD; most forms of parkinsonism
Presence of rest tremor	PD; secondary parkinsonism
Lack of rest tremor	Parkinson-plus syndromes
History of encephalitis	Postencephalitic parkinsonism
History of toxin exposure	Parkinsonism caused by the toxin
Taking neuroleptics	Drug-induced parkinsonism
Severe unilateral rigidity	CBGD
Cortical sensory signs	CBGD
Unilateral cortical myoclonus	CBGD
Unilateral apraxia	CBGD
Alien limb	CBGD
Early dementia	CBGD
Psychotic sensitivity to levodopa	Diffuse Lewy body disease; AD
Early loss of postural reflexes	Progressive supranuclear palsy
Impaired downgaze	Progressive supranuclear palsy
Deep nasolabial folds	Progressive supranuclear palsy
Furrowed forehead and eyebrows (procerus sign)	Progressive supranuclear palsy
Nuchal dystonia	Progressive supranuclear palsy
Abducted arms when walking	Progressive supranuclear palsy
Square wave jerks	Progressive supranuclear palsy
Pure freezing	Progressive supranuclear palsy
Meaningful orthostatic hypotension	Shy-Drager syndrome
Urinary or fecal incontinence	Shy-Drager syndrome
Cerebellar dysarthria and dysmetria	Olivopontocerebellar degeneration
Laryngeal stridor (vocal cord paresis)	Striatonigral degeneration
Lower motor neuron findings	Multiple system atrophy
Upper motor neuron findings	Multiple system atrophy

(continued)

TABLE 115.2

CLUES INDICATING THE LIKELY TYPE OF PARKINSONISM (*Continued*)

Clinical	Most likely form of parkinsonism
Laboratory	
Fresh blood smear: acanthocytes	Neuroacanthocytosis
Grossly elevated creatine kinase	Neuroacanthocytosis
MRI: many lacunes	Vascular parkinsonism
MRI: "tiger's eye" in pallidum	Hallervorden-Spatz disease
MRI: caudate atrophy	HD; neuroacanthocytosis
MRI: decreased T2 signal in striatum	Multiple system atrophy
MRI: midbrain atrophy	Progressive supranuclear palsy
MRI: huge ventricles	Normal pressure hydrocephalus
Abnormal autonomic function tests	Shy-Drager syndrome
Denervation on sphincter EMG	Shy-Drager syndrome

AD, Alzheimer disease; CBGD, corticobasal ganglionic degeneration; HP-HA, hemiparkinsonism-hemiatrophy; PD, Parkinson disease.

SYMPTOMS AND SIGNS

Insidious onset. Tremor: first symptom in 70%. Symptoms often unilateral at first, then bilateral.

Motor: signs as above.

Behavioral signs: reduced attention span, visuospatial impairment, personality change (more dependent, fearful, indecisive, passive). Depression frequent (2% per year).

Cognitive decline common: bradyphrenia (slow responses to questions), relative sparing of memory. Overt dementia in 15% to 20%.

Sensory symptoms: pain, burning, tingling. Sometimes akathisia (inability to sit still, restlessness), restless legs syndrome.

Autonomic disturbances: constipation, inadequate bladder emptying, impotence, low blood pressure.

Reflexes: nonextinguishing glabellar reflex (Myerson sign), snout reflex, palmomental reflexes common.

Sleep disturbances: REM-behavior sleep disorder; restless leg syndrome. Insomnia from: depression (early-morning awakening); insufficient dopaminergic treatments (difficulty finding comfortable position, feeling stiff); excessive dopaminergic treatment (nightmare, hallucinations).

GENETICS

Familial PD rare; mutations in genes for: α-synuclein (protein in Lewy bodies; autosomal dominant), parkin (protein abundant in substantia nigra; autosomal recessive).

ETIOLOGY, PATHOGENESIS

Steps responsible for initiation of neurodegeneration of substantia nigra neurons unknown. Two major pathogenic processes proposed as central to neurodegeneration: 1) misfolding, aggregation of proteins; 2) mitochondrial dysfunction, oxidative stress. Not mutually exclusive.

DIFFERENTIAL DIAGNOSIS

See Table 115.3.

DRUG-INDUCED PARKINSONISM

Drugs that block striatal dopamine D2 receptors (e.g., phenothiazines, butyrophenones) or deplete striatal dopamine (e.g., reserpine, tetrabenazine).

Reversible if offending agent withdrawn; may take weeks.

Antipsychotics least likely to cause parkinsonism: quetiapine, clozapine.

HEMIPARKINSONISM-HEMIATROPHY SYNDROME

Relatively benign, usually nonprogressive. Poor response to medication.

TABLE 115.3

THERAPEUTIC CHOICES FOR PARKINSON DISEASE

Medications
Dopamine precursor: levodopa $\pm$ carbidopa; standard, slow release
Dopamine agonists: bromocriptine, pramipexole, ropinirole, lisuride, apomorphine, cabergoline
Catechol-O-methyltransferase inhibitors: tolcapone, entacapone
Dopamine releaser: amantadine
Glutamate antagonist: amantadine
Monoamine oxidase type B inhibitor: selegiline, rasagiline
Anticholinergics: trihexyphenidyl, benztropine, ethopropazine, biperiden, cycrimine, procyclidine
Antihistamines: diphenhydramine, orphenadrine, phenindamine, chlorphenoxamine
Antidepressants: tricyclics, serotonin-reuptake inhibitors
Muscle relaxants: cyclobenzaprine, diazepam
Peripheral antidopaminergic: domperidone
Gut activator: cisapride
Antipsychotic: clozapine, quetiapine
Antianxiety agents: benzodiazepines

Surgery
Ablative surgery
  Thalamotomy, pallidotomy
Deep brain stimulation
  Subthalamic stimulation
  Thalamic stimulation
  Pallidal stimulation

NORMAL PRESSURE HYDROCEPHALUS

See Chapter 49.

VASCULAR PARKINSONISM

Multiple lacunar strokes in basal ganglia. Rare. Insidious onset, progressive. Gait profoundly affected; tremor rare. Poor response to antiparkinsonian drugs.

CORTICO-BASAL GANGLIONIC DEGENERATION

Typical onset: unilateral arm rigidity, dystonia. Cortical signs: apraxia, alien limb phenomenon, cortical sensory loss, reflex myoclonus. May be clinically indistinguishable from progressive supranuclear palsy (Chapter 116).

LYTICO-BODIG DISEASE

Also known as Parkinson–Dementia–ALS Complex of Guam.
  Combination of parkinsonism, dementia, motor neuron disease among Chamorro natives on Guam in the Western Pacific. Declining incidence. Cause uncertain, may be environmental, hereditary, or both.

MULTIPLE SYSTEM ATROPHY (MSA)

Striatonigral degeneration: pure parkinsonism, no tremor; unilateral or bilateral vocal cord paralysis sometimes. Neuronal loss, gliosis in nigrostriatal complex.

Shy-Drager syndrome: parkinsonism plus autonomic dysfunction: orthostatic hypotension, impotence, bladder-bowel dysfunction. Loss of preganglionic sympathetic neurons in intermediolateral horns.

Olivopontocerebellar atrophy (OPCA): includes many disorders. Familial OPCA: cerebellar syndrome. Sporadic OPCA: parkinsonism plus cerebellar syndrome. Degeneration of olives, pons, cerebellum.

Amyotrophy-parkinsonism: parkinsonism plus motor neuron disease. Degeneration of anterior horn cells, nigrostriatal complex. 18-FDG-PET: hypometabolism in striatum, frontal lobes.

OTHER PARKINSONIAN SYNDROMES

Progressive supranuclear palsy: see Chapter 116. Normal pressure hydrocephalus: see Chapter 49.

TREATMENT OF PD

No treatment prevents disease progression. Treatment symptomatic, individualized for symptoms, signs, response to drugs, social factors, disease stage (see below), degree of functional impairment.

TREATMENT MODALITIES

Drug Therapy
Typical drugs listed in Table 115.3. Choice discussed below ("Stages of PD"). All drug introductions, adjustments, discontinuation should be gradual.

Physiotherapy
Crucial role in PD: involves patient in own care, promotes exercise, keeps muscles active, preserves mobility.

Surgery
Reserved for those who do not respond satisfactorily to drugs, although responded to levodopa in past.

Surgical Lesions
Replaced by high-frequency electrical stimulation where available and affordable.

Thalamotomy: best for intractable contralateral tremor. About 15% to 20% risk of dysarthria if surgery bilateral.

Pallidotomy: for contralateral dopa-induced dystonia and chorea (dyskinesias).

Subthalamic nucleus (STN) lesion ("ablation"): may improve multiple parkinsonian signs. Hemichorea, hemiballism may result.

Deep-Brain Stimulation (DBS)
Indicated in patients with clear response to levodopa but with severe fluctuations or short duration of levodopa effectiveness, refractory to medication adjustments. No more effective, for a given patient, than treatment with levodopa in earlier stage of disease. Main goal is to increase proportion of time when symptoms are controlled.

Location of DBS: subthalamic nucleus (STN), internal segment of globus pallidum (GPi). STN placement may provide broadest improvement of symptoms.

Other Treatments

Fetal dopaminergic tissue implants: no more effective than placebo.

APPROACH TO TREATMENT

Stage of PD: major factor in treatment decisions.

Early Stage
No treatment needed until symptoms interfere with daily living.
 Delaying levodopa treatment may delay onset of levodopa-related complications (below). Other drugs used first.
 Selegiline, rasagiline: mild effect on symptoms; possible neuroprotective effect uncertain.

Symptomatic Treatment
Criteria: (a) threat to employability; (b) threat to domestic, financial, social affairs; (c) threat to activities daily living; (d) much worse gait or balance.

Amantadine: mild dopaminergic, anticholinergic effect. Adverse effects: livedo reticularis at knees, ankle edema, visual hallucinations. Also used in advanced stages: (a) as adjunctive drug; (b) to reduce severity of dopa-induced dyskinesias.

Anticholinergic (antimuscarinic) drugs: less effective than dopamine agonists. May improve tremor, e.g., trihexyphenidyl (Artane). Adverse effects: forgetfulness, decreased short-term memory, hallucinations, psychosis. Avoid after age 70. Peripheral side effects: blurred vision, glaucoma (try pilocarpine eye drops); dry mouth, urinary difficulties (try pyridostigmine).

Dopamine agonists: act on dopamine receptors in striatum. Ropinirole, pramipexole used as monotherapy or adjunct to levodopa. Less effective than levodopa. Use of pergolide in decline since cardiac valve fibrosis reported. Early use reduces time to complications of chronic levodopa therapy. Adverse effects: orthostatic hypotension, gastrointestinal upset, hallucinations, psychosis (all agonists); sleep attacks (pramipexole, ropinirole); inflamed skin, retroperitoneal and valvular fibrosis (pergolide). Increase dose slowly. Avoid in patients older than 70 or with cognitive problems.

Levodopa: dopamine precursor (crosses blood-brain barrier); most effective antiparkinsonian treatment. Usually given as carbidopa/levodopa (Sinemet) to avoid nausea, vomiting. Nearly all patients with PD respond quickly to levodopa; diagnosis questioned if ineffective. Usually started: (a) when milder drugs fail; (b) when rapid strong effect desired (e.g., patient falling); (c) initial monotherapy. Never discontinue levodopa suddenly (risk of neuroleptic malignant syndrome).

Treatment with Levodopa

Generally, use lowest dose required to control symptoms. Controlled release preparation for: (a) controlling symptoms through night; (b) avoiding high peak concentrations with drowsiness.

Bradykinesia, rigidity respond best. Tremor sometimes resistant. Inadequate response to levodopa: test adequate dose first (up to 2 g/d). If response nil or slight, probably not PD. Adequate response not necessarily PD.

Additional Drug Therapy

Catechol O-methyltransferase inhibitors (e.g., entacapone): prolong half-life levodopa.

Antidepressants: serotonin-reuptake inhibitors may aggravate parkinsonism if antiparkinsonian drugs not given concurrently.

Clozapine: can ameliorate levodopa-induced psychosis without worsening parkinsonism; monitoring white blood cell count weekly.

Quetiapine: blood counts not needed.

COMPLICATIONS OF LONG-TERM LEVODOPA THERAPY

Appear after 5 years levodopa therapy in 75% patients with PD. Usually irreversible, but severity may be ameliorated.

Response Fluctuations

Wearing off phenomenon: parkinsonian symptoms return less than 4 hours after last dose. Then "off state" lasts longer, starts more abruptly, more severe (including depression, dysphoria, anxiety, pain). "On" state shortens.

Strategies: add or substitute dopamine agonists for levodopa; add selegiline; substitute slow-release forms of carbidopa/levodopa (Sinemet CR) for standard form; shorten interval between levodopa doses; dissolve levodopa tablet in carbonated water or ascorbic acid solution for more rapid absorption, higher peaks; apomorphine injection; avoid high-protein meals; add entacapone. Surgical deep-brain stimulator placement.

Dyskinesias

Includes chorea, ballism, dystonia of limbs, neck, trunk. May be mild, unnoticed by patient.

Strategies: reduce each dose of levodopa, increase frequency or add selegiline, agonist if "off" period is worse.
Off dystonia: painful cramps in "off" state. Keep patient "on" as possible. Use agonist as major antiparkinsonian drug, with low doses of levodopa as adjunct.

Freezing

"Off-freezing": feature of parkinsonism itself. Treatment: keep patient from being "off."
"On-freezing": lessened by lower levodopa dose.
Combined fluctuations, dyskinesias, "off-freezing": consider subthalamic nucleus stimulation.

COURSE

Degenerative forms of parkinsonism, including PD, worsen with time.

Mortality reduced 50%, longevity extended by several years after introduction of levodopa.

TREATMENT OF OTHER PARKINSONIAN SYNDROMES

MSA, other parkinsonism syndromes sometimes respond (usually transiently) to levodopa. Drug treatment as for PD.

CHAPTER 116 ■ PROGRESSIVE SUPRANUCLEAR PALSY

SYMPTOMS AND SIGNS

Usually present: pseudobulbar palsy (emotional lability), supranuclear ocular palsy (vertical gaze), square-wave jerks, extrapyramidal rigidity, gait ataxia, loss of postural reflexes, dementia. Early: falls. Later: dysphagia, dysarthria.

Sometimes present: facial dystonia (appearance of surprise or concern; furrowed brow with vertical lines at nasion or procerus sign), freezing, rapid speech (tachyphemia). Rest tremor uncommon.

Aggressive course: unable to walk in 5 years; death in 6 to 10 years.

PATHOLOGY

Neuronal degeneration; "globose" neurofibrillary tangles (contain tau protein), chiefly in pons, midbrain.

TREATMENT

Antiparkinsonian drugs usually ineffective.

CHAPTER 117 ■ TARDIVE DYSKINESIA AND OTHER NEUROLEPTIC-INDUCED SYNDROMES

Adverse effects of drugs blocking D2 dopamine receptors (Table 117.1), especially antipsychotic agents (phenothiazines, butyrophenones); metoclopramide, flunarizine, cinnarizine.

Likelihood of these adverse effects for atypical neuroleptics: zero for clozapine (except acute akathisia); near zero for quetiapine; low but definite for olanzapine; unknown for newer agents.

Dopamine-depleting drugs (reserpine, tetrabenazine): acute akathisia, drug-induced parkinsonism.

Acute dystonic reaction: twisting postures of limbs, trunk, neck, tongue, face. Mostly in first few days; children, young adults, males. Easily reversed by parenteral antihistamines, anticholinergic drugs, diazepam.

Acute akathisia: defined in Chapter 9. Propranolol may help; disappears on discontinuing offending drug.

Drug-induced parkinsonism: levodopa not effective because dopamine receptors blocked. Anticholinergic drugs, amantadine help.

Neuroleptic malignant syndrome: fever, signs of autonomic dysfunction, movement disorder (akinesia, rigidity, dystonia); may be fatal. Treatment: hydration, cooling, dantrolene, bromocriptine.

Withdrawal emergent syndrome: chorea on abrupt cessation chronic therapy with antipsychotic drug; especially children; self-limited. Restart antipsychotic drug, then taper dosage slowly to eliminate chorea.

TARDIVE SYNDROMES

Often permanent.

Tardive dyskinesia: repetitive rapid movements, especially lower face (oral-buccal-lingual dyskinesia). Other movements: chewing; flexion-extension of trunk, fingers, toes.

TABLE 117.1

ADVERSE NEUROLOGIC EFFECTS OF D2 RECEPTOR BLOCKING AGENTS

Acute dystonic reaction
Oculogyric crisis
Acute akathisia
Drug-induced parkinsonism
Neuroleptic malignant syndrome
Withdrawal emergent syndrome
Persistent dyskinesias (tardive dyskinesia syndromes)
   Classic oral-buccal-lingual dyskinesia
   Tardive dystonia
   Tardive akathisia
   Tardive tics
   Tardive myoclonus
   Tardive tremor

Risk increases with age or longer duration of treatment with antipsychotic drugs. Movements often unmasked by lowering dose or stopping drug therapy; treat by restarting drug.

Other forms (often worse than tardive dyskinesia): tardive dystonia; tardive akathisia. Tardive tics, tardive myoclonus, tardive tremor less common.

Treatment: prevention (avoid older D2 receptor blockers); dopamine-depleting drugs (reserpine, tetrabenazine), may add α-methyltyrosine; clozapine. Deep brain stimulator placement sometimes effective for tardive dystonia (Chapter 113).

Section XVI
Spinal Cord Diseases

CHAPTER 118 ■ HEREDITARY AND ACQUIRED SPASTIC PARAPLEGIA

HEREDITARY SPASTIC PARAPLEGIA

Multiple inherited syndromes with prominent progressive leg weakness and spasticity. Complicated forms accompanied by additional clinical findings (Table 118.1).

GENETICS

Genetically heterogeneous. Affected proteins identified for several forms.

Autosomal dominant spastic paraplegias: SPG3A, SPG4, SPG6, SPG8, SPG9, SPG10, SPG12, SPG13, SPG17, SPG19.
Autosomal recessive: SPG5, SPG7, SPG11, SPG14, SPG15, SPG20, SPG21.
X-linked recessive: SPG1, SPG2, SPG16.

See Table 118.1.

CLINICAL FEATURES

Symptom-onset in childhood or adolescence. Spastic gait disorder; weakness may not be detectable. Sometimes starts in arms or hands. Usually overactive tendon reflexes, Babinski signs, clonus. Sensation usually normal.

LABORATORY DATA

Sensory evoked potentials may be abnormal. Magnetic stimulation of brain: abnormal central motor conduction.

DIAGNOSIS

Clinical, family data. Genetic testing for several forms.

TABLE 118.1

CLASSIFICATION OF THE HEREDITARY SPASTIC PARAPLEGIAS

Syndrome group	Syndrome	Inheritance	MIM no.
Pure Spastic Paraplegia	Autosomal dominant pure spastic paraplegias	AD	186200, 182601, 600363, 607152, 603563, 605280, 604805
	Autosomal recessive pure spastic paraplegia	AR	270800
Complicated spastic paraplegia with	Amyotrophy of hands (Silver syndrome)	AD	270685
	Mental retardation, motor neuropathy	AR	605229
	Thin corpus callosum, mental retardation, dysarthria	AR	604360
	Retinal degeneration	AR	270700
	CNS white matter abnormality or uncomplicated	XL	312920
	Spastic dysarthria and pseudobulbar signs	AR	248900
	Mitochondrial abnormalities or uncomplicated	AR	607259
	Amyotrophy of hands, Troyer syndrome	AR	275900
	Myoclonic epilepsy		270805
	Dementia, Mast syndrome		248900
	Peroneal muscular atrophy	AD	600361
	Mental retardation, aphasia, adducted thumbs	XL	303350
	Aphasia, poor vision, mental retardation	XL	30266
	Amyotrophy, juvenile primary lateral sclerosis	AR	606353
	Adrenomyeloneuropathy		300100

(continued)

TABLE 118.1			
CLASSIFICATION OF THE HEREDITARY SPASTIC PARAPLEGIAS (*Continued*)			
Syndrome group	Syndrome	Inheritance	MIM no.
	Ichthyosis, mental retardation, retinopathy (Sjögren-Larsson syndrome)		270200
	Ataxia, Charlevoix-Saguenay syndrome	AR	270550
	Pigmentary macular degeneration, mental retardation		270950
	Optic atrophy		182830
	Hypopigmentation		270750
	Deafness, nephropathy		182690
	Dementia (prion protein)		176640

MIM, Mendelian inheritance in man catalog; AD, autosomal dominant; AR, autosomal recessive; XL, X-linked.

TREATMENT

Symptomatic. Mainly aimed at reducing spasticity to maximize mobility: physical therapy, baclofen (oral or intrathecal), dantrolene, tizanidine. Oxybutynin may reduce urinary urgency.

ACQUIRED SPASTIC PARAPLEGIA

Most common cause: spinal multiple sclerosis (see Chapter 134).

TROPICAL MYELONEUROPATHIES

Disorders of spinal cord or peripheral nerves; tropical countries.

STRACHAN SYNDROME (NUTRITIONAL NEUROPATHY)

Predominantly sensory neuropathy. Presumably due to nutritional depletion. Numbness, burning limbs, girdling pains; impaired vision, hearing; muscle weakness, wasting, hyporeflexia, sensory ataxia, mucocutaneous lesions.

TROPICAL ATAXIC NEUROPATHY

Sensory ataxia; numbness; burning feet; deafness; visual loss; optic atrophy; mild spasticity with Babinski signs; wasting and weakness of legs. Attributed to eating cassava plant.

TROPICAL SPASTIC PARAPARESIS (TSP)

Infection with human T-cell lymphotrophic virus type 1 (HTLV-1). Pyramidal signs (spasticity), impaired posterior column sensation, bladder dysfunction, lumbar pain. Subacute. Sexually transmitted.

CSF: protein elevation, lymphocytic pleocytosis. Serum, CSF: antibodies to HTLV-1 in 80%. Sometimes with myopathy, peripheral neuropathy, leukoencephalopathy. Prednisone may help.

LATHYRISM

Attributed to ingestion of local chickpea in India, Bangladesh, Ethiopia. Clinically similar to TSP. Slowly progressive.

PRIMARY LATERAL SCLEROSIS

Disease of upper motor neurons; less than 5% all cases of motor neuron disease.

Clinical features: onset after age 40; slowly progressive spastic gait disorder, reaching stable plateau. Sometimes emotional lability; snout, jaw reflexes ("pseudobulbar signs"). Sensation normal; sphincter symptoms rare. After months or years, may terminate with lower motor neuron signs; then evident as ALS.

Laboratory data: MRI nonspecific. CSF protein content sometimes increased; normal γ-globulin, no oligoclonal bands. EMG may show signs of denervation before lower motor neuron signs appear. Magnetic resonance spectroscopy, magnetic brain stimulation of brain confirm corticospinal tract disorder.

Diagnosis: exclude MS, cervical cord compression, ALS, adrenoleukodystrophy, TSP, HIV-associated myelopathy, paraneoplastic myelopathy, combined system disease.

Treatment: Oral baclofen, tizanidine not usually helpful; intrathecal baclofen may help.

RARE CAUSES OF ADULT-ONSET PARAPARESIS

HIV myelopathy, adrenoleukodystrophy.

CHAPTER 119 ■ HEREDITARY AND ACQUIRED MOTOR NEURON DISEASES

DEFINITIONS

Diseases characterized by progressive degeneration and loss of motor neurons in spinal cord, motor nuclei of brainstem, motor cortex, or all three sites.

SPINAL MUSCULAR ATROPHIES (SMA) OF CHILDHOOD

SMA: lower motor neuron signs only.

Infantile, childhood, or juvenile forms differ in age at onset, severity. All autosomal recessive; all map to 5q11-q13 with mutations in survival motor neuron (SMN) gene (allelic heterogeneity).

Infantile SMA (type 1; Werdnig-Hoffmann disease): evident at birth or before age 6 months. Common cause of floppy infant syndrome. Sucking problems, feeble or no limb movements, tongue fasciculations, absent tendon reflexes. Proximal muscles affected before distal. Respiratory failure later. About 85% die before age 2 years. Survivors do not sit.

SMA type 2: onset age 6 to 12 months; can sit, not walk.

SMA type 3 (Kugelberg-Welander syndrome): onset in late childhood or adolescence; can walk, slowly progressive gait disorder, proximal arm weakness, absent tendon reflexes, fasciculation of limb muscles and tongue. Other cranial muscles spared.

LABORATORY DATA

EMG: denervation with normal nerve conduction. Serum CK may be increased. Diagnosis: DNA analysis.

FOCAL MUSCULAR ATROPHIES OF CHILDHOOD AND ADOLESCENCE

Lower motor neuron signs only. Most autosomal recessive.

Fazio-Londe disease: onset late childhood or adolescence; dysarthria, dysphagia, lingual fasciculation without limb weakness.

Scapuloperoneal, fascioscapulohumeral forms: distinction from corresponding muscular dystrophies depends on DNA analysis.

Childhood SMA with hexosaminidase deficiency: onset in childhood or adolescence. Autosomal recessive. Some have upper motor neuron signs as well.

MOTOR NEURON DISEASES OF ADULT ONSET

X-LINKED RECESSIVE SMA (KENNEDY SYNDROME)

Lower motor neuron signs only.

Onset after age 40; dysarthria, dysphagia. Limb weakness later; usually proximal; fasciculation of tongue, limbs. Tendon reflexes absent. Mutation: expansion of CAG repeat; longer repeat length associated with increased severity.

AMYOTROPHIC LATERAL SCLEROSIS (ALS)

Also known as Lou Gehrig's disease. Upper and lower motor neuron signs. In some patients, only lower motor neuron signs present; called "progressive muscular atrophy" (PMA) but more than half of these cases show degeneration of corticospinal tracts at autopsy.

Definition

Degeneration of both upper and lower motor neurons manifest by lower motor neuron signs (weakness, wasting, fasciculation) and upper motor neuron signs (hyperactive tendon reflexes, Hoffmann signs, Babinski signs, clonus).

Epidemiology

Prevalence 5:100,000. Increasing frequency after age 40; 10% begin before age 40; 5% before age 30. M:F ratio 1:1 to 2:1.

Autosomal dominant in 5%. About 20% of familial cases: mutations in superoxide dismutase gene (chromosome 21).

Pathogenesis

Basis of selective vulnerability of motor neurons unknown. Glutamate toxicity, oxidative stress, mitochondrial dysfunction may all play a role. Existence of paraneoplastic form debated. Clinical syndrome of ALS may be caused by radiotherapy, lead poisoning, lightning strike.

Clinical Features

Onset symptoms: weak legs (foot-drop), hands (common difficulty with buttons, keys), proximal arms, slurred speech, dysarthria, dysphagia; spastic gait disorder. Ultimately all skeletal muscles affected except sphincters, eye movement; respiration late, rarely early. Also, muscle cramps, weight loss.

Typical lower motor neuron signs: fasciculation in limbs or tongue; muscle wasting. Tendon reflexes increased or decreased. Unequivocal upper motor signs: Babinski signs, clonus, Hoffmann signs.

Cranial nerve signs: dysarthria, lingual wasting and fasciculation, impaired movement of uvula. Pseudobulbar palsy: dysarthria and dysphagia from upper motor neuron disease; hyperactive pharyngeal reflex; emotional lability (inappropriate laughing or crying); upper motor signs in limbs.

Dementia in 5% to 10% of cases.

TABLE 119.1

EL ESCORIAL CRITERIA (EEC) FOR RESEARCH DIAGNOSIS OF ALS TO PROVIDE HOMOGENOUS POPULATION FOR THERAPEUTIC TRIALS

Suspected ALS: pure LMN syndrome or pure UMN syndrome.

Possible ALS: UMN and LMN signs present together in 1 region, or UMN signs alone in 2 or more regions, or UMN signs caudal to LMN signs

Laboratory-supported ALS: UMN and LMN signs in 1 region, or UMN signs alone in 1 region with LMN signs identified by EMG in 2 limbs

Probable ALS: UMN and LMN signs in more than 2 regions, but some UMN signs must be rostral to LMN signs

Definite ALS: UMN and LMN signs in more than 3 regions

ALS, amyotrophic lateral sclerosis; EEC, El Escorial Criteria; EMG, electromyography; LMN, lower motor neuron; UMN, upper motor neuron.

Course: relentless, progressive, no remissions or relapses. Death from respiratory failure, aspiration pneumonitis, or pulmonary embolism. Mean duration of symptoms about 4 years; 20% live >5 years.

Laboratory Data

EMG: active denervation in at least three limbs; normal nerve conduction velocities. CSF: mild protein elevation. About 5% monoclonal gammopathy.

Diagnosis

Combination of widespread lower motor neuron signs plus any upper motor neuron signs (Babinski, clonus, hyperactive tendon reflexes) virtually diagnostic.

Diagnostic criteria: see Table 119.1.

Differential Diagnosis

Multifocal motor neuropathy with conduction block (MMNCB): asymmetric weakness of hands; conduction block in more than one nerve, not at site of entrapment neuropathy. Treatable: intravenous immunoglobulin therapy.

Myasthenia gravis (MG). Clues: ptosis, ophthalmoparesis, diurnal fluctuation, remissions differ from ALS. Prove MG: unequivocal response to edrophonium, EMG evidence (repetitive stimulation test or single-fiber EMG), antibodies to acetylcholine receptors (AChR), thymoma on CT or MRI.

Spastic paraplegia in middle life: see Chapter 118.

Pseudobulbar palsy: also in MS, bilateral strokes.

Peripheral neuropathy: abnormal nerve conduction studies; test for monoclonal gammopathy, conduction block, antibodies to GM_1 and MAG, lymphoproliferative disease.

Myopathy: excluded by fasciculations or upper motor neuron signs, EMG evidence of denervation.

Post-polio syndrome. Three forms: loss of ability to compensate for residual paresis with increasing age; addition of arthritis, nerve injury that impedes adaptation compensation; new weakness of muscles thought unaffected in childhood attack. Slow progression; upper motor neuron signs absent; clinically evident fasciculations exceptional.

Monomelic muscular atrophy (Hirayama disease): young men (much more often than women), about age 20; restricted to one limb. Slow progression for 1 to 2 years followed by arrest.

Reversible motor neuron disease: spontaneous recovery, rare.

Benign fasciculation and cramps: no weakness or wasting. ALS almost never starts with this syndrome.

Treatment

No effective drug therapy for ALS. Riluzole (glutamate inhibitor) said to prolong life by about 3 months; no visible effect on function or quality of life.

Symptomatic treatment, physical therapy, emotional support important. Antispastic agents not helpful for spastic gait except intrathecal. Major decision: tracheostomy and chronic mechanical ventilation.

CHAPTER 120 ◼
SYRINGOMYELIA

Tubular cavitation of spinal cord, usually cervical, then other segments; more frequent in men; sometimes familial.

Onset age 20 to 40. Slow progression; more rapid if brainstem affected (syringobulbia).

Chiari type 1 malformation in more than two thirds of cases; also seen with intramedullary spinal cord tumor or trauma.

CLINICAL FEATURES

Lower cervical region: loss of pain, temperature perception; preserved light touch, vibratory sense (dissociated sensory loss) in "shawl" distribution. Cavity may enlarge to posterior columns (loss of position and vibratory sense in feet), anterior horns (weakness, wasting of hand muscles, fasciculations, loss of tendon reflexes in arms), lateral columns (spastic paraparesis, hyperreflexia in legs, Babinski signs), autonomic tracts (sphincter symptoms). Deep, aching pain.

Brainstem (syringobulbia): dysphagia, pharyngeal and palatal weakness, atrophy of tongue, loss of pain and temperature sense in distribution of trigeminal nerve, nystagmus.

Associated clinical features: scoliosis, neurogenic arthropathy (Charcot joints) follows painless injuries, may have acute painful enlargement of shoulder, painless ulcers of hands.

Lumbar cord: atrophy of leg muscles; dissociated sensory loss in lumbar and sacral dermatomes (loss of cutaneous sensation, preserve position and vibration sense); tendon reflexes absent in legs; impaired sphincter function; usually no upper motor neuron signs.

Syringomyelia and pregnancy: symptoms may worsen during childbirth.

PATHOLOGY AND PATHOGENESIS

Hypothesis: abnormal CSF hydrodynamics. Obstruction or atresia of fourth ventricle outlets leads to build-up of pressure in central canal, formation of syrinx. Herniated cerebellar tonsils in Arnold-Chiari malformation may cause obstruction.

Problem: at autopsy, syrinx usually does not communicate with fourth ventricle.

LABORATORY DATA

CSF: mild elevation of pressure, protein, cells sometimes seen. Complete subarachnoid block may occur.

MRI: cystic enlargement of spinal cord over several segments. MRI of brain, craniovertebral junction to identify associated anomalies.

DIFFERENTIAL DIAGNOSIS

ALS, MS, anomalies of craniovertebral junction, cervical ribs.

TREATMENT

Drainage (via shunt catheter draining into pleural or peritoneal space). Treatment of etiology of syrinx sometimes possible (e.g., removal of tumor).

Section XVII
Disorders of the
Neuromuscular Junction

CHAPTER 121 ■ MYASTHENIA GRAVIS

Disorder of neuromuscular transmission from antibody-mediated attack on nicotinic AChR at neuromuscular junctions. Fluctuating weakness improved by inhibitors of cholinesterase.

ETIOLOGY AND PATHOGENESIS

Polyclonal IgG antibodies to AChR saturate 80% of AChR sites on muscle. Major damage to end-plates from actual loss of receptors due to complement-mediated lysis. Amplitude of miniature end-plate potentials reduced to 20% of normal. Increased sensitivity to nondepolarizing blocker curare.

FORMS OF MYASTHENIA GRAVIS (MG)

Juvenile and Adult Forms
Typical MG. Most common ages 10 to 40. Circulating AChR antibodies usually present (see below). Patients without demonstrable antibodies respond identically to treatment.

Neonatal Myasthenia
Placental transmission of AChR antibodies by affected mother. Affects 12% of infants born to myasthenic mothers. Onset in first 48 hours of impaired sucking, weak cry, limp limbs. Respiratory insufficiency rare; recovery inevitable if child supported. Antibodies demonstrable in baby and mother. Duration limited to life span of antibodies (days or weeks). Only supportive treatment needed.

Congenital Myasthenia
Due to abnormalities of motor end-plate, including abnormal AChR subunits. Usually autosomal recessive. No antibodies to AChR.

Mothers asymptomatic, lack anti-AChR antibodies. Often infantile onset with ophthalmoplegia; sometimes later onset with limb.

Anticholinesterase drugs sometimes helpful. Warn parents: sudden apneic spells may be induced by mild infections.

Drug-Induced Myasthenia
Most common cause: D-penicillamine. Clinical manifestations: AChR antibody titers similar to those of typical adult MG. Symptoms, antibodies disappear with discontinuation of drug.

PATHOLOGY

Thymus: lymphoid hyperplasia in 70%; thymoma in 10% to 15% after age 40.

INCIDENCE

Prevalence 14:100,000 in United States. M:F ratio 1:3 before age 40; 1:1 after 40. Familial cases rare.

SYMPTOMS

Weakness (not fatigue) major symptom, with following features:

1. **Fluctuating nature:** varies in single day, sometimes within minutes; varies from day to day, or longer periods. Major variations: remissions, exacerbations.
2. **Distribution:** ocular muscles first (ptosis, diplopia) in 40%; ultimately involved in 85%. Other common symptoms: dysarthria, dysphagia, facial paresis. Limb, neck weakness common.
3. Clinical response to cholinergic drugs.

SIGNS

Ptosis, weakness of isolated ocular muscles or conjugate gaze; dysarthria ("nasal" voice), dysphagia; weakness of face, neck, or limbs; respiratory muscle weakness. Sensation normal; reflexes preserved.

MYASTHENIC CRISIS

Exacerbation with respiratory insufficiency, defined by intubation for mechanical ventilation. Occurs in 15% to 20% of patients; one third of these have two or more episodes of crisis. Mortality approaching zero with improved intensive care.

Common precipitants: (a) infection (40%; pneumonia, viral upper respiratory infection); (b) no obvious cause (30%); (c) aspiration (10%). About 25% of patients in crisis extubated after 1 week, 50% after 2 weeks, 75% after 1 month.

LABORATORY DATA

EMG: more than 10% decrement in amplitude of muscle action potentials evoked by repetitive nerve stimulation at 3 to 5 Hz in 90% of patients with generalized MG.

Single-fiber EMG: increased jitter (interval between evoked potentials of muscle fibers in same motor unit), blocking (failure of expected potential).

Antibodies to AChR: 85% of patients with generalized MG; 50% to 60% of ocular MG. Half of the seronegative patients have antibodies to muscle-specific tyrosine kinase (MuSK).

Chest CT or MRI: thymoma in 15% adults.

DIAGNOSIS

Formal diagnosis depends on demonstration of:

Response to cholinergic drugs. Neostigmine test: 1.5 to 2 mg with 0.4 mg atropine sulfate intramuscularly; muscle strength recorded at 20-minute intervals up to 2 hours. Edrophonium test: 1 to 10 mg intravenously (e.g., 1 mg followed in 15 seconds by additional 3 mg, and then in another 15 seconds by 5 mg, to maximum of 10 mg); improvement within 30 seconds, lasting a few minutes. Positive response to either test practically diagnostic of MG.

Demonstration of circulating antibodies to AChR. Specificity >99.9%, sensitivity 88%.

Electrophysiologic evidence of abnormal neuromuscular transmission (see above).

DIFFERENTIAL DIAGNOSIS

Muscular dystrophies, ALS, progressive bulbar palsy, ophthalmoplegia of other cause.

Other disorders of neuromuscular transmission: botulinum intoxication, snake bite, organophosphate intoxication; rarely clinical features and antibodies of both MG and Lambert-Eaton syndrome.

COURSE

Not progressive disease. If restricted to ocular muscles for 2 years, likely to remain restricted. Spontaneous remissions in 25%, especially in first 2 years.

Mortality of MG crisis: previously 25%; now near zero in intensive care units.

TREATMENT

Anticholinesterase drug therapy: early institution recommended. Pyridostigmine most commonly used; neostigmine, ambenonium also available. Side effects: abdominal cramps, diarrhea. Some symptoms usually remain, especially ocular.

Thymectomy: recommended for most patients with generalized MG. About 80% of patients without thymoma become asymptomatic within 5 years of thymectomy, some with continued medication. Thymoma itself indication for removal. Thymectomy not usually recommended for ocular myasthenia unless concomitant thymoma. Beneficial effects usually delayed for months or years.

Immunomodulating therapies: prednisone, plasmapheresis, intravenous immunoglobulin. Often used in preparation for thymectomy. Not proven value for crisis.

Prednisone: used if disability persists after thymectomy. No controlled trial performed. Treatment with azathioprine or cyclophosphamide if no improvement with steroids in 6 months.

Treatment of myasthenic crisis: as for respiratory failure in general. Cholinergic drug therapy discontinued once endotracheal tube in place.

CHAPTER 122 ■
LAMBERT-EATON MYASTHENIC SYNDROME

Lambert-Eaton myasthenic syndrome (LEMS): autoimmune disease of peripheral cholinergic synapses. Small-cell lung carcinoma in 60%; other tumors in 7%. Neurologic symptoms precede those of tumor.

Pathogenesis: antibodies against voltage-gated calcium channels in peripheral nerve terminals impair release of acetylcholine at nicotinic and muscarinic sites. Cells from associated lung cancer bear voltage-gated calcium channels displaying antigenic sites. LEMS-affected tumor-free individuals often have HLA-B8, DR3 haplotype.

Clinical features: proximal limb weakness, loss of knee and ankle jerks, dry mouth, myalgia. Less common: other autonomic symptoms (impotence, constipation, hypohidrosis). Diplopia, dysarthria, dysphagia, dyspnea absent (vs. myasthenia).

Laboratory data: much decreased amplitude of evoked motor unit potential, followed by incremental response to repetitive nerve stimulation at rates above 10 Hz. Some patients with LEMS have ptosis with antibodies to acetylcholine receptor, have two autoimmune disorders ("combined" myasthenia plus LEMS).

Treatment: directed to concomitant tumor. Neuromuscular disorder treated with drugs that facilitate release of acetylcholine (e.g., pyridostigmine). Plasmapheresis, intravenous immunoglobulin help. Treatment with 3,4-diaminopyridine sometimes effective.

CHAPTER 123 ■ BOTULISM AND ANTIBIOTIC-INDUCED NEUROMUSCULAR DISORDERS

BOTULISM

Toxin blocks nicotinic and muscarinic cholinergic synapses by impeding presynaptic release of acetylcholine. Blocks fusion of vesicles with surface membrane.

Epidemiology: toxin produced by spores of *Clostridium botulinum*. Exposure risks: inadequately cooked food; contamination of anaerobic wounds; ingestion or inhalation of spores; intestinal surgery; gastric achlorhydria; antibiotic therapy. May appear at any age.

Pathogenesis: toxin disrupts exocytosis without causing cell death. Effects slowly disappear over several months.

Laboratory data: EMG: abnormally small single muscle action potential evoked in response to supramaximal nerve stimulus; potentiation of response with repetitive stimulation at high rates (20 to 50 Hz), similar to Lambert-Eaton myasthenic syndrome.

Clinical features: dry, sore mouth and throat; nausea, vomiting; blurred vision, diplopia, total external ophthalmoplegia, pupillary paralysis (not invariable); symmetric descending facial, oropharyngeal, limb, respiratory paralysis.

Infantile botulism: reduced spontaneous movements, lethargy, poor sucking, drooling; sucking, gag reflexes decreased or absent; facial diplegia, lethargy, ptosis, ophthalmoparesis. From ingestion of contaminated food, especially honey.

Diagnosis: symmetry of signs, dry mouth, pupillary paralysis. EMG: characteristic incremental response to repetitive nerve stimulation.

Differential diagnosis: acute anterior poliomyelitis excluded by normal CSF and EMG with repetitive stimulation. MG excluded by dilated pupils, incremental response to repetitive nerve stimulation (rather than decremental pattern).

Treatment: respiratory support in intensive care facility; antitoxin (may cause serum sickness, anaphylaxis); guanidine hydrochloride.

Prevention: proper precautions in preparing canned foods; discarding (without sampling) any canned food with rancid odor or in which gas has formed. Toxin destroyed by cooking. Avoid honey before age 1 year.

ANTIBIOTIC-INDUCED NEUROMUSCULAR BLOCKADE

May be caused by aminoglycoside antibiotics (neomycin, streptomycin, kanamycin, gentamicin, amikacin), polypeptide antibiotics (colistin, polymyxin B).

Avoid these drugs in patients with myasthenia.

CHAPTER 124 ■ ACUTE QUADRIPLEGIC MYOPATHY

Also known as "critical illness myopathy."

Corticosteroids, nondepolarizing neuromuscular blocking agents, or both considered the prime inciting factors. Condition may appear in critically ill patients without exposure to either agent. Particularly vulnerable: patients being treated for status asthmaticus, organ transplantation, severe trauma, all likely to have received high doses of steroids in addition to blocking agents.

Clinical features: severe quadriplegia and muscle wasting 4 to 105 days after starting intensive care. Limb weakness usually diffuse, plus respiratory; tendon reflexes often lost. Diagnosis suspected when weaning patient from mechanical ventilation proves difficult (respiratory muscle weakness). Improvement: generally occurs over several months, but may be more protracted.

Laboratory data: normal or high serum creatine kinase levels.

Nerve conduction studies: absent or low-amplitude compound motor action potentials. Sensory nerve action potentials normal, reduced, or absent.

EMG: signs of denervation from muscle necrosis and myopathic or normal motor unit action potentials; motor unit recruitment analysis frequently suboptimal due to confounding factors (severe weakness, encephalopathy, sedation).

Muscle biopsy: predominantly myopathy; loss of myosin filaments in electron microscopy.

Differential diagnosis: 1) persistent weakness may follow administration of nondepolarizing blocking agents to patient with impaired hepatic metabolism, reduced renal excretion, or both. 2) *Critical-illness neuropathy* (axonal neuropathy with gram-negative sepsis, multiorgan failure, or both); may coexist with acute quadriplegic myopathy.

Section XVIII
Myopathies

CHAPTER 125 ■ IDENTIFYING DISORDERS OF THE MOTOR UNIT

Motor unit: anterior horn cell, peripheral motor nerve, muscle. Manifestations: flaccid weakness, wasting, depression of tendon reflexes (Table 125.1).

Tests to distinguish neurogenic from myopathic disorders: EMG, nerve conduction studies (see Chapter 15); muscle biopsy, serum levels sarcoplasmic enzymes (especially creatine kinase).

DEFINITIONS

Atrophy: word with three meanings: (a) visible wasting of muscle from any cause; (b) small muscle fibers under light microscope; (c) name of neurogenic diseases.

Myopathy: symptoms due to dysfunction of muscle with no clinical, EMG, or muscle biopsy signs of denervation.

Dystrophies: myopathies with five characteristics: (a) inherited; (b) all symptoms due to limb or cranial muscle weakness; (c) weakness progressively more severe; (d) symptoms result from dysfunction in voluntary muscles (heart, viscera may also be involved); (e) no histologic abnormalities in muscle other than degeneration, regeneration, or inflammatory-fibrous reaction to muscle changes.

TABLE 125.1

IDENTIFICATION OF DISORDERS OF THE MOTOR UNIT

	Anterior horn cell	Peripheral nerve	Neuro-muscular junction	Muscle
Clinical				
Symptoms				
Persistent weakness	Yes	Yes	Yes	Yes
Variable weakness	No	No	Yes	No
Painful cramps	Often	Rare	No	Rare
Myoglobinuria	No	No	No	Rare
Paresthesias	No	Yes	No	No
Bladder disorder	No	Occasional	No	No
Signs				
Weakness	Yes	Yes	Yes	Yes
Wasting	Yes	Yes	No	Yes
Reflexes lost	Yes	Yes	No (MG)	Yes
Reflexes increased	Sometimes (ALS)	No	No	No
Babinski, Hoffman signs	Often (ALS)	No	No	No
Distal sensory loss	No	Yes	No	No
Fasciculation	Common	No	No	No
Laboratory				
Serum enzymes ↑	No or mild	No	No	Yes
CSF protein ↑	Yes or mild	Yes	No	No
Motor nerve conduction				
Velocity slow	No or mild	Often	No	No
↑ or ↓ amplitude (repetitive stimulation)	No	No	Yes	No
EMG				
Denervation	Yes	Yes	No	No
Myopathic	No	No	No	Yes
Biopsy				
Neurogenic features	Yes	Yes	No	No
Myopathic features	No	No	No	Yes

CHAPTER 126 ■ PROGRESSIVE MUSCULAR DYSTROPHIES

GENERAL CONSIDERATIONS

Definition

Characteristics of progressive muscular dystrophy: (1) myopathy (by clinical, histologic, and EMG criteria); (2) all symptoms are effects of muscle weakness; (3) symptoms become progressively worse; (4) histologic changes imply degeneration and regeneration of muscle, but no abnormal storage of a metabolic product is evident; (5) inheritable condition, even if no other cases identified in a particular family.

Other features: pathophysiologic basis of weakness unknown; no specific therapy exists.

CLASSIFICATION

Based on clinical, genetic characteristics. Three main types (Table 126.1): Duchenne muscular dystrophy (DMD), facioscapulohumeral muscular dystrophy (FSHD), and myotonic muscular dystrophy (MMD). Fourth category, limb-girdle muscular dystrophy (LGMD) being depleted with improved diagnosis of metabolic, congenital, inflammatory myopathies and refined with discovery of new mutations.

PATHOGENESIS

Progressive muscular dystrophies result from diverse defects in proteins of different muscle cell compartments.

INVESTIGATIONS

DNA diagnosis available for Duchenne, Becker, facioscapulohumeral, scapuloperoneal, myotonic, and about half of LGMDs.

TABLE 126.1
FEATURES OF THE MOST COMMON MUSCULAR DYSTROPHIES

Features	Duchenne (DMD)	Facioscapulohumeral (FSHD)	Myotonic dystrophy (DM1), Proximal myotonic myopathy (PROMM, DM2)
Incidence estimates	1 in 3,500 live male births	1 in 20,000 people	1 in 8,000 live births
Mode of inheritance	X-linked recessive	Autosomal dominant	Autosomal dominant
Gene defect	Deletion or point mutation in gene for dystrophin	Reduced number of tandem repeats in D4Z4 1 to 8 repeats (normal 10 to >100 repeats)	DM1: CTG expansion in protein kinase gene; 50 to >2000 repeats (normal 5–37 repeats) DM2: CCTG repeat expansion in zinc finger protein 9 gene
Gene location	Xp21.2	4q35	DM1 19q13; DM2 3q21
Expressivity	Complete	Variable	Variable
Age of onset	Childhood	Adolescence, rarely childhood	DM1: broad range (infancy to adult life) DM2: adolescence to adult life
Site of onset	Pelvic girdle	Shoulder girdle	DM1: face and distal limbs; congenital form: hypotonia, club feet, dysphagia, dysmorphism, respiratory distress, mental retardation DM2: pelvic girdle, neck flexors

Calf hypertrophy	Common	Never	DM1: never DM2: some
Rate of progression	Relatively rapid	Slow	Variable
Facial weakness	Rare and mild	Common	Common
Contractures	Common	Rare	Rare
Cardiac disease	Usually late (cardiomyopathy)	None	Common (conduction defect)
Other clinical features	Respiratory insufficiency; scoliosis; cognitive function variably impaired sometimes (high function)	High-frequency hearing loss and retinal vasculopathy (rare)	Cataracts, endocrine dysfunction DM1 compared to PROMM patients usually have more: facial weakness, dysphagia, and distal weakness and wasting.
Genetic heterogeneity	Duchenne and Becker allelic Becker resembles Duchenne, but onset later and less severe	Not all FSHD phenotypes linked to 4q35	Some PROMM patients not linked to 3q21

Diagnosis sometimes confirmed by immunohistochemistry or Western blot of muscle tissue, or sequencing white blood cell DNA.

Muscle biopsy: 1) can improve prognostic accuracy in some syndromes; 2) needed for histochemical, electrophoresis of abnormal proteins (such as dystrophin) if no defining mutation found in a limb-girdle syndrome; 3) needed to characterize most congenital, metabolic myopathies.

Serum CK determination, ECG included for all patients with any kind of myopathy.

SPECIFIC CONDITIONS

X-LINKED MUSCULAR DYSTROPHIES (DUCHENNE, BECKER)

Definitions
Duchenne muscular dystrophy (DMD), Becker muscular dystrophy (BMD).

Mutations in gene for dystrophin at Xp21 (dystrophinopathies). X-linked recessive inheritance (manifest in boys). Carriers (girls and women) may have mild symptoms or high CK.

Prevalence and Incidence
Duchenne: incidence 1 in 3,500 male births; prevalence 1 in 18,000 boys. Becker: one in 20,000.

Pathogenesis
Dystrophin: cytoskeletal protein located at plasma membrane, associated with glycoproteins linking cytoskeleton to plasma membrane.

Mutation in dystrophin gene leads to absence of dystrophin in DMD; smaller size, reduced levels in BMD. Sarcolemma unstable in contraction and relaxation, liable to breakage, excessive influx of calcium, causing muscle necrosis.

Deletions in Xp21 in 66%; point mutations in others. New mutations in 33%.

Specific Features
Duchenne Muscular Dystrophy
See Table 126.1. Proximal weakness with delayed walking, difficulty running, toe-walking, waddling gait. Progression to

overt symptoms before age 5: difficulty walking, climbing stairs, rising from chairs. Exaggerated lordosis, falls, use of arms to push up on rising from ground (Gower sign). Calf hypertrophy. Knee jerks lost before ankle jerks.

Speech, swallowing, ocular movements spared. Wheelchair by age 9 to 12. Scoliosis, contractures at elbows and knees.

Onset of respiratory function decline around age 8. Mechanical ventilation by age 20.

ECG abnormal in most patients. Often cardiomyopathy with congestive heart failure. Mental retardation in 33%.

Other possible manifestations: intestinal hypomotility, acute gastric dilatation; osteoporosis; intellectual impairment.

Anesthetic catastrophes may occur (analogous to malignant hyperthermia): hyperkalemia, extremely high CK levels, acidosis, cardiac failure, hyperthermia, rigidity. Risk decreased by avoiding inhaled general anesthetics, depolarizing muscle relaxants.

Becker Muscular Dystrophy
Two differences from Duchenne: age at onset (usually after age 12); rate of progression slower (walk after age 12, often later). Otherwise syndrome nearly identical.

Intermediate Phenotype
Ambulatory after age 12; wheelchair bound before age 16. Anti-gravity strength in neck flexors preserved longer than typical DMD patients.

Manifesting carriers: DMD X-linked recessive. Women carrying gene show mild limb weakness, calf hypertrophy, cardiomyopathy or high serum CK levels.

Investigations
Serum CK elevated (usually at least 20 times normal). DNA test for Xp21 mutation.

EMG: myopathic pattern.

Dystrophin assay by immunoprecipitation of muscle proteins from biopsy or immunocytochemistry on frozen muscle section.

Diagnosis
Usually evident from clinical features. CK values 20 times higher than normal characteristic. Blood DNA testing usually

confirmatory. If not, muscle biopsy performed (immunocyto-chemistry for dystrophin; Western blot for quantitative dystrophin analysis).

Differential diagnosis: spinal muscular atrophy. Conditions causing great elevation of CK: Xp21 gene carrier state, idiopathic or asymptomatic hyperCKemia, dysferlinopathies (Miyoshi myopathy or LGMD), caveolin-3 mutations.

Treatment
Prednisone therapy beneficial in controlled trials; limited by side effects of chronic administration.

Rehabilitation critical to: 1) maximize function based on preserved muscle strength; 2) prevent contractures.

Braces, surgery for spine or limb deformity; social, emotional support; genetic counseling. Respiratory support when needed. May need special instruction for learning disorders.

Other Xp21 Myopathies
Some due to dystrophin abnormalities (dystrophinopathies); dystrophin normal in others.

Dystrophinopathies: dystrophin abnormality with large deletion in neighboring gene extending into dystrophin gene; myopathy with congenital adrenal insufficiency, glycerol kinase deficiency.

Non–dystrophin-related Xp21 myopathies: McLeod syndrome. Mild or asymptomatic myopathy, abnormally shaped red blood cells (acanthocytes), serum CK >29 times normal. Dystrophin normal.

EMERY-DREIFUSS MUSCULAR DYSTROPHY

Distinct features: (a) humeroperoneal distribution of weakness; (b) severe contractures at elbows, knees before symptomatic weakness; (c) heart block common. Myopathy mild or severe.

X-linked mutation in gene for emerin (Xq28). Emerin absent in muscle nuclei, circulating white blood cells, skin. Diagnostic test: emerin assay in mucosal cells from cheek swab.

Clinical presentation: Onset before age 5 with difficulty walking. Symmetric contractures; weakness without pseudohypertrophy. Tendon reflexes hypoactive or absent. Serum CK activity often mildly elevated (less than 10 times normal).

Diagnosis usually confirmed by DNA testing. Absence of emerin can be demonstrated by immunocytochemical study of muscle biopsy.

Cardiac surveillance (including 24 hour ECG, echocardiography) crucial.

Differential diagnosis: rigid spine syndrome; Bethlem myopathy (clinically similar except no cardiac disease).

Management: symptomatic, including pacemaker implantation. Female carriers are at risk for arrhythmias.

FACIOSCAPULOHUMERAL MUSCULAR DYSTROPHY

Clinical Features
Facioscapulohumeral distribution of weakness. Limited movements of lips, wide eyes. Prominent scapular winging with characteristic shoulder girdle appearance (sagging clavicles, elevated tips of scapulae). Leg weakness usually involves anterior tibials, peroneals.

Onset in adolescence. Slow progression; wheelchair rarely needed; respiration spared.

Molecular Genetics
Autosomal-dominant inheritance. Due to deletions at 4q35 locus. Penetrance nearly complete. Diagnosis: DNA analysis.

Laboratory Studies
Serum enzyme levels normal or near normal. ECG normal.

Treatment
Albuterol may be helpful.

MYOTONIC MUSCULAR DYSTROPHY (MMD)

Myotonic dystrophy (DM1): autosomal dominant, multisystem disease including muscular dystrophy of unique distribution, myotonia, cardiomyopathy, cataracts, endocrinopathy.

Proximal myotonic myopathy (DM2): shares many characteristics with DM1, but differs genetically.

Epidemiology

Prevalence 5:100,000; incidence 13.5:100,000 live births.

Clinical Features

Myotonic Dystrophy (DM1)

Multisystem disease; variation in age at onset, severity.

Unique distribution of myopathy. (a) Cranial, facial muscles affected: ptosis, ophthalmoplegia, dysarthria, dysphagia; small temporalis muscles; distinctive appearance (long lean face, ptosis; frontal baldness in men). (b) Distal limb myopathy affecting hands and feet equally: prominent weakness of finger flexors; foot-drop; "steppage" gait.

Tendon reflexes lost in proportion to weakness.

Myotonia: (a) clinically, impaired relaxation; (b) EMG waxing and waning of high frequency discharge after relaxation begins. Difficulty letting go after shaking hands, turning doorknob. Examination: forceful grasp followed by slow relaxation; elicited also by percussion of thenar eminence, finger extensors, tongue.

Other features: cataracts, endocrinopathy (frontal baldness, testicular atrophy, diabetes mellitus), cardiac disorder (mostly conduction abnormalities), gastrointestinal disorders (pseudo-obstruction, megacolon). Cognitive impairment common in congenital form of DM1; mild cognitive impairment may occur in adult-onset form.

Slow progression. Compatible with long life.

Congenital myotonic dystrophy: about 5% of children born to person with DM1 have symptoms at birth. Mother is the affected parent in almost all cases. Manifestations: difficulty feeding and breathing in newborn period, delayed development, mental retardation, developmental anomalies of face and jaws, severe limb weakness, clubfeet. EMG evidence of myotonia may be absent in child, but present in mother.

Proximal Myotonic Myopathy (PROMM, DM2)

Like DM1: autosomal dominant myopathy, myotonia, cataracts, weakness of sternocleidomastoids.

Unlike DM1: weakness of pelvic girdle muscles more pronounced than distal leg weakness. DM1 mutation absent; disease maps to chromosome 3q. Other differences: myotonia more difficult to elicit; symptoms less severe; calf hypertrophy sometimes present.

DNA diagnosis available but may miss 20% of affected people, indicating need for more reliable test.

Molecular Genetics and Pathophysiology

DM1: Autosomal dominant; penetrance almost 100%. Expansion of CTG triplet repeat within dystrophia myotonica protein kinase (DMPK) gene. Correlation between number of repeats, age onset, severity: anticipation (earlier onset succeeding generations), potentiation (more severe in next generation).

DM2: Mutation is unstable four-nucleotide repeat expansion, CCTG, in gene for zinc finger protein 9 gene on chromosome 3q21.

Investigations

Normal serum CK level. EMG: evidence of myopathy; waxing and waning after-discharge. ECG: conduction abnormalities.

Diagnosis

Usually evident at presentation: long lean face, baldness in men, small sternomastoids, distal myopathy, myotonia. DNA analysis confirmatory.

Differential diagnosis. Nondystrophic myotonias: hyperkalemic periodic paralysis, paramyotonia congenita (Chapter 127); myotonia congenita, Schwartz-Jampel syndrome (Chapter 128). "Pseudomyotonia," (impaired relaxation without true myotonic discharges), seen in Isaacs syndrome or neuromyotonia (Chapter 130). Myotonic-like discharges but not clinical myotonia seen in patients with acid maltase deficiency.

Management and Genetic Counseling

Myotonia rarely bothersome: can use mexiletine, phenytoin, other anticonvulsants. Rehabilitation measures, orthosis. Periodic slit-lamp examination, ECG. Prenatal testing available.

General anesthesia should be avoided if possible because of increased postoperative pulmonary complications.

LIMB-GIRDLE MUSCULAR DYSTROPHY

Heterogeneous group of progressive muscular dystrophies primarily involving shoulder and hip girdle muscles, with autosomal dominant or recessive inheritance, and normal dystrophin gene product.

TABLE 126.2

CONDITIONS SIMULATING LIMB-GIRDLE MUSCULAR DYSTROPHY

Acquired Diseases
Inflammatory
  Polymyositis, dermatomyositis, inclusion body myositis, sarcoidosis
Toxic myopathies
  Chloroquine, steroid myopathy, vincristine, statins, ethanol abuse, phenytoin
Endocrinopathies
  Hyperthyroidism, hypothyroidism, hyperadrenocorticism (Cushing syndrome), hyperparathyroidism, hyperaldosteronism
Vitamin deficiency
  Vitamin D, vitamin E malabsorption
Paraneoplastic
  Lambert-Eaton syndrome, carcinomatous myopathy

Heritable Diseases
Becker muscular dystrophy
Manifesting carrier of Duchenne or Becker gene
Emery-Dreifuss muscular dystrophy
Facioscapulohumeral or scapulohumeral dystrophy
Myotonic muscular dystrophy
Congenital myopathies
  Centronuclear, central core, nemaline, tubular aggregates, cytoplasmic body
Metabolic myopathies
  Glycogen storage diseases (phosphorylase deficiency, acid maltase deficiency, debrancher deficiency), lipid storage diseases (carnitine deficiency), mitochondrial myopathies
Myopathy of periodic paralysis

Previously included metabolic myopathies (including acid maltase and debrancher enzyme deficiencies), other myopathies later identified as BMD, mitochondrial myopathies, polymyositis, inclusion body myositis, or other diseases (Table 126.2).

Remaining group: diverse genetic causes; specific mutations located or identified for 17. Divided into autosomal dominant, recessive groups. Usually not clinically distinguishable, due to marked variability in severity and onset age. Characteristic features seen with specific defects (Table 126.3).

Clinical Manifestations

Recessive forms more common, more severe, with earlier onset. None can be conclusively diagnosed on clinical grounds alone. All characterized by proximal weakness of pelvic or shoulder

TABLE 126.3
LIMB-GIRDLE MUSCULAR DYSTROPHIES

Syndrome	Map position	Gene product	Features	Diagnosis method
Autosomal Dominant				
LGMD1A	5q31	Myoflin		
LGMD1B	1q11-21	Lamin A/C	Nasal speech	DNA
LGMD1C	3p25	Caveolin-3	HyperCKemia	Muscle
LGMD1D	6q23	Unknown	Dilated cardiomyopathy, conduction disease, myopathy	
LGMD1E	7q	Unknown		
Other		Unknown		
Autosomal Recessive				
LGMD2A	15q15	Calpain-3	HyperCKemia	DNA
LGMD2B	2p13	Dysferlin	High CK	Blood, muscle and DNA
LGMD2C	13q12	γ-sarcoglycan	Early onset, severe [~10 % of LGMD are sarcoglycanopathies]	Muscle and DNA
LGMD2D	17q12-21	α-sarcoglycan (adhalin)		Muscle and DNA
LGMD2E	4q12	β-sarcoglycan		Muscle and DNA
LGMD2F	5q33-34	δ-sarcoglycan		Muscle and DNA
LGMD2G	17q11-12	Telethonin	Rimmed vacuoles	
LGMD2H	9q31-34	TRIM32	Manitoba Hutterites	
LGMD2I	19q13.4	Fukutin-related protein	Congenital MD1C	
LGMD2J	2q	Titin	Tibial muscular dystrophy	Blood

LGMD, limb-girdle muscular dystrophy; hyperCKemia, asymptomatic increased creatine kinase; TRIM32, Tripartite motif protein 32 (E3-ubiquitin ligase); Muscle, diagnostic muscle biopsy immunostaining; DNA, genetic screening; Blood, lymphocyte immunoblot analysis.

girdle muscles, dystrophic signs on muscle biopsy; some include cardiomyopathy.

Severity may vary between and within families. Common early symptoms: difficulty with stair climbing and rising from chair. Waddling gait then develops. Cranial muscles usually spared.

Investigations
Serum CK levels almost always high in recessive types; often elevated in dominant forms. Slow progression. EMG, muscle biopsy: nondiagnostic myopathic, dystrophic changes.

Diagnosis
Clinical features, genetic testing (Table 126.3). Differential diagnosis: Table 126.2.

CONGENITAL MUSCULAR DYSTROPHIES

See Chapter 128.

DISTAL MYOPATHIES (DISTAL MUSCULAR DYSTROPHIES)

Defined by involvement of feet and hands before proximal limb muscles. Characterized by myopathy, slow progression.

Welander distal myopathy: most common form; autosomal dominant. Symptom onset in adolescence or adult years. Legs affected before hands. Mild histologic changes. Serum CK slightly elevated.

Nonaka variant: autosomal recessive; gastrocnemius muscles spared; serum CK slightly elevated. Histology: vacuolar myopathy.

Miyoshi distal myopathy: autosomal recessive; gastrocnemius muscles affected first; elevated serum CK; nonspecific histologic changes (no vacuoles).

Other variants exist.

CHAPTER 127 ■ FAMILIAL PERIODIC PARALYSIS

Episodic bouts of limb weakness. Inherited "channelopathies" (inherited abnormalities of ion channels). Clinical features in Table 127.1.

HYPOKALEMIC PERIODIC PARALYSIS (HoPP)

Serum potassium decreases in spontaneous attack to <3.0 mEq/L.

Usually maps to gene for dihydropyridine-sensitive L-type calcium channel of muscle (CACNL1A3, chromosome 1q31); sometimes maps to same gene as hyperkalemic periodic paralysis (SCN4A; see below).

EPIDEMIOLOGY

Rare. M:F ratio 1:1 to 3:2.

SYMPTOMS AND SIGNS

Attack starts after period of rest or ingestion of meal high in carbohydrates. Paralysis ranges from slight weakness of legs to complete paralysis of all limb muscles. Tendon reflexes may be absent. Oropharyngeal, respiratory muscles usually spared. Lasts 1 to 48 hours.

Frequency: one attack per year to several per day.
Between attacks: usually normal strength, normal serum potassium. Mild-to-severe proximal limb weakness persists in some patients.

COURSE

First attack usually around puberty (range 4 to 70 years). Frequency decreases with time; may cease after age 40. Rarely fatal.

531

TABLE 127.1

CLINICAL FEATURES OF HYPOKALEMIC AND HYPERKALEMIC PERIODIC PARALYSIS AND PARAMYOTONIA

	Hypokalemic periodic paralysis (HoPP)	Hyperkalemic periodic paralysis (HyPP)	Paramyotonia congenita
Age of onset	Usually second or latter part of first decade	First decade	First decade
Sex	Male preponderance	Equal	Equal
Incidence of paralysis	Interval of weeks or months	Interval of hours or days	May not be present; otherwise, interval of weeks or months
Degrees of paralysis	Tends to be severe	Tends to be mild but can be severe	Tends to be mild but can be severe
Effect of cold	May induce an attack	May induce an attack	Tends to induce an attack
Effect of food (especially glucose)	May induce an attack	Relieves an attack	Relieves an attack
Serum potassium	Low	High	Tends to be high
Oral potassium	Prevents an attack	Precipitates an attack	Precipitates an attack
Precipitants	Food, cold	Fasting, stress, rest after exercise, potassium-rich foods	Fasting, stress, rest after exercise
Myotonia	Absent	Present	Present

Modified from Hudson AJ. *Brain* 1963;86:811.

TABLE 127.2
POTASSIUM AND PARALYSIS: NONINHERITED FORMS

Hypokalemia
Excessive urinary loss
  Hyperaldosteronism
  Drugs: glycyrrhizate (licorice), thiazides, furosemide,
    chlorthalidone, ethacrynic acid, amphotericin, duogastrone
  Pyelonephritis, renal tubular acidosis
  Recovery from diabetic acidosis
  Ureterocolostomy
Excessive gastrointestinal loss
  Malabsorption syndrome
  Laxative abuse
  Diarrhea
  Fistulas, vomiting, villous adenoma
  Pancreatic tumor, diarrhea
Thyrotoxicosis

Hyperkalemia
Uremia
Addison disease
Spironolactone excess
Excessive intake
  Iatrogenic
  Geophagia (eating sand)

DIAGNOSIS

DNA test obviates need for provocative tests. Can measure serum potassium during spontaneous attack. Attacks can be induced by injection of glucose, insulin, epinephrine, fludrocortisone.

Differential diagnosis: noninherited causes of hypokalemia (Table 127.2). Hyperthyroidism a cause of hypokalemic periodic paralysis, especially in Japanese and Chinese people.

TREATMENT

Attacks: 20 to 100 mEq potassium salts by mouth.

Prophylactic therapy: acetazolamide prevents attacks in about 90%, also improves interictal weakness. Alternatives: triamterene, spironolactone, dichlorphenamide.

HYPERKALEMIC PERIODIC PARALYSIS (HyPP)

Serum potassium normal or increased during attack.

Maps to gene for alpha subunit of sodium channel (SCN4A, chromosome 17q13). Autosomal dominant.

SYMPTOMS AND SIGNS

Onset before age 10. Attacks in daytime; shorter, less severe than in HoPP. Precipitated by hunger, rest, cold, or by administration of potassium chloride. Myotonia demonstrable by EMG; myotonic lid-lag (myotonia of upper lid when looking downward), lingual percussion.

TREATMENT

Attacks: calcium gluconate, glucose, insulin.

Prophylactic therapy: (a) acetazolamide, other diuretics that promote urinary excretion of potassium (thiazides, fludrocortisone); (b) β-adrenergic drugs.

PARAMYOTONIA CONGENITA

Probably allelic variation of HyPP with paucity of paralytic attacks. Autosomal dominant (SCN4A gene).

Myotonia precipitated by cold (as in other forms of myotonia but more so), worsened by exercise ("myotonia paradoxica" differs from other myotonias that lessen with warming up).

PERIODIC PARALYSIS WITH CARDIAC ARRHYTHMIA (ANDERSEN SYNDROME)

Potassium high, low, or normal during attacks. Attack may be precipitated by administration of potassium (but avoided as risk of cardiac arrhythmia).

Gene for inwardly rectifying potassium channel (KCNJ2, chromosome 17q23).

Features: dysmorphism, periodic paralysis, potassium sensitivity, myotonia (usually mild), cardiac arrhythmia.

CHAPTER 128 ■ CONGENITAL MYOPATHIES

Primary manifestation: delayed motor milestones.

CONGENITAL MUSCULAR DYSTROPHIES

Congenital myotonic dystrophy, congenital muscular dystrophies: muscle destruction, replacement by fat and connective tissue on muscle biopsy.

Congenital muscular dystrophies vs. congenital myopathies: previously distinguished by progressive vs. static course. Distinction obsolete, as both groups include static and progressive disorders.

Specific disorders listed in Table 128.1.

CONGENITAL MYOPATHIES

GENERAL FEATURES

Classification: historically defined by distinctive structural, histochemical features on muscle biopsy (Table 128.2). Often marked by aggregation of defective, mutant proteins, leading to gene- and protein-based nosology (Table 128.3). Most are familial.

Clinical features: delayed motor developmental milestones; child moves less than expected in neonatal period ("floppy baby syndrome"). Symptom onset sometimes delayed until adult years. Weakness may progress slowly or not at all. Heart occasionally affected.

Investigations: serum CK normal or mildly elevated. EMG: normal or mild myopathic features.

Diagnosis: based on muscle pathology. Other congenital syndromes include MG, congenital myotonic dystrophy, spinal muscular atrophy.

Treatment: symptomatic.

TABLE 128.1

CONGENITAL MUSCULAR DYSTROPHIES

Merosin-deficient congenital muscular dystrophy
Merosin-positive congenital muscular dystrophy
Fukuyama type congenital muscular dystrophy
Muscle-eye-brain disease (Santavuori disease)
Walker-Warburg syndrome and congenital muscular
  dystrophy

Modified from Griggs RC, Mendell JR, Miller RG. Evaluation and treatment of myopathies. Philadelphia: FA Davis Co, 1995; Tome FMS, Guicheney P, Fardeau M. Congenital muscular dystrophies. In: Emery AEH, ed. Neuromuscular disorders: clinical and molecular genetics. New York: John Wiley & Sons, 1998:21–58; Goebel HH, Anderson JR. *Neuromuscul Disord* 1999;9:50–57.

CENTRAL CORE DISEASE

Typically autosomal dominant with variable penetrance.

Proximal limb weakness, hypotonia, absent tendon reflexes, delayed motor milestones. Normal examination in up to one third. Less common: dysmorphic features (club feet, scoliosis, hip dislocation, finger contractures). Bulbar muscles spared. Increased risk for malignant hyperthermia.

TABLE 128.2

MORPHOLOGIC CLASSIFICATION OF CONGENITAL MYOPATHIES

Chief structure involved	Myopathy
Sarcomere	Central core, multicore, trilaminar, hyaline body (lysis of myofibrils)
Z-Disc	Nemaline rod, desmin-related
Nuclear abnormalities, inclusions	Myotubular, centronuclear, fingerprint, reducing body
Organelle	Tubular aggregate myopathy
Abnormality of fiber size/number	Congenital fiber type disproportion; uniform type 1 fiber myopathy

Adapted from Bodensteiner JB. *Muscle Nerve* 1994;17:133.

TABLE 128.3
MOLECULAR GENETICS OF CONGENITAL MYOPATHIES

Myopathy	Gene locus	Protein product
Nemaline myopathy	1q21-23	α-Tropomyosin 3 [TPM3]
	2q21.2-22	Nebulin [NEB]
	1q42.1	Sarcomeric actin [ACTA]1
Central core disease	9p13.2	β-Tropomyosin [TPM2]
	19q13.4	Troponin T1 [TNNT1]
	19q13.1	Ryanodine receptor 1 [RYR1]
	14q11.2	Cardiac β-myosin [MYH7] heavy chain
Myotubular myopathy	X28q	Myotubularin [MTMX]
Desminopathy	2q35	Desmin [DES]
α B-crystallinopathy	11q22	α B-crystallin [CRYAB]
Desmin-related myopathies	2q21	Unknown
	10q22.3	Unknown
	12	Unknown
	15q22	Unknown

From Goebel HH. Congenital myopathies at their molecular dawning. *Muscle Nerve* 2003;27:528.

Serum CK level normal or slightly elevated. EMG: increased terminal innervation ratio (average number of fibers innervated by single anterior horn cell).

Muscle biopsy: circumscribed circular regions in center of most type 1 fibers.

NEMALINE MYOPATHY

Autosomal dominant, autosomal recessive, sporadic forms. At least five different gene loci (Table 128.3).

Clinical forms range from floppy infant with dysmorphism, to adult-onset with "dropped head" sign and monoclonal gammopathy. Sometimes present: skeletal abnormalities, congenital hip dislocation, arthrogryposis congenita multiplex (flexion contractures of limbs), cardiomyopathy, ophthalmoplegia, rigid spine. Increased susceptibility to malignant hyperthermia.

Muscle biopsy (using a modified trichrome stain): dark red-staining rod-shaped material in type 1 fibers.

MYOTUBULAR MYOPATHY

141 different disease-associated mutations described. Autosomal dominant, X-linked.

Severe hypotonia, weakness, poor suck and swallow, prominent respiratory failure often present at birth. Nonprogressive. X-linked form so severe that survival is not possible without ventilatory support.

Muscle biopsy: pathologically small muscle fibers with central nuclei resembling fetal myotubes.

MULTIMINICORE MYOPATHY

Usually autosomal recessive.

Phenotypes: a) axial weakness, scoliosis, respiratory insufficiency, distal joint laxity; b) ophthalmoplegia, severe facial, limb weakness; c) early-onset form with arthrogryposis; d) slowly progressive form with weakness, hand amyotrophy.

Other clinical features: cardiomyopathy, septal cardiac defects, malignant hyperthermia.

Muscle biopsy: cores like those of central core disease, but not extending full length of fiber.

DESMIN-RELATED MYOPATHIES

Also known as myofibrillar myopathies, "surplus protein myopathies." Includes cytoplasmic body myopathy, sarcoplasmic body myopathy, spheroid body myopathy, Mallory body-like myopathy, granulofilamentous myopathy.

Autosomal dominant, autosomal recessive.

Broad clinical spectrum.

Muscle biopsy: aggregation of desmin into inclusion bodies or granulofilamentous material.

CONGENITAL MUSCLE FIBER TYPE DISPROPORTION

Predominance of type 1 fibers smaller than type 2 fibers.

Neonatal weakness, hypotonia, dysmorphism, contractures.

MYOPATHIES WITH ABNORMAL INCLUSIONS OF UNKNOWN ORIGIN

Other myopathies with abnormal inclusions include fingerprint, reducing, zebra, hyaline, cylindrical body myopathies. Rare disorders requiring further characterization.

MYOTONIA CONGENITA (THOMSEN DISEASE)

Channelopathy characterized by myotonia without weakness; abnormality of chloride channel.

Autosomal dominant form: Thomsen disease. Autosomal recessive: Becker disease.

CLINICAL FEATURES

Contrast with myotonic muscular dystrophy (Chapter 126): only myotonia; no weakness or wasting, no systemic disorder. Myotonia more severe and widespread: orbicularis oculi (difficulty opening eyes after forceful closure), leg muscles (difficulty starting to walk or run), pharyngeal muscles (dysphagia). Respiratory muscles spared. Improves with exercise. Muscles tend to hypertrophy.

Becker disease: more common; starts earlier.

Risk of severe muscle spasms from administration of depolarizing muscle relaxants (suxamethonium) for surgery.

INVESTIGATIONS

EMG: profuse myotonic discharges.

Muscle biopsy: tubular aggregates, absence of type 2b fibers.

TREATMENT

Phenytoin, quinine, mexiletine; acetazolamide sometimes effective.

CHONDRODYSTROPHIC MYOTONIA (SCHWARTZ-JAMPEL SYNDROME)

Stiff, often hypertrophied limb muscles; facial abnormalities (narrow palpebral fissures, pinched nose, micrognathia); other skeletal anomalies. Inheritance, onset age variable.

EMG: myotonia often continuous.
Differential diagnosis: Isaacs syndrome (see Chapter 130).

Myotonia can be treated with phenytoin, carbamazepine, or mexiletine. Procainamide relieves myotonia but risks lupus erythematosus.

CHAPTER 129 ■
MYOGLOBINURIA

Acute muscle necrosis leads to gross pigmenturia (brown) with myoglobin in urine. Also termed rhabdomyolysis. Most important syndromes in Table 129.1.

HEREDITARY MYOGLOBINURIA

IDENTIFIED ENZYME DEFICIENCIES

Genetic defect identified in six forms (first six entries in Table 129.1). Impaired metabolism of a fuel (glycogen or lipid) necessary for muscular work (see also Chapter 85).

Exercise limited by myalgia after exertion. Myoglobinuria follows strenuous activity. Clinical diagnosis of glycogen disorders: failure of venous lactate to rise after ischemic exercise.

Phosphoglycerate kinase deficiency X-linked; others are autosomal recessive.

TABLE 129.1

CLASSIFICATION OF HUMAN MYOGLOBINURIA

I. Hereditary Myoglobinuria
Myophosphorylase deficiency (McArdle)
Phosphofructokinase deficiency (Tarui)
Carnitine palmitoyl transferase deficiency (DiMauro)
Phosphoglycerate kinase (DiMauro)
Phosphoglycerate mutase (DiMauro)
Lactate dehydrogenase (Kanno)
Incompletely characterized syndromes
Excess lactate production (Larsson)
Uncharacterized
Familial; biochemical defect unknown
Provoked by diarrhea or infection
Provoked by exercise
Malignant hyperthermia
Repeated attacks in an individual; biochemical defect
unknown

II. Sporadic Myoglobinuria
Exertion in untrained individuals
"Squat-jump" and related syndromes
Anterior tibial syndrome
Convulsions
High-voltage electric shock, lightning strike
Agitated delirium, restraints
Status asthmaticus
Prolonged myoclonus or acute dystonia
Crush syndrome
Compression by fallen weights
Compression by body in prolonged coma
Ischemia
Arterial occlusion
Cardioversion
Coagulopathy in sickle-cell disease or disseminated
intravascular coagulation
Ischemia in compression and anterior tibial syndromes
Laparoscopic nephrectomy
Ligation of vena cava
Surgery on morbidly obese people, including bariatric
surgery
Mitochondrial Myopathies
Cytochrome oxidase-1 mutation
Mitochondrial tRNA mutation
Trifunctional protein deficiency
Metabolic depression
Barbiturate, carbon monoxide, narcotic coma
Cold exposure
Diabetic acidosis
General anesthesia
Hyperglycemic, hyperosmolar coma
Hypothermia

(continued)

TABLE 129.1

CLASSIFICATION OF HUMAN MYOGLOBINURIA
(Continued)

Exogenous toxins and drugs
  Alcohol abuse
  Amphotericin B
  Carbenoxolone
  Clopidogrel (and heart transplant)
  Gemfibrozil (plus statin)
  Glycyrrhizate
  Haff disease
  Heat stroke
  Heroin
  Hypokalemia, chronic (any cause)
  Interferon alpha2B
  Isoretinoin
  Malayan sea-snake bite poison
  Malignant neuroleptic syndrome
  Plasmocid
  Phenylpropanolamine
  Statin drugs
  Succinylcholine
  Toxic shock syndrome
  Wasp sting
Progressive muscle disease
  Alcoholic myopathy
  Dystrophinopathy
  Polymyositis or dermatomyositis
Cause unknown

MALIGNANT HYPERTHERMIA

Precipitated by succinylcholine, halothane. Widespread muscular rigidity (not always present), rapid rise in body temperature, myoglobinuria, arrhythmia, metabolic acidosis.

Autosomal dominant; sometimes sporadic. Gene mapped to 19q12–13.2 in some families. Pathogenesis may involve abnormal influx of calcium into muscle cells.

ACQUIRED MYOGLOBINURIA

Causes listed in Table 129.1. Common ones include vigorous exercise in untrained people (e.g., military recruits), crush injury, ischemia.

CLINICAL SYNDROMES

Syndrome regardless of cause: widespread myalgia, weakness, malaise, renal pain, fever, highly elevated serum CK. Main hazard: heme-induced nephropathy with renal failure.

Neuroleptic malignant syndrome: clinically similar to malignant hyperthermia; offending drugs differ. See Chapter 117.

Heat cramps: arise after heavy sweating during vigorous exercise if water is replaced but not salt.

Heat exhaustion: syndrome of salt or water depletion after exercise in hot environments. Malaise, collapse. No tissue damage.

Heat stroke: life-threatening disorder with similarities to malignant hyperthermia. Two major forms seen: a) exercise-induced myoglobinuria in hot weather; b) excessive heat (with or without exercise) during heat waves, likely to affect young children or the elderly. Increased core temperature, cerebral symptoms (inappropriate behavior, delirium, seizures, encephalopathy, coma). Multiple organ dysfunction. Fatality 10% to 50%.

Statin myopathy: abnormally high CK, sometimes more than 10 times upper limit of normal; myalgia, cramps; attacks of myoglobinuria, sometimes with renal failure.

TREATMENT

Acute attack: treatment directed to kidneys. Aggressive hydration; promote diuresis (if oliguria present), correct hyperkalemia.

Malignant hyperthermia: stop administration of offending agent; cooling; correct acidosis or arrhythmias. Intravenous dantrolene may relieve rigidity.

Neuroleptic malignant syndrome: stop administration of offending agent. Bromocriptine, carbamazepine reportedly beneficial (Chapter 117).

Statin-induced hyperCKemia: stop statin therapy if CK levels sustained at more than 10 times normal.

Attack prevention (lifelong conditions): patient learns limit of exercise tolerance. Diet therapy ineffective.

CHAPTER 130 ■ MUSCLE CRAMPS AND STIFFNESS

Stiffness: continuous muscle contraction at rest.
Cramps (spasms): transient, painful, involuntary contraction of muscle or group of muscles; lasts seconds to minutes. Causes listed in Table 130.1.

ORDINARY MUSCLE CRAMPS

Provoked by trivial movement or by contracting already shortened muscle. Predisposing factors: during or after vigorous exercise, pregnancy, hypothyroidism, uremia, profuse sweating or diarrhea, hemodialysis, lower motor neuron disorders (especially anterior horn cell diseases); often occur in bed at night or on waking in the morning.

EMG: brief, periodic bursts of motor unit potentials discharging at 200 to 300 Hz. Activity arises within anterior horn cell, distally along motor nerve, or both.
Treatment: stretching affected muscle usually terminates cramp; e.g., walking for gastrocnemius cramp. Nocturnal leg cramps prevented by bedtime dose of quinine, phenytoin, carbamazepine, or diazepam. Frequent daytime cramps: carbamazepine or phenytoin.
Benign fasciculation with cramps (Denny-Brown, Foley syndrome): inordinately frequent cramps, often with fasciculations. No weakness or upper motor neuron signs; almost never transforms to motor neuron disease.
Contracture: painful shortening of muscle with no electrical activity on EMG. Seen in McArdle disease (phosphorylase deficiency); attributed to depletion of adenosine triphosphate (ATP).

TABLE 130.1

MOTOR UNIT DISORDERS CAUSING CRAMPS AND STIFFNESS

Location of abnormality	Name of disorder	Principal manifestations	Treatment
Spinal cord and brain stem	Stiff-person syndrome	Rigidity, reflex spasms	Diazepam
	Tetanus	Rigidity, reflex spasms	Diazepam
	Progressive encephalomyelitis with rigidity and spasms	Rigidity, reflex spasms, focal neurologic deficits	None
	Myelopathy with alpha rigidity	Extensor rigidity	Clonazepam
	Spinal myoclonus	Segmental repetitive myoclonic jerks	
Peripheral nerves	Tetany	Carpopedal spasm	Correction of calcium, magnesium, or acid-base derangement
	Neuromyotonia	Stiffness, myokymia, delayed relaxation	Phenytoin, carbamazepine
Muscle	Myotonic disorders	Delayed relaxation, percussion myotonia	Phenytoin, carbamazepine, procainamide
	Schwartz-Jampel syndrome	Stiffness and myotonia	Phenytoin, carbamazepine
	Phosphorylase deficiency, phosphofructokinase deficiency	Cramps with intense or ischemic exercise	None
	Malignant hyperthermia	Rigidity, acidosis, myoglobinuria with general anesthesia	Dantrolene
Unknown	Ordinary muscle cramps	Cramps during sleep or ordinary activity	Quinine, phenytoin, carbamazepine

NEUROMYOTONIA (ISAACS SYNDROME)

Syndrome of continuous muscle fiber activity. Sometimes paraneoplastic. May be one in group of syndromes with autoimmune peripheral nerve hyperexcitability.

CLINICAL FEATURES

Myokymia: clinically visible, continuous muscle twitching, may be difficult to distinguish from vigorous fasciculation. EMG features of myokymia: spontaneous activity at rest includes fasciculations, doublets, multiplets, prolonged trains of discharges at rate up to 60 Hz.

Pseudomyotonia: difficulty relaxing without myotonic discharges on EMG. No percussion myotonia. Seen in Isaacs syndrome; also in hypothyroidism with muscle hypertrophy (Hoffmann syndrome).

Characteristic abnormal posture of limbs in Isaacs syndrome: identical to carpal or pedal spasm but fixed; persistent or intermittent. Liability to superimposed cramps. Hyperhidrosis.

Insidious onset in children or young adults. Slow movements, clawing of fingers, toe-walking, followed by stiffness of proximal limb and axial muscles. Stiffness, myokymia seen at rest; persist in sleep.

INVESTIGATIONS

EMG: continuous spontaneous activity at rest in one of two forms: a) *electrical myokymia* (grouped discharges at rates up to 60 Hz); b) electrical neuromyotonia (continuous discharges at 150 to 300 Hz, usually with abrupt onset, offset).

Consider checking for possible associated tumor (paraneoplastic antibodies) or autoimmune disease.

TREATMENT

Carbamazepine, phenytoin, plasmapheresis, intravenous immunoglobulin therapy reported helpful.

TETANY

Hyperexcitability of peripheral nerves, convulsions, paresthesias, prolonged spasm of limb muscles, or laryngospasm. Caused by hypocalcemia, hypomagnesemia, alkalosis; hyperventilation.

Clinical features: intense circumoral and digital paresthesias, then carpopedal spasm. Trousseau sign (carpal spasm induced by ischemia distal to pressure cuff) and Chvostek sign (twitching at angle of lips on percussion of facial nerve).

Treatment: correct underlying metabolic disorder. In hypomagnesemia, tetany does not respond to correction of accompanying hypocalcemia unless magnesium deficit also corrected.

Hyperventilation tetany reversed by rebreathing into paper bag.

STIFF-PERSON SYNDROME (MOERSCH-WOLTMAN SYNDROME)

CLINICAL FEATURES

Progressive muscular rigidity, painful spasms, aching discomfort; predominantly in axial and proximal limb muscles; awkward gait, slow movement. May become stable. Stiffness diminishes in sleep or general anesthesia. Painful reflex spasms in response to movement, loud noise, emotion.

Sometimes paraneoplastic. Diabetes mellitus in 30 percent of patients.

INVESTIGATIONS

EMG of stiff muscles: continuous discharge of motor unit potentials resembling normal voluntary contraction.

CSF: immunoglobulin G (IgG) may be increased; oligoclonal IgG bands sometimes.

Antibodies to glutamic acid decarboxylase (GAD) in serum of about 60% of patients. When associated with breast cancer, anti-amphiphysin antibodies (rather than anti-GAD) sometimes elevated.

TREATMENT

Diazepam frequently effective. Baclofen (oral or intrathecal), phenytoin, clonidine, tizanidine, may also help. IVIG beneficial in most patients.

CHAPTER 131 ■
DERMATOMYOSITIS

PATHOLOGY AND PATHOGENESIS

Autoimmune disease of skin and muscle. Degeneration, regeneration, edema, infiltration by lymphocytes in both tissues. Inflammatory cells (predominantly B cells) around small vessels or in perimysium; absent in 25% of biopsies. Complement deposits in capillaries (vasculopathy). Muscle degeneration and regeneration most marked at periphery of muscle bundles (perifascicular atrophy).

INCIDENCE

Incidence, together with polymyositis: seven cases per year per million people.

Occurs in all decades of life; peaks before puberty and age 40. About 10% of cases starting after age 40 associated with malignant neoplasm.

SYMPTOMS AND SIGNS

Rash: butterfly distribution nose and cheeks; eyelids; periungual skin (base of finger nails); extensor surfaces of knuckles, elbows, knees; upper chest. Gottron sign: red-purple scaly macules on extensor surfaces of finger joints. Subcutaneous calcinosis palpable or visible later.

Muscles: proximal limb weakness, with aching and tenderness. Cranial muscles spared except for dysphagia. Weakness alone almost never first symptom.

Maximum severity within weeks.

INVESTIGATIONS

Serum CK elevated. EMG: myopathic abnormalities; increased irritability of muscle. Tests for occult tumor.

PROGNOSIS

Inactive after 5 to 10 years. Mortality much reduced by modern treatment; recovery may be complete or with permanent disability.

TREATMENT

Prednisone, reducing as symptoms improve or immunosuppressive drug is added. Improvement in 50% to 80%. Plasmapheresis of no value; IVIG beneficial (small controlled trials). Also used: mycophenolate, cyclophosphamide.

CHAPTER 132 ■ POLYMYOSITIS, INCLUSION BODY MYOSITIS, AND RELATED MYOPATHIES

POLYMYOSITIS

DEFINITION

Polymyositis: acute or subacute onset; sometimes spontaneous improvement; infiltration of muscle by lymphocytes. Occurs alone or as part of systemic disease (including collagen-vascular disease, HIV infection).

CLINICAL FEATURES

Symptoms of proximal limb myopathy: difficulty climbing stairs, rising from low seats, lifting packages or dishes, working with arms overhead.

Difficulty holding head erect ("dropped head" syndrome) due to neck muscle weakness. Cranial muscles spared except for dysphagia.

Usually subacute, nadir in months. Rare before puberty. Often seen with collagen vascular diseases: systemic lupus erythematosus, rheumatoid arthritis, Sjögren disease, systemic sclerosis.

INVESTIGATIONS

EMG: myopathic pattern fibrillations, positive waves may be present.

Serum CK: usually increased 10 times normal.

Muscle biopsy: lymphocytic infiltrate (predominantly T cells) around healthy muscle fibers. Differs from dermatomyositis: no vascular lesions or perifascicular atrophy and less likely to be associated with malignancy.

PATHOGENESIS

Autoimmune disease of disordered cellular immunity.

TREATMENT

As for dermatomyositis (Chapter 131).

INCLUSION BODY MYOSITIS (IBM)

Features of IBM different from polymyositis:

Clinical: slower progression. Distal muscles affected early; especially weakness of finger-flexors. Affects men after age 50. Usually without collagen-vascular or other autoimmune disorders. Some familial, autosomal recessive with consanguinity.

Investigations: may show mixed neurogenic-myopathic EMG. Serum CK values normal or only slightly increased.

Pathology: rimmed vacuoles, cellular inclusions on muscle biopsy (besides inflammation). Stain for amyloid diagnostic. Ragged red muscle fibers, cytochrome *c* oxidase negative.

Treatment: no response to steroid therapy or plasmapheresis; intravenous immunoglobulin reported to help but not consistently.

Familial IBM: inclusion body "myopathy," not "myositis." Autosomal recessive and dominant forms, chromosome 9p12-13. Quadriceps spared. Usually little inflammation seen in biopsy.

RELATED MYOPATHIES

Eosinophilic myositis (eosinophilia-myalgia syndrome), AIDS-related myopathy.

CHAPTER 133 ■ MYOSITIS OSSIFICANS

Deposition of bone in subcutaneous tissue and along fascial planes in muscle. Probably sporadic appearance of an unidentified mutation. Primary disorder may be in connective tissue (fibrodysplasia ossificans).

Onset: transient localized swellings of neck and trunk in infancy. Later, minor bruises followed by deposition of solid material beneath skin and within muscles of limbs, paraspinal tissues, abdominal wall.

Myopathic changes in muscle biopsy or EMG. Serum CK levels sometimes increased.

Treatment: excision of masses followed by recurrence but may help joint deformity. Diphosphonate therapy attempted without clear benefit.

Section XIX
Demyelinating Diseases

CHAPTER 134 ■ MULTIPLE SCLEROSIS

DEFINITION

Chronic disease of young adults; characterized pathologically by multiple central nervous system white matter lesions.

EPIDEMIOLOGY

Age at onset: peaks at 20 to 30 years; rare before age 10 or after 60. M:F ratio 1:1.4 to 1:3.1.

Prevalence related to geographic latitude. High-prevalence regions (>30/100,000 population): northern Europe, northern United States, southern Canada, southern Australia, New Zealand.

Prevalence related to geographic latitude: increases with increasing distance from Equator, up to 65 degrees north or south. Relevant latitude is place of residence before age 15. Prevalence up to 30/100,000 population in northern Europe, northern United States, southern Canada, southern Australia, New Zealand.

ETIOLOGY AND PATHOGENESIS

Cause unknown. Postulated combination of genetic susceptibility and environment: initial trigger early in life (probably viral infection) leads to autoimmune mechanisms causing demyelination.

Genetic Susceptibility
Whites most susceptible. Lifetime risk of developing MS: 0.00125% in general population; 2.6% in siblings of MS patients; 1.8% in parents; 1.5% in children. Concordance rate 25% in monozygotic twins, 2.4% for same-sex dizygotic twins. Multiple genes suspected.

Immunology

Peripheral blood: no specific changes. CSF: pleocytosis, oligoclonal immunoglobulin G bands common. Histopathology: perivascular lymphocyte and macrophage infiltration.

Autoimmunity supported by animal model, experimental allergic encephalomyelitis.

Viruses

Environmental exposure implied by epidemiology. Epstein-Barr virus, Herpes simplex type 6 virus suggested as candidates.

PATHOLOGY

Macroscopic: diffuse brain atrophy common in long-standing cases. Brain sections: numerous small irregular gray areas in older lesions; pink areas in acute lesions (plaques), particularly in white matter tracts. Also periventricular.

Microscopic: myelin sheath stains show areas of demyelination in plaques. Sharply circumscribed, diffusely scattered throughout brain and spinal cord. Size varies. Acute lesion: marked hypercellularity, macrophage infiltration, astrocytosis, perivenous lymphocytes, plasma cells. Myelin sheaths disintegrate. Inactive plaque: prominent demyelination, severe loss oligodendrocytes, extensive gliosis.

SYMPTOMS AND SIGNS

MS usually manifests as one of three major clinical syndromes: relapsing-remitting, secondary progressive, or primary progressive.

Manifestations in All MS Types

Symptoms and signs (Table 134.1 and 134.2): determined by location of plaque. Frequently involved structures include optic nerves, corticospinal tracts, brainstem, cerebellum, spinal cord (especially lateral and posterior columns), giving rise to characteristic syndromes.

Common clinical features: optic neuritis (characteristically producing pain on eye movement); internuclear ophthalmoplegia (lesion of medial longitudinal fasciculus); hemiparesis or monoparesis; urinary incontinence or retention.

TABLE 134.1

COMMON SYMPTOMS AND SIGNS IN CHRONIC MULTIPLE SCLEROSIS

Functional system	% Frequency[a]
Motor	
Muscle weakness	65–100
Spasticity	73–100
Reflexes (hyperreflexia, Babinski, absent abdominals)	62–98
Sensory	
Impairment of vibratory and position sense	48–82
Impairment of pain, temperature, or touch	16–72
Pain (moderate to severe)	11–37
Lhermitte symptom	1–42
Cerebellar	
Ataxia (limb/gait/trunk)	37–78
Tremor	36–81
Nystagmus (brainstem or cerebellar)	54–73
Dysarthria (brainstem or cerebellar)	29–62
Cranial nerve/brain stem	
Vision affected	27–55[b]
Ocular disturbances (excluding nystagmus)	18–39
Cranial nerves V, VII, VIII	5–52
Bulbar signs	9–49
Vertigo	7–27
Autonomic	
Bladder dysfunction	49–93
Bowel dysfunction	39–64
Sexual dysfunction	33–59
Others (sweating and vascular abnormalities)	38–43
Psychiatric	
Depression	8–55
Euphoria	4–18
Cognitive abnormalities	11–59
Miscellaneous	
Fatigue	59–85

[a]Frequency values derived from the lowest and highest published rates. The higher frequency values are obtained mostly from studies with older patients with long-standing disease.
[b]Visual-evoked response abnormalities not included in these figures. Earlier studies suggested a much higher frequency, but these rates are not reproducible using current psychometric tests and therefore are excluded.

TABLE 134.2

SYMPTOMS AND SIGNS SEEN INFREQUENTLY IN MULTIPLE SCLEROSIS

Well-recognized associations	Rare associations
Generalized seizures	Aphasia
Tonic seizure	Anosmia
Headache	Hiccoughs
Trigeminal neuralgia	Deafness
Paroxysmal dysarthria/ataxia	Horner syndrome
Paroxysmal itching	Cardiac arrhythmias
Chorea/athetosis	Acute pulmonary edema
Myoclonus	Hypothalamic dysfunction
Facial hemispasm	Narcolepsy
Myokymia	
Spasmodic torticollis/focal dystonia	
Lower motor neuron signs—wasting, decreased tone, areflexia	
Restless legs	

Clinical manifestations multiple in time and space. Often, complete remission of first symptoms. Later, remissions incomplete or absent.

Symptoms sometimes evanescent; precipitated by heat (Uhthoff phenomenon), exercise, stress. Increased risk of exacerbation in postpartum period long debated.

MAIN TYPES OF MS

RELAPSING-REMITTING MS

Episodes (days to weeks) of clinical manifestations separated by asymptomatic intervals (weeks to years). Maximum symptom severity for a given episode reached within days.

Variable course for decades; rarely silent for decades or fatal within months. Exacerbations followed by variable improvement from complete remission to symptomatic residual dysfunction. About 10% have few attacks throughout life, accrue minimal disability.

Disease-modifying treatment improves prognosis. Approximately 85% become secondary progressive type.

Isolated optic neuritis: if brain MRI normal, chance of developing MS <10%.

SECONDARY PROGRESSIVE MS

Progresses slowly between discrete attacks or without abrupt episodes.

Prognostic indicators not reliable. After 10 years, 70% not working full-time. Average survival: 35 years after onset.

PRIMARY PROGRESSIVE MS

Progressive from outset; no distinct exacerbations. May be fatal in 10 years.

10% to 15% of cases; more common in older men. Mainly a spinal cord syndrome.

INVESTIGATIONS

MRI, CSF, evoked potentials most helpful (Table 134.3).

DIFFERENTIAL DIAGNOSIS

See Table 134.4.

VARIANTS OF MS

Marburg variant: rapidly progressive; severe disability; may be fatal in first year.
Devic disease: fulminant transverse myelitis with optic neuritis.
Schilder disease: fulminant MS in children. Confluent lesions in both hemispheres (see Chapter 95).
Concentric sclerosis of Balo: primarily children; concentric rings of inflammation and demyelination.

MANAGEMENT

Acute Attack
If symptoms severe enough: intravenous methylprednisolone, 1 g daily for 7 to 10 days; follow with oral prednisone in tapering schedule. Steroids hasten recovery from acute attack, do not affect long-term outcome.

TABLE 134.3

LABORATORY FINDINGS IN MULTIPLE SCLEROSIS

MRI

Appropriate T2-weighted scans abnormal in approximately 90% of patients.

MRI interpretation should be conservative and correlate with the clinical findings.

Typically, at least four white matter areas of increased signal of >3 mm diameter or three areas if at least one is periventricular should be seen.

False-positive scans are common in patients with one or two white matter lesions, particularly in patients older than age 50 yr.

Cerebrospinal fluid findings

Protein	Normal or mildly increased in 50%
Glucose	Normal
Lymphocytes	Normal in 66%. In others show 5 to 20 cells/mm^3 T/B lymphocyte ratio 80:20 CD4$^+$/CD8$^+$ 2:1
IgG	Increased in about 70%
Increased IgG synthesis	3.3 mg/day in 90% of patients
High IgG index	0.7 in 90% of patients
Oligoclonal IgG bands	90% of cases immunoelectrophoresis and silver staining
Light chains	Increased ratio of κ/λ and free κ light chains
Myelin basic protein	Normally <1 ng/mL. Increased in acute relapses to 4 ng/mL in 80% of cases

Evoked potentials

Visual-evoked responses	Very sensitive for detecting plaques in optic nerves, chiasm, or tracts Abnormal responses in 85% of those with definite and 58% of those with probable MS Interocular P$_{100}$ latency difference is common feature
Brainstem auditory	Most useful in detecting suspected pontine lesions Abnormal responses in 67% of patients with definite and 41% of those with probable MS
Somatosensory	Useful to document sensory abnormalities in patients with MS and normal clinical sensory examination Abnormal in 77% of patients with definite and 67% of patients with probable MS

IgG, immunoglobulin G.

TABLE 134.4

DIFFERENTIAL DIAGNOSIS OF MULTIPLE SCLEROSIS

Disorder	Distinguishing clinical/ Laboratory features
Acute disseminated encephalomyelitis	Follows infections or vaccination in children; fever, headaches, and meningism common
Lyme disease	Antibodies to *Borrelia* antigens in serum and CSF by ELISA and Western blot
HIV-associated myelopathy	HIV serology
HTLV-I myelopathy	HTLV-1 serology in serum/CSF
Neurosyphilis	Serum/CSF serology
Progressive multifocal leukoencephalopathy	Immunosuppressed patients; biopsy of lesions demonstrates virus by electron microscopy
Systemic lupus erythematosus	Non-CNS manifestations of lupus; antinuclear antibodies, anti-dsDNA and anti-Sm antibodies
Polyarteritis nodosa	Systemic signs; angiography shows microaneuryms; biopsy of involved areas shows vasculitis
Sjögren syndrome	Dry eyes and mouth; anti-Ro and anti-La antibodies; lower lip biopsy helpful
Behçet disease	Oral/genital ulcers, antibodies to oral mucosa
Sarcoidosis	Non-CNS signs; increased protein in CSF; biopsy shows granuloma
Paraneoplastic syndromes	Older age group; anti-Yo antibodies; identify neoplasm
Subacute combined degeneration of cord	Peripheral neuropathy, vitamin B_{12} levels
Subacute myelo-optic neuritis (SMON)	Mainly in Japanese; adverse reaction to chlorhydroxyquinoline
Adrenomyeloneuropathy	Adrenal dysfunction; neuropathy; plasma very-long-chain fatty acids increased
Spinocerebellar syndromes	Familial; pes cavus; scoliosis; absent reflexes; normal CSF IgG and no bands
Hereditary spastic paraparesis/primary lateral sclerosis	Normal CSF studies
Miscellaneous	Strokes, tumors, arteriovenous malformations, arachnoid cysts, Arnold-Chiari malformations, and cervical spondylosis all may lead to diagnostic dilemmas on occasion. These conditions may coexist; differentiation based on history, clinical followup and MRI features.

ELISA, enzyme-linked immunosorbent assay; HTLV, human T-lymphotrophic virus type I; IgG, immunoglobulin G.

Adverse effects: psychological agitation; avascular necrosis of hips after chronic steroid therapy; calcium carbonate supplements used to forestall osteoporosis.

Disease-Modifying Treatment
All patients with clinically definite exacerbating disease should take disease-modifying medication.

β-**interferons (IFNs):** IFN-β1b (Betaseron, Rebif), IFN-β1a (Avonex): synthetic variants of naturally occurring interferons; thought to have multiple immunomodulatory actions. Reduce frequency of attacks in relapsing-remitting phase by 30%. Other benefits: reduced severity of attacks; favorable effects on MRI changes; likely less disability; may retard transition to progressive form. Adverse effects: "flu-like" syndrome early; abnormal liver function tests; bone marrow depression; contraindicated in pregnancy. Neutralizing antibodies may develop, make treatment ineffective.

Glatiramer acetate (Copaxone or Copolymer 1): peptide fragment of myelin basic protein. Effects: similar effects to β IFNs on exacerbation frequency, attack severity. Sometimes brief severe pain with injections.

Mitoxantrone (Novantrone): antineoplastic agent thought to inhibit B-cell function, antibody production, macrophage-mediated myelin degradation; also thought to enhance T-cell suppressor function. Indicated for severe, frequent relapsing or progressive MS. Therapy limited to 8 to 10 cycles over lifetime due to cumulative cardiac toxicity. Echocardiogram warranted before starting therapy to ensure left ventricular ejection fraction >50%. Risk of acute, fatal leukemia.

Treatment of Severe and Frequent Relapses or Rapidly Progressive MS
Poor response to high-dose intravenous steroids.

Cyclophosphamide, azathioprine, methotrexate sometimes used. Limited by toxicity. Benefit not proven.

Combinations of regimens may be helpful, including corticosteroids, IVIG, mitoxantrone.

OTHER SYMPTOMATIC TREATMENT

Spasticity: baclofen, diazepam, dantrolene, tizanidine, injections of botulinum toxin. Intrathecal baclofen for severe cases.

Atonic bladder (post-voiding residual volume >100 mL): clean intermittent self-catheterization. Urine acidifiers (e.g., vitamin C), urinary antiseptics (e.g., methenamine mandelate) may help prevent urinary infection.

Spastic bladder: detrusor muscle hyperexcitability; most common cause of urinary urgency and incontinence in MS. Oxybutinin (most effective), propantheline, hycosamine, imipramine, tolterodine (Detrol). Synthetic antidiuretic hormone (desmopressin acetate intranasal spray) useful for nocturia.

Painful radiculopathy or neuralgia, painful paresthesias: carbamazepine, phenytoin, amitriptyline.

Fatigue: amantadine, pemoline, methylphenidate.

Constipation: change diet, bulk-providing food, stool softeners. Laxatives reserved for resistant cases.

Sexual dysfunction: counseling, sildenafil (Viagra), lubricating agents.

Severe paraparesis: skin care to prevent decubitus ulcers.

Physical therapy, adequate nutrition and hydration protect against decubitus ulcers, renal and bladder calculi, contractures, intercurrent infections. Physical therapy helps maintain mobility. Occupational therapy important for activities of daily living.

CHAPTER 135 ■
MARCHIAFAVA-BIGNAMI DISEASE

Demyelination of corpus callosum without inflammation; other CNS areas may be involved.

ETIOLOGY AND PATHOGENESIS

Primary degeneration of corpus callosum; may extend to anterior commissure, posterior commissure, centrum semiovale, other tracts.

Cause not known. First noted in elderly Italian men who consumed red wine.

CLINICAL FEATURES

Dementia, depression, extreme apathy, seizures, multifocal neurologic signs. Also, confusion, mania, paranoia, delusions.

MRI: typical callosal lesions plus symmetric demyelinating lesions in other areas.

DIFFERENTIAL DIAGNOSIS

Wernicke encephalopathy: may occur simultaneously; ataxia, ophthalmoplegia, nystagmus, dementia, delirium.

COURSE

Usually slowly progressive, results in death in 3 to 6 years. Spontaneous recovery reported. Some patients improve with thiamine or corticosteroid therapy.

CHAPTER 136 ■ CENTRAL PONTINE MYELINOLYSIS

Symmetric destruction of myelin in basis pontis, precipitated by rapid correction of hyponatremia. Often with chronic alcoholism, malnutrition.

Signs and symptoms 2 to 3 days after rapid correction of low sodium levels. Range from asymptomatic to comatose. Include: dysarthria or mutism, behavioral abnormalities, ophthalmoparesis, bulbar and pseudobulbar palsy, hyperreflexia, quadriplegia, seizures, coma, locked-in state.

May be fatal within days, but full recovery possible.

Extrapontine myelinolysis in about 10%: cerebellum, putamen, thalamus, corpus callosum, subcortical white matter, claustrum, caudate, hypothalamus, lateral geniculate bodies, amygdala, subthalamic nuclei, substantia nigra, medial lemnisci. Always bilaterally symmetric. Manifestations include ataxia, irregular behavior, visual field deficits, parkinsonism, choreoathetosis, dystonia.

MRI: hyperintense lesions on T2-weighted images, hypointense on T1 images; typically do not enhance. Pontine abnormalities in BAER.

Pathology: demyelination without inflammation.

Prevention: judicious correction of hyponatremia, no faster than 12 mmol/L in 24 hours.

Variants: pontine myelinolysis without hyponatremia in binge-drinking of alcohol or in anorexia nervosa; good recovery. Pontine myelinolysis in chronic alcohol users with profound hypophosphatemia.

Section XX
Autonomic Disorders

CHAPTER 137 ▪ NEUROGENIC ORTHOSTATIC HYPOTENSION AND AUTONOMIC FAILURE

Orthostatic hypotension (OH): fall of 20 mmHg in systolic blood pressure or 10 mmHg diastolic within 3 minutes after changing position from supine to standing or similar orthostatic challenge, such as $\geq 60°$ upright tilt. May be asymptomatic, especially in elderly. Marker of advanced autonomic failure.

MULTIPLE SYSTEM ATROPHY (MSA)

Autonomic failure present in 97% patients with any form of MSA (see Chapter 115). When present early in course, condition also referred to as Shy-Drager syndrome. (Other forms of MSA: striatonigral degeneration; olivopontocerebellar atrophy.)

Clinical features: OH or syncope often first and most disabling symptom. Parkinsonism sometimes mild or absent for years after onset of autonomic failure. Other features: inspiratory stridor from vocal fold paralysis; urinary incontinence; sleep disturbance.

Laboratory data: abnormal autonomic tests (Table 137.1), anal sphincter EMG (denervation), sleep tests (e.g., sleep apnea). Supine blood levels of norepinephrine (NE) normal or slightly reduced; does not increase on head-up tilt.

Pathology: argyrophilic glial cytoplasmic inclusions in oligodendroglia, especially in CNS autonomic control centers.

Prognosis: progression to severe disability in several years. Worse prognosis than Parkinson disease with autonomic features.

TABLE 137.1

TESTS OF AUTONOMIC FUNCTION

Well Established
Cardiovagal (Parasympathetic)
  HR variability to cyclic deep breathing
  HR response to Valsalva maneuver (Valsalva ratio)
  HR response to standing (30:15 ratio)
Adrenergic (Sympathetic)
  BP response to Valsalva maneuver (phases IV and late II)
  BP response to orthostatic stress
    Head-up tilt
    Standing
Sudomotor
  Quantitative sudomotor axon reflex test
  Thermoregulatory sweat test
  Silastic sweat imprint testing
  Sympathetic skin response

Additional or Investigational Methods
Serum norepinephrine levels, supine and upright
BP or HR response to alternate stressors
  Lower body negative pressure
  Sustained handgrip
  Mental arithmetic
  Diving reflex
  Cold pressor test
  Cough
Spectral analysis of HR and BP signals
Pharmacologic challenges
Pupillary testing (pharmacologic, pupillometry, pupil cycle time)
Urodynamics/sphincter EMG
GI motility and manometry studies
Salivary testing/Schirmer test
Microneurography
Vasomotor testing

BP, blood pressure; GI, gastrointestinal; HR, heart rate.

PURE AUTONOMIC FAILURE

Profound, slowly progressive disorder with disabling OH. Onset usually after age 50. Marked autonomic testing abnormalities with no other neurologic impairment.

Clinical features: multisymptom autonomic failure with prominent, often disabling orthostatic hypotension.

Laboratory data: low supine NE levels that fail to rise with head-up tilt; excessive response to NE infusion (denervation supersensitivity).

TABLE 137.2

SELECTED DISORDERS OF AUTONOMIC FUNCTION

Pure autonomic failure

Multisystem disorders
  Multiple system atrophy
    Shy-Drager syndrome
    Striatonigral degeneration
    Sporadic OPCA
  Parkinson disease with autonomic failure
  Machado-Joseph disease

Central
  Brain tumors (posterior fossa, third ventricle, hypothalamus),
    syringobulbia, multiple sclerosis, tetanus, Wernicke-Korsakoff
    syndrome, fatal familial insomnia

Spinal cord
  MS, syringomyelia, transverse myelitis, transection/trauma,
    tumor

Peripheral
  Immune mediated
    GBS (Chap. 106), acute and subacute pandysautonomia,
      acute cholinergic neuropathy, Sjögren syndrome, SLE,
      rheumatoid arthritis, Holmes-Adie syndrome
  Metabolic
    Diabetes, vitamin B_{12} and thiamine deficiency, uremia
  Paraneoplastic
    Paraneoplastic autonomic neuropathy, sensory neuronopathy
      with autonomic failure (ANNA antibodies), enteric
      neuropathy, Lambert-Eaton myasthenic syndrome
      (cholinergic)
  Infectious
    Chagas disease (cholinergic), tabes, leprosy, HIV, Lyme
      disease, diphtheria
  Hereditary
    Familial amyloidosis, hereditary sensory and autonomic
      neuropathies (Chap. 105), dopamine β-hydroxylase
      deficiency, porphyria, Fabry disease
  Toxins
    Botulism, vincristine, cisplatin, taxol, amiodarone, vacor,
      hexacarbon, carbon disulfide, heavy metals, podophyllin,
      alcohol
  Drug and medication effects

Reduced orthostatic tolerance
  Neurocardiogenic syncope, postural orthostatic, tachycardia
    syndrome (POTS), mitral valve prolapse syndrome, prolonged
    bed rest or weightlessness

Other
  Acquired amyloidosis, chronic idiopathic autonomic
    neuropathies, small fiber neuropathy, idiopathic
    hyperhidrosis, idiopathic anhidrosis, Ross syndrome
    (anhidrosis, hyporeflexia, Adie pupil).

ANNA, antineuronal antibody; OPCA, olivopontocerebellar atrophy;
POTS, postural orthostatic tachycardia syndrome; GBS,
Guillain-Barré syndrome; SLE, systemic lupus erythematosus.

Pathology: degeneration of postganglionic sympathetic neurons.

DOPAMINE β-HYDROXYLASE DEFICIENCY

Rare but treatable entity with severe OH, syncope, nearly undetectable NE, epinephrine.

Treatment: NE precursor L-threo-dihydroxyphenylserine (L-DOPS); not yet approved in US.

OTHER CAUSES OF AUTONOMIC FAILURE

See Table 137.2.

Chronic peripheral neuropathies: autonomic involvement typically seen in diabetic or amyloid polyneuropathy, paraneoplastic neuropathy, other hereditary or toxic neuropathy.

TREATMENT

OH: maintain head and trunk 15 to 20 degrees above legs in bed, squatting, cross legs; supplemental dietary sodium chloride; fludrocortisone, midodrine. 3,4-Dihydroxyphenylserine for hereditary dopamine hydroxylase deficiency.

Symptomatic treatment for other autonomic manifestations.

Severe inspiratory stridor: tracheostomy. Sleep apnea: nocturnal positive pressure ventilation.

CHAPTER 138 ■ ACUTE AUTONOMIC NEUROPATHY

Generalized autonomic dysfunction of unknown etiology. Also known as *acute pandysautonomia*. May be subacute.

Often preceded by acute illness of presumed viral origin as in Guillain-Barré syndrome. Paraneoplastic forms reported.

Pathogenesis: primarily affects peripheral autonomic nerves. May be immune-mediated.

Clinical features: orthostatic hypotension (absent in 25%), nausea, vomiting, constipation or diarrhea, bladder atony, impotence, anhidrosis, impaired lacrimation and salivation, pupillary abnormalities. Sometimes gastroparesis, impaired sensation.

Laboratory data: abnormalities in tests of autonomic dysfunction. Antibodies to nicotinic ganglionic acetylcholine receptor (AChR) α-3 subunits correlate with disease severity.

Treatment: symptomatic. Intravenous immunoglobulin therapy may be effective.

Course: recovery slow, often incomplete.

CHAPTER 139 ■ FAMILIAL DYSAUTONOMIA

Inherited disorder of autonomic and peripheral nervous systems plus somatic growth.

Genetics: autosomal recessive, almost exclusively in Eastern European Ashkenazi Jewish people. One of two possible mutations in IKBKAP gene on chromosome 9.

Pathogenesis: impaired synthesis of NE.

Clinical features in infancy: low birth weight, breech presentation, hypotonia, diminished tendon reflexes, no corneal responses, poor Moro reflex, weak cry and suck, breath-holding spells. Tongue tip lacks fungiform papillae, appears smooth. Risk aspiration pneumonia from impaired swallowing, gastroesophageal reflux. Lack of overflow tears risks corneal ulceration.

Clinical features after age 3: dysautonomic crises (irritability, self-mutilation, negativistic behavior, diaphoresis, tachycardia, hypertension, thermal instability); episodic vomiting. Short stature, awkward gait, nasal speech, scoliosis. Later: orthostatic hypotension, vasovagal responses exaggerated.

Other features: no ventilatory response to hypercapnia, hypoxia; cardiovascular instability; excessive drooling, dysphagia.

Laboratory data: (a) little pain, lack of erythema after intradermal histamine injection; (b) pupillary miosis (instead of no effect in normals) after one drop 2.5% metacholine or dilute pilocarpine.

Treatment: surgery to prevent gastroesophageal reflux. Midodrine for orthostatic hypotension. For dysautonomic crisis: parenteral fluids, sedation, antiemetics, midodrine, clonidine.

Prognosis: long-term survival possible if survive infantile, adolescent crises.

Section XXI
Paroxysmal Disorders

CHAPTER 140 ■ MIGRAINE AND OTHER HEADACHES

MIGRAINE

Benign recurring headache, neurologic dysfunction, or both, with pain-free interludes.

Provoked by stereotyped stimuli (specific foods, relief of stress, exercise). Far more common in women. Hereditary predisposition. Head pain lateralized in about 60% of cases.

Severe attacks likely to be throbbing, associated with vomiting and scalp tenderness. Milder headaches nondescript—tight, band-like discomfort involving entire head.

CLINICAL SUBTYPES

Migraine without Aura
Previously called "common" migraine. Benign periodic headache lasting several hours, without preceding focal neurologic symptoms; most frequent type of headache; includes "tension headache."

Unilateral pain, nausea or vomiting, positive family history, response to ergotamine, scalp tenderness in 60% to 80%.

Migraine with Aura
Previously "classic" migraine. Headache associated with characteristic premonitory sensory, motor, or visual symptoms. Focal symptoms in small proportion of attacks, more common during headache than as prodromal symptoms.

Most common premonitory symptoms: visual—scotomas or hallucinations (usually in central visual field) in about 33%. "Fortification spectrum" in 10%; paracentral scotoma expands into "C" shape, with luminous angles at outer edge. Duration 20 to 25 minutes. Pathognomonic of migraine.

"Complicated" migraine: term previously used for migraine with dramatic focal neurologic features, such as hemiplegia. Overlaps with classic migraine. Also used for persistent focal signs after migraine attack.

Basilar Migraine

Brainstem signs, including vertigo, dysarthria, diplopia; occur as sole neurologic symptoms of migraine in 25%.

Severe form: episodes of total blindness and sensorial clouding, with or followed by vertigo, ataxia, dysarthria, tinnitus, distal and perioral paresthesias. Confusion follows in 25%. Duration about 30 minutes. Episode followed by throbbing occipital headache. Most common in adolescent women. Sensorial alterations, including confusion, may last as long as 5 days.

Carotidynia (Facial Migraine)

Older patients. Continuous deep, dull, aching pain in jaw or neck, episodically throbbing. Sharp, ice pick–like jabs superimposed. Attacks one to several times a week, each lasting minutes to hours. Ipsilateral tenderness, prominent pulsations of cervical carotid artery, swelling of soft tissues. Commonly precipitated by dental trauma.

Differential diagnosis: carotid dissection.

Hemiplegic Migraine

Hemiparesis may occur during prodrome; lasts 20 to 30 minutes.

More severe form: hemiplegia for days to weeks after headache subsides. Accompanying findings: dysarthria, aphasia, hemisensory loss, CSF pleocytosis, CSF protein content increased.

Familial form autosomal dominant; CACNLIA4 gene, chromosome 19, encoding calcium channel.

Ophthalmoplegic Migraine

Attacks of periorbital pain and vomiting for 1 to 4 days. Complete third nerve palsy follows, often including pupillary dilation, loss of light response. May persist days to 2 months. Onset in childhood.

Migraine Equivalents

Episodic focal neurologic symptoms without headache or vomiting.

PATHOGENESIS

Cortical "spreading depression" of electrical activity suspected: wave of excitation followed by wave of complete inhibition of activity across areas of cerebral cortex. Neurologic symptoms attributed to neuronal dysfunction from spreading inhibition. Vasoconstriction, vasodilation, secretion of vasoactive peptides likely to play role.

Three-phase sequence model: (a) brainstem generation; (b) "vasomotor activation" (arteries within and outside the brain may contract or dilate); (c) release of vasoactive neuropeptides at terminations of trigeminal nerve on blood vessels.

Role of serotonin receptors supported by efficacy of sumatriptan.

TREATMENT

Acute Treatment
Immediate administration of full dose of agent at attack onset.

Mild headache: aspirin, acetaminophen. Butalbital and caffeine added if necessary. Ibuprofen, naproxen often useful. Isometheptene compounds effective for mild-to-moderate "stress headaches."

Moderate-to-severe headache: ergotamine (oral or suppository); sumatriptan (oral, intranasal, subcutaneous dose), rizatriptan, zolmitriptan, naratriptan. Triptans indicated for attack frequency >2 to 3 per month.

Severe headache: dihydroergotamine (parenteral, nasal spray). Intravenous prochlorperazine, metoclopramide, dihydroergotamine.

Chronic daily headache: amitriptyline, nortriptyline, other antidepressants, valproate, phenelzine, topiramate, zonisamide. Restrict opiate-type analgesics to 2 days out of 7.

Prophylaxis
Daily administration required. Effect lags 2 weeks. Major drugs listed in Table 140.1. Additional drugs include doxepin, topiramate, zonisamide.

Phenelzine (a monoamine oxidase inhibitor) reserved for recalcitrant headaches because of adverse effects. Tyramine-free diet required.

Probability of success 60% to 75%. Once effective, drug may be tapered after 6 months.

TABLE 140.1
DRUG STABILIZATION OF MIGRAINE

Drug	Tablet size (mg)	Daily dose range (mg)	Most common side effects
Propranolol	10, 20, 40, 60, 80, 90; sustained release: 60, 80, 120, 160	40–320	Fatigue, insomnia, light-headedness, impotence
Amitriptyline	10, 25, 50, 75, 100	10–175	Sedation, dry mouth, appetite stimulation
Ergonovine	0.2	0.4–2.0	Nausea, abdominal pain, leg tiredness, diarrhea
Verapamil	40, 80, 120; sustained release: 120–480	120–480; sustained release: 320–960	Constipation, nausea, fluid retention, light-headedness, hypotension
Valproate	125, 250, 500	500–2,000	Nausea, tremor, alopecia, appetite stimulation
Phenelzine	15	30–90	Sedation, orthostatic hypotension, constipation, urinary retention

CLUSTER HEADACHE

Episodic: most common type. One to three short-lived attacks of periorbital pain daily for 4 to 8 weeks, then pain-free interval for about 1 year.

Chronic: begins de novo or evolves from episodic type. Attacks similar; no sustained remission. M:F ratio 8:1. Prevalence 69:100,000 people. Onset ages 20 to 50.

CLINICAL FEATURES

Periorbital, temporal, or maxillary pain begins without warning, peaks within 5 minutes. Often excruciating, deep, nonfluctuating, explosive. Strictly unilateral. Attacks last 30 to 120 minutes. Frequently with ipsilateral lacrimation, red eye, nasal stuffiness, lid ptosis, nausea.

Alcohol provokes attacks in 70% during bout of attacks, but may not during prolonged remission. During bout, attacks may recur at same hour each day.

TREATMENT

To abort attack: oxygen inhalation (10 mL/min via non-rebreathing mask), intranasal topical lidocaine, sumatriptan. Sumatriptan contraindicated within 24 hours of ergotamine use. To prevent further attacks during bout: prednisone, lithium, methysergide, ergotamine, verapamil. Lithium effective for chronic form.

CHRONIC PAROXYSMAL HEMICRANIA

Similar to cluster headaches, but briefer, more frequent attacks. Female preponderance. Pain: boring quality reaching full intensity very rapidly. Ipsilateral lacrimation, nasal congestion, eyelid edema, partial Horner's syndrome.

Remarkably responsive to indomethacin therapy (50–250 mg daily); sometimes to COX-II inhibitors.

SUNCT SYNDROME

SUNCT: *S*hort-lasting *u*nilateral *n*euralgiform headache with *c*onjunctival injection and *t*earing. Rare. Male preponderance. Multiple attacks per hour. lasting seconds.

Pain: stabbing or throbbing. Same autonomic symptoms as cluster headaches. Lamotrigine, gabapentin sometimes effective.

HEMICRANIA CONTINUA

Continuous unilateral headache, fluctuating in severity. Same autonomic symptoms as cluster headaches. Dramatic response to indomethacin.

COUGH HEADACHE

Transient, severe head pain on coughing, bending, lifting, sneezing, stooping. Persists seconds to minutes. Headache diffuse; may be lateralized in 33%. M:F ratio 4:1.

Intracranial structural anomalies (e.g., Arnold-Chiari malformation) in 25%; MRI indicated.

Idiopathic form responds to indomethacin. Large volume LP terminates syndrome in 50%.

COITAL HEADACHE

Headache during coitus, usually close to orgasm. Abrupt onset; subsides few minutes after interruption of coitus.

Differential diagnosis: (a) subarachnoid hemorrhage (persistence for hours; presence of vomiting, confusion, focal neurologic signs); (b) unruptured aneurysm (can be indistinguishable from benign coital headache at first but not repetitive).

NOCTURNAL HEADACHES

Most commonly migraine; less frequently, cluster headache.

Hypnic headaches: elderly; awakening due to headache, lasting 15–60 minutes. MRI to exclude intracranial neoplasms, giant cell arteritis. Treatment: lithium (150–300 mg) or caffeine (if tolerated) at bedtime.

POST-CONCUSSION HEADACHE

Follows severe or trivial head injury (including head trauma without loss of consciousness). Often with vertigo, impaired memory and concentration, mood changes for months or years (post-concussion syndrome). Eventually remits.

GIANT CELL ARTERITIS (TEMPORAL ARTERITIS)

Onset after 60. Annual incidence 77:100,000 people aged ≥50. Results in blindness in 50%.

Most common initial symptoms: headache, polymyalgia rheumatica, jaw claudication, fever, weight loss (see Chapter 155). Headache unilateral or bilateral; temporal in 50%. Peaks in few hours. Quality dull, boring with superimposed episodic ice pick–like lancinating pain. Scalp tenderness common.

ESR almost always elevated. After temporal artery biopsy, prednisone for 4 to 6 weeks.

IDIOPATHIC INTRACRANIAL HYPERTENSION AND HYPOTENSION

See Chapter 50.

LUMBAR PUNCTURE (POST-LP) HEADACHE

Onset within 48 hours; may be delayed for up to 12 days. Mean incidence 30%. Present only on sitting or standing. Worsened by head shaking, jugular vein compression. Quality usually dull; location occipitofrontal. Other symptoms: nausea, stiff neck. Duration usually few days; may persist weeks to months.

Prevention: small styletted or round-point needle ($\geq$20-gauge); avoid multiple puncture holes.

Management: bed rest; adequate hydration; simple analgesics. Intravenous caffeine sodium benzoate terminates headache in 75%; may be repeated 1 hour later. Epidural blood patch (epidural injection of patient's blood) highly effective.

BRAIN TUMOR HEADACHE

Chief complaint in 30% of patients with brain tumor. Deep, dull aching quality, moderate intensity, intermittent, worsened by exertion or change in position, associated with nausea and vomiting. Headache disturbs sleep in about 10%. Vomiting precedes headache by weeks in posterior fossa brain tumors.

CHAPTER 141 ■ EPILEPSY

DEFINITIONS

Epileptic seizure: temporary dysfunction of brain caused by self-limited, abnormal hypersynchronous electrical discharge of cortical neurons (see also Chapter 3).

Epilepsy: group of chronic disorders characterized by recurrence of unprovoked, usually unpredictable seizures. Approximately 40 million people affected worldwide.

CLASSIFICATION

SEIZURES

Developed by International League Against Epilepsy (ILAE; Table 141.1). Seizure type most reliably indicated by initial events of seizure.

Partial Seizures

Ictal discharge in limited, circumscribed area of cortex (epileptogenic focus). Diverse symptoms may be subjective ("aura") or overt (e.g., focal limb jerks, head turning, sensory disturbance, complex emotional phenomena).

Simple partial seizure: no confusion or impairment of consciousness.

Complex partial seizure: impaired awareness; bilateral spread of seizure discharge (at least to basal forebrain and limbic areas). Frequent auras: visceral sensation, motionless stare, automatisms (lip-smacking, buttoning shirt). Postictal confusion common. About 70% to 80% arise in temporal lobe.

Generalized Seizures

Generalized tonic-clonic (grand mal) seizures: abrupt loss of consciousness with bilateral tonic extension of trunk and limbs (tonic phase), followed by synchronous muscle jerking (clonic phase). Brief postictal stupor followed by lethargy,

TABLE 141.1

CLASSIFICATION OF EPILEPTIC SEIZURES (INTERNATIONAL LEAGUE AGAINST EPILEPSY)

Partial (focal) seizures
A. Simple partial seizures (consciousness not impaired)
  1. With motor signs (including jacksonian, versive, and postural)
  2. With sensory symptoms (including visual, somatosensory, auditory, olfactory, gustatory, and vertiginous)
  3. With psychic symptoms (including dysphasia, hallucinations, affective changes)
  4. With autonomic symptoms (including epigastric sensation, pallor, flushing, pupillary changes)
B. Comlex partial seizures (consciousness is impaired)
  1. Simple partial onset followed by impaired consciousness
  2. With impairment of consciousness at onset
  3. With automatisms
C. Partial seizures evolving to secondarily generalized seizures

Generalized seizures of nonfocal origin (convulsive or nonconvulsive)
A. Absence seizures
  1. With impaired consciousness only
  2. With one or more of the following: atonic components, tonic components, automatisms, autonomic components
B. Myoclonic seizures, myoclonic jerks (single or multiple)
C. Tonic-clonic seizures (may include clonic-tonic-clonic seizures)
D. Tonic seizures
E. Atonic seizures

Unclassified epileptic seizures

From Commission on Classification and Terminology of the International League Against Epilepsy. Proposal for revised clinical and electroencephalographic classification of epileptic seizures. *Epilepsia* 1981;22:489–501.

confusion. Vague, variable prodromal symptoms may precede seizure for hours.

Absence (petit mal) seizures: momentary lapse of awareness, motionless stare, arrest of any ongoing activity. Abrupt onset (without prodromal symptoms) and abrupt end.

Myoclonic seizures: rapid, brief unilateral or bilateral muscle jerks, may be bilateral.

Atonic (astatic) seizures (drop attacks): sudden loss of muscle tone: may be fragmentary (e.g., head drop) or generalized, resulting in a fall.

TABLE 141.2

MODIFIED CLASSIFICATION OF EPILEPTIC SYNDROMES

I. Idiopathic epilepsy syndromes (focal or generalized)
A. Benign neonatal convulsions
   1. Familial
   2. Nonfamilial
B. Benign childhood epilepsy
   1. With central midtemporal spikes
   2. With occipital spikes
C. Childhood/juvenile absence epilepsy
D. Juvenile myoclonic epilepsy (including generalized tonic-clonic seizures on awakening)
E. Idiopathic epilepsy, otherwise unspecified

II. Symptomatic epilepsy syndromes (focal or generalized)
A. West syndrome (infantile spasms)
B. Lennox-Gastaut syndrome
C. Early myoclonic encephalopathy
D. Epilepsia partialis continua
   1. Rasmussen syndrome (encephalitic form)
   2. Restricted form
E. Acquired epileptic aphasia (Landau-Kleffner syndrome)
F. Temporal lobe epilepsy
G. Frontal lobe epilepsy
H. Posttraumatic epilepsy
I. Other symptomatic epilepsy, focal or generalized, not specified

III. Other epilepsy syndromes of uncertain or mixed classification
A. Neonatal seizures
B. Febrile seizures
C. Reflex epilepsy
D. Other unspecified

EPILEPSY (EPILEPTIC SYNDROMES)

See Table 141.2. Syndromes mainly associated with partial seizures (localization-related epilepsies) or generalized seizures (generalized epilepsies).

Specific Generalized Epilepsy Syndromes

Infantile Spasms (West Syndrome)

Seizures characterized by sudden flexor or extensor spasms involving head, trunk, and limbs simultaneously. Onset before age 6 months. EEG: chaotic, high-voltage slow activity with multifocal spikes (hypsarrhythmia).

Causes: cerebral dysgenesis, tuberous sclerosis, phenylketonuria, intrauterine infections, hypoxic-ischemic injury. About 15% idiopathic.

Treatment: corticotropin (ACTH), prednisone, topiramate, zonisamide, vigabatrin. No effect on long-term prognosis. Severe long-term disabilities in >66%.

Childhood Absence (Petit Mal) Epilepsy

Onset at age 4 to 12 years. Recurrent absence seizures (up to hundreds a day). EEG during attack: stereotyped, bilateral 3-Hz spike-wave discharges. Generalized tonic-clonic seizures additionally in 30% to 50%. Most children otherwise normal. Treatment: ethosuximide, valproate, lamotrigine, topiramate, zonisamide.

Lennox-Gastaut Syndrome

Childhood epileptic encephalopathies characterized by mental retardation, uncontrolled seizures, distinctive EEG (slow spike wave, 1.5 to 2.5 Hz). Causes include brain malformations, perinatal asphyxia, severe head injury, CNS infection. Seizures persist into adult years in 80%.

Treatment: valproate, lamotrigine, topiramate, zonisamide, vagus nerve stimulation, corpus callosotomy. Felbamate often the only effective agent.

Juvenile Myoclonic Epilepsy

Onset usually 8 to 20 years. Morning myoclonic jerks, generalized tonic-clonic seizures just after waking, normal intelligence, family history of similar seizures. EEG: generalized spikes, 4- to 6-Hz spike-wave, "polyspike" discharges. Valproate controls seizures, myoclonus in >80%; also lamotrigine (may exacerbate myoclonus), zonisamide, levetiracetam, topiramate.

Specific Localization-Related Epilepsy Syndromes

Benign Focal Epilepsy of Childhood

Most common: benign rolandic epilepsy; central to midtemporal spikes on EEG. Onset 4 to 13 years. Attacks mainly or exclusively at night, often with secondary generalization. Seizures uniformly disappear in adolescence. If treatment needed: carbamazepine or gabapentin in low doses.

Temporal Lobe Epilepsy

Most common epilepsy syndrome of adults. Epileptogenic region in medial temporal lobe. Seizure type almost universally complex partial. Interictal EEG: focal temporal slowing, epileptiform discharges (sharp waves or spikes) over anterior temporal region. Surgical resection far superior to medical treatment; anterior temporal lobe resection effective in 80%.

Frontal Lobe Epilepsy
Seizure types vary but characterized by: brief duration, abrupt onset, nighttime occurrence; bizarre motor manifestations (e.g., bilateral limb thrashing); no postictal confusion; minimal EEG abnormality; history of status epilepticus.

Post-traumatic Seizures
Follow 7% of head injuries in general population. Injury severe, associated with brain contusion, intracerebral or intracranial hematoma, unconsciousness or amnesia for >24 hours, or persistent neurologic signs.

Types: impact (immediately with injury), early (within 2 weeks), late. Risk of posttraumatic epilepsy (recurrent late seizures) raised by early seizures. Seizures partial or secondarily generalized in 70%.

Treatment: prophylactic phenytoin for 1 week after any severe head injury. Overt seizures treated as outlined later in chapter.

Epilepsia Partialis Continua (EPC)
Unremitting motor seizures involving part or all of one side of body.

Causes: inflammatory brain diseases, stroke, metastasis, metabolic encephalopathy (especially hyperosmolar nonketotic hyperglycemia).

Rasmussen syndrome: chronic focal encephalitis with EPC. Onset before age 10. About 20% begin with episode of convulsive status epilepticus. Slowly progressive hemiparesis, mental impairment, hemianopia typically follow. MRI: unilateral cortical atrophy, evidence of gliosis. IVIG possibly helpful. Hemispherectomy often the only effective treatment.

EPIDEMIOLOGY

U.S. prevalence of active epilepsy (recurrent unprovoked seizures): about 6.5 persons per 1,000. Annual incidence: 31 to 57 new cases per 100,000. M:F ratio 1.1 to 1.5:1. Lifetime risk of epilepsy 3%.

TABLE 141.3

PREDICTORS OF INTRACTABILITY

Very young age at onset (<2 yr)
Frequent generalized seizures
Failure to achieve control readily
Evidence of brain damage
A specific cause of the seizures
Severe EEG abnormality
Low IQ
Atonic atypical absence seizures

Most common etiologies: idiopathic (largest group), cerebrovascular disease, developmental neurologic disorders, head trauma.

Risk of recurrence: 40% in 2 years after first unprovoked seizure; >80% after second unprovoked seizure.

Factors predicting recurrence: seizure of partial type; epileptiform discharges on EEG; preceding brain injury or neurologic syndrome.

Factors predicting response to treatment: idiopathic epilepsy; normal neurologic examination; onset in early to middle childhood (except neonatal seizures). Unfavorable prognostic factors listed in Table 141.3.

INITIAL DIAGNOSTIC EVALUATION

History: risk factors (Table 141.4); age at seizure onset; developmental history; nature of aura; presence of automatisms, sustained postures, myoclonus.

Examination: hand or face asymmetry; skin lesions.

EEG: epileptiform discharges (spikes and sharp waves) highly correlated with seizure susceptibility. Recorded on first EEG in about 50% of patients with epilepsy; in 60% to 90% with multiple EEGs.

MRI: for all patients over age 18 years and children with abnormal development, abnormal findings on examination, or seizure types suggesting symptomatic epilepsy. Hippocampal atrophy and gliosis highly correlated with mesial temporal sclerosis and epileptogenic temporal lobe.

Other tests: LP if meningitis or encephalitis suspected. Urine or blood toxicologic screens for otherwise unexplained new-onset generalized seizures.

TABLE 141.4

RISK FACTORS FOR EPILEPSY[a]

Family history of seizures	2.5
Severe military head trauma	580
Severe civilian head trauma	25
Moderate head trauma	4
Mild head trauma[b]	1.5
Stroke	22
Alzheimer disease	10
Viral encephalitis	16.2
Bacterial meningitis	4.2
Aseptic meningitis	2.3
Multiple sclerosis	3.6
Alcohol[c]	10.1
Heroin	2.6
Marijuana	0.36
No adverse exposure	1.0

[a]Relative to people without these adverse exposures.
[b]Not statistically significant.
[c]One pint of 80 proof, 2.5 bottles of wine.
From Hauser WA, Hesdorffer DC. *Epilepsy: frequency, causes and consequences.* New York: Demos, 1990.

Long-term monitoring: recording electrographic seizure discharge during typical behavioral attack. Indicated by ambiguous history, nonspecific interictal EEG, treatment failure. Methods: (a) ambulatory EEG; (b) simultaneous closed circuit television and EEG (CCTV/EEG) monitoring.

MEDICAL TREATMENT

Drug treatment risks adverse effects, approaches 30% for first treatment.

ACUTE SYMPTOMATIC SEIZURES

Caused by or associated with acute medical or neurologic illness. Usually self-limited. Treatment generally not needed after recovery.

THE SINGLE SEIZURE

Need for treatment questionable. Reasonable to defer treatment until second seizure.

BENIGN EPILEPSY SYNDROMES

Treatment not always necessary, used for frequent or severe seizures, wishes of child or parents.

ANTIEPILEPTIC DRUGS (AEDs)

Selection of AEDs

See Table 141.5. Valproate: drug of choice for generalized-onset seizures. Absence seizures: ethosuximide if no other seizure types present; otherwise valproate. Carbamazepine, phenytoin, gabapentin, lamotrigine can aggravate myoclonic seizures; all but lamotrigine can also exacerbate absence seizures. Tiagabine can aggravate or induce absence seizures.

TABLE 141.5

DRUGS USED IN TREATING DIFFERENT TYPES OF SEIZURES

Type of seizure	Drugs[a]
Simple and complex partial	Carbamazepine, valproate; gabapentin, lamotrigine, topiramate, oxcarbazepine, zonisamide, levetiracetam, phenytoin, primidone, phenobarbital
Secondarily generalized	Carbamazepine, valproate, gabapentin, lamotrigine, topiramate, oxcarbazepine, zonisamide, levetiracetam, phenytoin, phenobarbital, primidone
Primary generalized seizures	
Tonic-clonic	Valproate; lamotrigine, topiramate, zonisamide, carbamazepine, oxcarbazepine, phenytoin
Absence	valproate, lamotrigine ethosuximide, zonisamide
Myoclonic	valproate; clonazepam, levetiracetam
Tonic	valproate, felbamate; clonazepam, zonisamide

[a]Not all drugs have FDA approval for listed uses.

Adverse Effects of AEDs

Common to virtually all AEDs, especially when treatment started: sedation, mental dulling, impaired memory and concentration, mood changes, gastrointestinal upset, dizziness. May be dose-related or idiosyncratic.

Selected idiosyncratic reactions: (a) agranulocytosis or aplastic anemia: 2:575,000 for carbamazepine; up to 1:5,000 for felbamate; (b) fatal hepatotoxicity in children for valproate, especially if <2 years of age and with polytherapy.

Increased risk of serious adverse drug reactions: metabolic or biochemical disorders, history of previous drug reactions, illness affecting hematopoiesis or liver and kidney function.

AED Pharmacology

Therapy starts with single AED chosen with regard to type of seizure or epilepsy syndrome, modified for side effects, required dosing schedule, cost. Combination treatment with two drugs attempted only when monotherapy with primary AEDs fails. Published "therapeutic ranges" are only guidelines.

Felbamate has high risk of serious adverse reactions, including aplastic anemia and hepatic failure. Use restricted to patients refractory to other agents and those with risk of continued seizures outweighing risk of side effects.

AEDS and Reproductive Health

Relationship of seizures to menstrual cycle (catamenial seizures) in about one third of women with epilepsy. Possibly related to proconvulsant action of estrogen, anticonvulsant action of progesterone.

Epilepsy associated with higher frequency of reproductive endocrine disturbance, lower fertility rates, higher rates of sexual dysfunction.

Discontinuing AEDs

About 60% to 70% of people with epilepsy become free of seizures for at least 5 years within 10 years of diagnosis. Attempt to discontinue AED (via taper) after 2 years without seizures.

Risk of seizure relapse after AED discontinuation **higher** if: (a) patient required more than one AED to control seizures; (b) seizure control difficult to establish; (c) patient had history of generalized tonic-clonic seizures; (d) EEG significantly abnormal when drug withdrawal was considered.

Lower risk with: (a) longer seizure-free intervals before drug withdrawal; (b) few seizures before remission;

(c) monotherapy; (d) normal EEG and examination; (e) no difficulty establishing seizure control.

SURGICAL TREATMENT

Indicated when seizures refractory to optimal medical management (usually, two trials of high-dose monotherapy using two appropriate drugs and one trial of combination therapy).

RESECTION PROCEDURES

Appropriate if: (a) seizures begin in identifiable and restricted cortical area; (b) surgical excision encompasses all or most of epileptogenic tissue; (c) resection will not impair neurologic function. Include anterior temporal resection, lesion resection.

CORPUS CALLOSOTOMY

Indicated for uncontrolled atonic or tonic seizures without identifiable focus suitable for resection. Palliative, not curative. Up to 80% effective for generalized seizures.

HEMISPHERECTOMY

Indicated when epileptogenic lesion involves most or all of one hemisphere. Considered only in children with unilateral structural lesion that has already resulted in hemiplegia, hemisensory loss, hemianopia.

PREOPERATIVE EVALUATION

Objective: to demonstrate that all seizures originate in limited cortical area that can be removed safely. May include video-EEG monitoring, MRI, PET, ictal SPECT, neuropsychologic testing, intracarotid injection of amobarbital (Wada test) to determine hemisphere dominant for speech, intracranial electrode placement.

VAGAL NERVE STIMULATION

Palliative. About 30% to 35% of patients have ≥50% reduction in seizure frequency.

STATUS EPILEPTICUS

A medical emergency. Seizure lasting >10 minutes, or 2 or more seizures in close succession without intervening recovery of consciousness.

Convulsive: clear outward motor manifestations; the most life-threatening pattern.

Nonconvulsive: "twilight" confusion caused by continuing generalized absence seizures or CPS.

No prior history of epilepsy in >50% of cases. First manifestation of epilepsy in about 10% of patients with epilepsy. Acute cause or precipitating factor identified in 66%.

CONVULSIVE STATUS EPILEPTICUS

Causes: stroke, drug change, noncompliance, intake of alcohol or other drugs, CNS infection, hypoxia, metabolic disorders, tumor, trauma, fever, infection, congenital malformation of brain. Mortality 2% to 3% in children, 7% to 10% in adults.

EEG monitoring necessary: electrographic ictal discharges continue in 20% of patients after motor activity stops completely.

Goals of treatment: eliminate all seizure activity; identify and treat underlying medical or neurologic disorder (Table 141.6).

NONCONVULSIVE STATUS EPILEPTICUS

Patients most often middle-aged or elderly, usually no history of seizures. Manifestations: alert; bizarre behavior; change in affect; memory loss; hallucinations; paranoia; catatonia. Underlying seizures: focal or generalized.

Diagnosis: ictal patterns in EEG while patient symptomatic. Most common pattern: continuous or nearly continuous 1- to 2.5-Hz generalized spike-wave ("atypical spike-wave") activity. Diagnosis confirmed by EEG and clinical response to intravenous diazepam or lorazepam.

TABLE 141.6

PROTOCOL AND TIMETABLE FOR TREATING STATUS
EPILEPTICUS IN ADULTS AT THE NEUROLOGICAL
INSTITUTE OF NEW YORK, COLUMBIA UNIVERSITY
MEDICAL CENTER

Time (min)	Action
0–5	Diagnose; give O_2; ABCs; obtain IV access; begin ECG monitoring; draw blood for chem-7, Mg, Ca, CBC count, AED levels, ABG; toxicology screen
6–10	Thiamine 100 mg IV; 50 mL of D50 IV unless adequate glucose level known Lorazepam 4 mg IV over 2 min; repeat once in 8–10 min p.r.n. *Or* Diazepam 10 mg IV over 2 min; repeat once in 3–5 min p.r.n.
10–20	If status persists or if it was stopped with diazepam immediately begin fosphenytoin 20 mg/kg IV at 150 mg/min, with blood pressure and ECG monitoring
20–30	If status persists, give additional 5 mg/kg fosphenytoin two times (total 30 mg/kg)
30+	If status persists, intubate and give one of the following (in order of our preference), preferably with EEG monitoring: Phenobarbital 20 mg/kg IV at 50–100 mg/min. Additional 5-mg/kg boluses can be given as needed; *or* Midazolam continuous infusion, 0.2 mg/kg slow bolus, then 0.1–2.0 mg/kg/h; *or* Propofol continuous infusion, 1–5 mg/kg bolus over 5 min, then 2–4 mg/kg/h

ABCs, airway, blood pressure, cardiac function; ABG, arterial
blood gas; AED, antiepileptic drug; CBC; complete blood cell;
D50, 50% dextrose in water; IV, intravenous; p.r.n., as needed.
From Dodson et al. (1993), Lowenstein and Alldredge (1998),
and Treiman et al. (1998).

GENE DEFECTS IN EPILEPSY

Genes identified for increasingly long list of epilepsy syndromes, regularly updated in online databases (e.g., OMIM).

TABLE 141.7	
FACTORS THAT LOWER THE SEIZURE THRESHOLD	
Common	**Occasional**
Sleep deprivation	Barbiturate withdrawal
Alcohol withdrawal	Hyperventilation
Stress	Flashing lights
Dehydration	Diet and missed meals
Drugs and drug interactions	Specific "reflex" triggers
Systemic infection	
Trauma	
Malnutrition	

PSYCHOSOCIAL AND PSYCHIATRIC ISSUES

Common factors that increase likelihood of seizure in Table 141.7. Legal proscription (e.g., on driving); varies by state and country.

Most common cause of breakthrough seizures: medication noncompliance.

Postictal psychosis: 24–72 hours after lucid interval following prolonged seizure or cluster of seizures. Delusions, paranoia common. Self-limited, usually to a few days.
Treatment: antipsychotic medications.

CHAPTER 142 ■ FEBRILE SEIZURES

Generalized seizures with febrile illness (not meningitis or encephalitis). Even if recurrent, do not warrant designation of epilepsy. Usually occur between ages 3 months and 5 years.

About 2% to 5% of all children in United States and Europe have at least one febrile seizure before age 5 years. Increased risk of syndrome in siblings and offspring of affected probands.

CLINICAL FEATURES

Most seizures occur during first 24 hours of febrile illness. Subdivided into simple and complex types:

Simple: brief, isolated, no focal manifestations (80 to 90%).

Complex: focal onset, longer than 15 minutes, or recurrent within 24 hours.

PROGNOSIS AND TREATMENT

Probability of recurrence about 33%. Risk factors for recurrence: age <1 year; family history of febrile seizures; complex type.

Risk of later epilepsy: 2% to 3% for simple type (similar to general population); 10% to 13% if complex type, family history of afebrile seizures, or neurologic abnormality before first febrile seizure. Up to 49% if all 3 features of complex febrile seizures present (see above).

Chronic prophylactic treatment with anticonvulsant medications not indicated. For acute attack: rectal diazepam, parental reassurance.

CHAPTER 143 ■ TRANSIENT GLOBAL AMNESIA

Sudden inability to form new memory traces (anterograde amnesia) plus retrograde memory loss for preceding days or weeks. Accompanied by bewilderment, anxiety, repeated questions (e.g., "Where am I?"). Immediate registration of events intact; self-identification preserved. No other abnormality on examination.

Duration minutes to hours. Patients usually middle-aged or elderly. Recurrent attacks occur in <25%; >3 attacks in <3%; no clear association with seizure disorders, stroke, migraine but all implicated in some case-control studies.

Cause unknown. No drug treatment required; reassure family.

CHAPTER 144 ■ MÉNIÈRE SYNDROME

Attacks of vertigo lasting hours to days. Hearing loss, tinnitus occur within attacks early in course; permanent later. Sense of fullness in affected ear often accompanies attacks.

Prevalence 1:500. Women may be more affected. Vertigo absent in 10%.

ETIOLOGY AND PATHOGENESIS

Due to pressure surges in endolymphatic compartment of inner ear (*endolymphatic hydrops*).

May be idiopathic (Ménière disease) or secondary to specific causes (Ménière syndrome): post-traumatic (inner ear concussion, temporal bone fracture), endolymphatic fistula, postinfectious or inflammatory (labyrinthitis, meningitis, Lyme disease, otosyphilis), congenital (anatomic abnormality of inner ear), tumor (e.g., vestibular Schwannoma), vertebrobasilar insufficiency, autoimmune.

SYMPTOMS AND SIGNS

Onset unilateral in 95%. If bilateral: consider autoimmune cause.

Tinnitus: roaring, machinery-like; fluctuating. Vertigo: nausea, vomiting, sweating, pallor often present, due to peripheral origin.

Examination: during attack, horizontal nystagmus beating toward affected ear.

Course: attacks typically become less frequent and less severe, with or without medical management. Hearing loss progressive.

INVESTIGATIONS

Audiometry: normal early; then low-frequency loss; then loss at all frequencies.

Electronystagmography: normal early; then vestibular weakness in affected ear.

MRI: for vestibular Schwannoma, stroke, demyelination.

Bilateral symptoms: blood tests for autoimmune inner ear disease, infections (including CBC, ESR, rheumatoid factor, 68-kilodalton protein, ANA, anti-double-stranded DNA, Lyme titer, fluorescent treponemal antigen).

Onset after age 60: neck Doppler examinations for cerebrovascular disease.

TREATMENT

Medical treatment decreases attack frequency, severity; minimizes permanent hearing loss or disequilibrium. Surgery in 5%.

Medical Therapy

Low-sodium diet (1500 mg/day); diuretic therapy (e.g., hydrochlorothiazide 37.5 mg/triamterene 25 mg once daily). Monitor electrolytes, renal function.

During attack: anticholinergic drugs (glycopyrrolate 2 mg orally twice per day), vestibular suppressants, (meclizine 12.5, 25, or 50 mg orally up to three times daily; diazepam 5 mg orally three times daily).

Intractable vertigo with nausea and vomiting: intravenous hydration; promethazine 75 mg intramuscularly or droperidol 0.625 mg intravenously.

Surgical Therapy
Vestibular neurectomy successful in >90%. Labyrinthectomy only if hearing already permanently lost. Endolymphatic shunt rarely performed due to hearing loss.

Other Methods of Treatment
Middle ear perfusion with gentamicin (preferentially destroys vestibular hair cells): significant incidence of sensorineural hearing loss.

Meniett device: micropressure pulses to inner ear. Effectiveness unknown.

Intramuscular streptomycin: end-stage patients with bilateral disease, vertigo, no hearing. Eradicates remaining vestibular function.

CHAPTER 145 ■ SLEEP DISORDERS

SLEEP PHYSIOLOGY

Sleep cycle: sequence of stages 1, 2, 3, 4, followed by the reverse (4, 3, 2), followed by rapid eye movement (REM) period. Typical cycle duration 80 to 120 minutes. Normal sleep pattern: 3 to 5 repetitions of sleep cycle.

Excessive daytime sleepiness may result from insufficient quantity of sleep or poor sleep quality from sleep disorder.

DIAGNOSTIC PROCEDURES

Clinical polysomnography: simultaneous recording of sleep and physiologic variables (EEG, electrooculogram, EMG, ECG, respiratory effort, oxygen saturation).

Multiple sleep latency test: useful for evaluation of daytime sleepiness (time taken to fall asleep, normal >10 mins); also to detect sleep-onset REM (narcolepsy, REM sleep rebound).

SELECTED DISORDERS OF SLEEP

DISORDERS WITH INSOMNIA

Transient insomnia: duration <3 weeks; usually situational.

Psychophysiologic insomnia: multiple contributing factors: initiating stressor, maladaptive habits perpetuate problem. Treatment: behavioral therapy, sleep hygiene (Table 145.1).

Persistent, chronic insomnia: many underlying causes, including medical and psychiatric diorders. Treatment directed at cause.

Insomnia may be a complaint in patients with sleep disruption due to obstructive sleep apnea, narcolepsy, restless legs syndrome (see below).

SLEEP-RELATED RESPIRATORY DISORDERS

Obstructive Sleep Apnea (OSA) Syndrome

Repeated apneas due to collapse, obstruction of upper airway. Predominantly ages 30 to 50. M:F ratio 2.5:1. Risk factors:

TABLE 145.1

PRINCIPLES OF SLEEP HYGIENE

Regulate sleep-wake cycle
Wake regularly at a fixed time
Regulate the amount of sleep obtained each night
Exercise daily and regularly but not in the late evening
Sleep in a quiet environment
Avoid caffeinated beverages
Avoid alcohol within 3 hours of bedtime
Avoid hypnotic drugs
Do something relaxing before bedtime

habitual snoring, obesity, upper airway abnormalities. In children, often associated with adenotonsillar hypertrophy.

Symptoms: snoring, witnessed apneas, excessive daytime sleepiness, insomnia, impairment of daytime performance, headache, irritability, depression.

Polysomnography differentiates OSA from central sleep apnea syndrome (much less common).

Treatment: nasal continuous positive airway pressure.

Alveolar Hypoventilation Syndrome
Failure to adequately ventilate, especially during REM sleep. Idiopathic or with other disorders, including respiratory muscle weakness, brainstem dysfunction, extreme obesity.

RESTLESS LEGS SYNDROME (RLS); PERIODIC LIMB MOVEMENT DISORDER (PLMD)

RLS: irresistible urge to move legs, especially sitting or supine. Discomfort deep inside leg relieved by walking.
PLMS (periodic limb movements in sleep): stereotyped periodic movements of one or both legs and feet. Often with RLS.

Movements lead to disturbed sleep, sometimes daytime drowsiness.

Treatment: start with dopamine agonist (ropinirole, pramipexole, pergolide). Other medications: levodopa + carbidopa; opiates for severe cases.

NARCOLEPSY

Characterized by: (a) excessive daytime sleepiness, (b) cataplexy, (c) sleep paralysis, (d) hypnagogic hallucinations. Features represent intrusion of REM sleep into wakefulness. Prevalence 20 to 100 per 100,000 individuals in North America and Europe. Onset age: 12 to 30 years.

Cataplexy: few seconds of paralysis or weakness of voluntary muscles without change in consciousness. Precipitated by strong emotions. Pathognomonic of narcolepsy.
Sleep paralysis: global paralysis of voluntary muscles on falling asleep or waking.

Hypnagogic hallucinations: vivid dream-like images at sleep onset and arousal.

Treatment: stimulant drugs (modafinil, methylphenidate, amphetamines). Cataplexy: tricyclic compounds, selective serotonin reuptake inhibitors.

DISORDERS OF SLEEP-WAKE SCHEDULE

Transient: acute phase-shift syndromes (e.g., jet lag, sleep deprivation). Persistent: medical condition, occupational schedule (e.g., shift worker).

Specific sleep disorders: delayed-sleep-phase syndrome (sleeping late, waking late), advanced-sleep-phase syndrome (sleeping early, waking early), non–24-hour sleep-wake disorder, irregular sleep-wake pattern.

PARASOMNIAS

Disorders of arousal, partial arousal, sleep stage transition with undesirable sleep behaviors that are manifestations of CNS activation.

Sleep-walking, sleep terrors, confusional arousals: more common in children, occur during deeper stages of non-REM sleep. Confusion during and following arousal; amnesia for episode. Treatment: small nightly doses of benzodiazepine.

REM sleep behavior disorder: intermittent loss of REM sleep atonia accompanied by motor activity consistent with dream enactment. Tend to occur in later half of the night. More common in older men; may be precede degenerative neurologic disorder, especially Parkinson disease, multisystem atrophy, Lewy body dementia. Injury to self or bed partner a complication. Treatment: small doses of clonazepam at bedtime.

SLEEP DISORDERS ASSOCIATED WITH NEUROLOGIC DISORDERS

Examples: dementia, parkinsonism, fatal familial insomnia (Chapter 34).

Systemic Diseases and General Medicine

CHAPTER 146 ▪ ENDOCRINE DISEASES

PITUITARY

HYPOPITUITARISM

Common causes: tumors, infection, vascular lesions, trauma. Lesion in pituitary gland, stalk, or hypothalamus.

Evaluation: thyroid function tests, prolactin level, assess adrenal reserve (corticotropin [ACTH] stimulation for cortisol responses). Pituitary stimulation tests sometimes useful.

Pituitary Tumors

Most common cause of neurologic symptoms of hypopituitarism. Headache, visual loss, cavernous sinus syndromes with large tumors.

Symptoms only from secreted hormone for microadenomas (<10 mm) or general pituitary dysfunction for macroadenomas (>10 mm).

Prolactinoma: most common cause of clinically manifest hyperprolactinemia. Women: amenorrhea, galactorrhea. Men: impotence, infertility, galactorrhea (rare). Prolactin >200 ng/mL diagnostic of prolactinoma.

Treatment: dopaminergic agonists (e.g., bromocriptine, cabergoline), trans-sphenoidal adenomectomy, radiotherapy.

Other Causes of Hypopituitarism

Pituitary apoplexy: hemorrhage into pituitary tumor. Acute headache, meningismus, visual loss, ocular palsies, altered level of consciousness.

Sheehan syndrome: postpartum necrosis of pituitary. Obtundation, hypotension, tachycardia, hypoglycemia, amenorrhea, failure to lactate. Acute or chronic.

EXCESSIVE GROWTH HORMONE AND ACROMEGALY

Acromegaly: slowly progressive, excessive growth of skeleton, soft tissues. Coarse facial features, large hands and feet; gigantism if onset at young age. Usually growth hormone (GH)–secreting pituitary tumor.

Diagnosis: sustained elevation of GH, cannot be suppressed by physiologic stimuli (e.g., glucose); MRI shows tumor.

Treatment: somatostatin analogues, surgical removal.

EXCESSIVE ADRENOCORTICOTROPIC HORMONE

Cushing disease: hypersecretion of ACTH by pituitary tumor. Plethoric round face, centripetal obesity, abdominal striae, hypertension, diabetes mellitus, amenorrhea, hirsutism, acne, osteoporosis. Mental status changes, myopathy sometimes.

Laboratory data: elevated urinary free cortisol levels; cortisol secretion suppressed by dexamethasone.

Treatment: trans-sphenoidal pituitary adenomectomy.

DIABETES INSIPIDUS (DI)

Excessive excretion of urine (polyuria), abnormally large fluid intake (polydipsia) from diminished antidiuretic hormone (vasopressin) in posterior pituitary. Hypothalamic dysfunction primary (idiopathic) or secondary (tumor, aneurysm, xanthomatosis, sarcoid, trauma, infections, stroke).

Laboratory data: low urine specific gravity; decreased urine output after vasopressin injection (vs. nephrogenic DI); urine-specific gravity increases with water restriction (vs. psychogenic polydipsia).

Treatment: tumor resection; desmopressin (1-desamino-8-d-arginine vasopressin, DDAVP).

EXCESSIVE SECRETION OF ANTIDIURETIC HORMONE (ADH)

Syndrome of inappropriate ADH secretion (SIADH). Hypothalamo-hypophyseal pathology (head injury, infection, tumor). Also with remote lung carcinoma, other lung disease, drugs (e.g., carbamazepine).

Clinical features: headache, confusion, somnolence, coma, seizures, transient focal neurologic signs, abnormal EEG.

Laboratory data: hyponatremia, hypotonic body fluids, excessive urinary excretion of sodium despite hyponatremia, improves with fluid restriction.

Treatment: restrict fluids; furosemide diuresis; replace electrolytes. Avoid rapid correction hyponatremia; risk of central pontine demyelination.

THYROID

HYPOTHYROIDISM

Cretinism (thyroid deficiency in utero or congenital): delayed physical and mental development, thick subcutaneous tissue, hoarse cry, large tongue, widely spaced eyes, pot-belly, umbilical hernia. Neurologic signs: mental retardation, proximal pyramidal and extrapyramidal signs, strabismus, deafness, primitive reflexes. Thyroid hormone replacement within first two weeks of life may result in nearly complete recovery restoration of normal physical and mental function.

Adult myxedema: lethargy, weakness, slow speech, nonpitting edema, coarse pale skin, dry brittle hair, thick lips, macroglossia, sensitivity to cold. Neurologic complications: headache, peripheral neuropathy, nerves, changes in cognition, level of consciousness. Specific signs: slow relaxation of tendon reflexes, myopathic weakness, cerebellar ataxia, lethargy, delirium, psychosis. Euthyroid encephalopathy with Hashimoto thyroiditis.

Laboratory data: low circulating T4 and T3, high thyrotropin (TSH), low radioiodine uptake by thyroid; high CSF protein.

Treatment: increasing doses oral levothyroxine; intravenous for myxedema coma.

Subacute encephalopathy (Hashimoto encephalopathy): see Chapter 158.

HYPERTHYROIDISM

Increased metabolic rate, abnormal cardiovascular and autonomic functions, tremor, myopathy, mental symptoms; ocular signs (infrequent blinking, lid lag, impaired convergence).

Graves ophthalmopathy: eyelid retraction in 75%; edema, hypertrophy, infiltration, fibrosis extraocular muscles, ophthalmoparesis. Treatment controversial. Prednisone may help.

Limb myopathy common; weakness of pelvic girdle muscles. Tendon reflexes normal or hyperactive. Improves with treatment of hyperthyroidism.

Other associations: periodic paralysis, MG.

PARATHYROID

HYPOPARATHYROIDISM; PSEUDOHYPOPARATHYROIDISM

Low serum calcium levels, manifest by tetany. Causes: thyroidectomy with parathyroid injury; idiopathic autoimmune syndrome.

Pseudohypoparathyroidism: ineffective action of parathyroid hormone at cellular receptors; abnormal skeletal growth.

Common clinical features: mental deficiency, tetany, seizures, cataracts, scaly skin, alopecia, atrophic finger nails. Other findings: intracranial calcifications, increased intracranial pressure, ECG changes.

Tetany: lower threshold of electrical excitability of nerve; carpopedal spasm, facial muscles contract after tapping facial nerve in front of ear (Chvostek sign), carpal spasm on inflating blood pressure cuff above systolic pressure (Trousseau sign).

Treatment: vitamin D, calcium supplements.

HYPERPARATHYROIDISM

Most common cause: parathyroid gland adenoma.

Clinical features: hypercalcemia with renal lithiasis, osteitis, peptic ulcer. Neurologic symptoms: proximal limb weakness, memory loss, irritability, depression.

PANCREAS

HYPOGLYCEMIA

Causes: insulin overdose, pancreatic hyperinsulinism, impaired liver function, pathology in pituitary or adrenal, metabolic disease in infants.

Neurologic symptoms: anxiety, tremulousness, diplopia, focal neurologic abnormalities, seizures, abnormal behavior, encephalopathy, coma. Paroxysmal if glucose level fluctuates.

Early treatment crucial: oral sugar (conscious patient), intravenous glucose (comatose patient).

DIABETES MELLITUS

Neurologic complications similar in types I and II. Neurologic disorder related to duration, severity of diabetes.

Peripheral neuropathy: mononeuropathy of peripheral or cranial nerves, sensorimotor polyneuropathy, trunk pain caused by neuropathy of cutaneous terminals; autonomic neuropathy, radiculopathy; see also Chapter 106.

Mononeuropathy, radiculopathy: rapid onset, painful; recovery. Oculomotor (sparing pupil), abducens nerves.

Polyneuropathy: numbness, burning common; symmetric. CSF protein high.

Autonomic neuropathy: arrhythmia, orthostatic hypotension, nausea, diarrhea, bladder dysfunction, erectile-ejaculatory failure.

Entrapment neuropathy: median, ulnar, peroneal.

CNS complications: stroke, hyperglycemic coma, hypoglycemia.

ADRENAL

HYPOADRENALISM

Causes: idiopathic adrenal atrophy; tuberculosis, neoplasms, amyloidosis, hemochromatosis, fungal or HIV infection, autoimmunity, adrenoleukodystrophy.

Chronic adrenocortical insufficiency (Addison disease): weight loss, skin pigmentation, hypotension, behavioral change, cognitive change, hypoglycemia.

Treatment: glucocorticoids; replace mineralocorticoids with sodium.

HYPERADRENALISM

Cushing syndrome from hyperfunction of adrenal cortex, administration of corticosteroids. Symptoms as in Cushing disease (see above). Memory problems, myopathy most common neurologic symptoms.

PRIMARY HYPERALDOSTERONISM

Sometimes from tumor of adrenal cortex. Recurrent attacks of muscular weakness, tetany, polyuria, hypertension, electrolyte imbalance.

GONADS

Fluctuating gonadal secretion (menses, pregnancy) linked to migraine, epilepsy (see also Chapter 141). Oral contraceptive use increases risk of stroke, especially with cigarette smoking and age >35.

Pregnancy also associated with chorea gravidarum, enlargement of meningioma.

CHAPTER 147 ■ HEMATOLOGIC AND RELATED DISEASES

ERYTHROCYTE DISORDERS

SICKLE-CELL DISEASE

Neurologic disorders with hemoglobin (Hb)-SS, Hb-SC genotypes, or sickle-β-thalassemia syndromes.

Stroke

7% to 15% of homozygous children (250 to 400 times higher risk for stroke than in general population). Cumulative risk of stroke by age 45 about 24% for SS patients, 10% for SC patients. Transcranial Doppler ultrasonography identifies children at risk for stroke.

Approximately 60% ischemic, 40% hemorrhagic. Thrombosis of large and small arteries; less common, dural sinus thrombosis. Often watershed distribution. Subarachnoid hemorrhage more common in children; intraparenchymal in adults.

Risk factors include: prior TIA, low hemoglobin content, frequent acute chest syndrome episodes or one within last two weeks, high systolic blood pressure, family history. Recurrent strokes more frequently in younger patients.

Incidence of stroke recurrence lower if patients given transfusions regularly: 10% vs. 46% to 90% within 3 years of first stroke. Goal of transfusion: Hb-S concentration <30% of total Hb. Repeated thrombosis in ~65% untreated children.

Cerebrovascular complications less common in sickle Hb-C disease. Risk in sickle cell trait same as in general population.

Other Manifestations

Seizures: 6% to 12% from stroke, meningitis, dehydration, medications (e.g., meperidine).

Headache (28%); myelopathy; acute mononeuropathy; meningitis.

THALASSEMIA

Transient dizziness, blurred vision (20%); headache (13%); seizures (13%); peripheral neuropathy (mainly motor; 20%); stroke; spinal cord, cauda equina, optic nerve compression (extramedullary hematopoiesis).

POLYCYTHEMIA

Risk of cerebral infarction increased by hyperviscosity (accelerated atherosclerosis, thrombosis); reduced by aspirin. Peripheral neuropathy (mainly sensory axonal) in 50%.

Headache, dizziness, tinnitus, visual disturbances, cognitive impairment also seen. Improve with lowering red blood cell count by phlebotomy, chemotherapy.

PLATELET DISORDERS

ESSENTIAL THROMBOCYTOSIS (THROMBOCYTHEMIA)

Headache, paresthesias, TIAs, cerebral infarction, seizures. Bleeding complications seen paradoxically at very high platelet counts ($>1,500,000/\mu$L).

Treatment: lower platelet count. (hydroxyurea, platelet pheresis).

THROMBOTIC THROMBOCYTOPENIC PURPURA

Neurologic symptoms in 70%: hemiparesis (25%), encephalopathy (50%). Symptoms transient, fluctuating, usually <48 hours. MRI may show reversible posterior leukoencephalopathy.

Treatment: plasma exchange with fresh frozen plasma infusion.

HEPARIN-INDUCED THROMBOCYTOPENIA (HIT)

Incidence 2.5%. Thrombocytosis associated with 2% of HIT cases; thrombosis may precede thrombocytopenia.

Consider HIT in heparin-treated patients with cerebral ischemia, cerebral venous thrombosis, transient confusion, whether platelet count decreased.

BLOOD CELL DYSCRASIAS

LEUKEMIA

Acute myelogenous leukemia: CNS involvement uncommon early in course. Risk factors for CNS symptoms: high circulating blast counts, monocytic M4 subtype. Leptomeningeal, intracerebral lesions seen. LP deferred until peripheral blood clear of blast cells to avoid CNS seeding. Chloroma (granulocytic sarcoma) may compress cranial nerves, spinal cord.

Acute lymphocytic leukemia: CNS involved at time of diagnosis in 5% to 10%. Risk factors for CNS leukemia: high lymphocyte count, T-cell acute lymphoblastic leukemia phenotype, L3 (Burkitt) morphology. Leptomeningeal metastases: manifestations at all levels of CNS (cranial nerve signs, seizures, cognitive deficit, hydrocephalus).

Chronic leukemia rarely affects CNS.

Neurologic symptoms from therapy (hemorrhage due to thrombocytopenia, infection from low white blood cell counts), vessel occlusion, or vessel wall infiltration by white cells.

PLASMA CELL DYSCRASIAS

Monoclonal gammopathy of unknown significance (MUGUS): peripheral neuropathy common. Antibodies against myelin-associated glycoprotein in 50% (see Chapter 106).

Multiple myeloma: thoracic or lumbosacral radiculopathy from nerve compression by vertebral lesion or collapsed bone; intracranial plasmacytomas; leptomeningeal invasion. Spinal cord compression from extramedullary plasmacytoma in 5%; requires emergency high-dose steroids, radiotherapy.

Waldenström macroglobulinemia: peripheral neuropathy, often with antibodies to myelin-associated glycoprotein (MAG) antibodies, anti-GM1 ganglioside, asialo-GM1 ganglioside; leukoencephalopathy; hyperviscosity syndrome (headache, blurred vision, tinnitus, vertigo, ataxia). *Bing-Neel syndrome*: Waldenström disease with CNS infiltration, diffuse or focal manifestations (personality change, altered alertness, seizures, focal neurologic signs).

Treatment of neuropathy: immunosuppressive drugs, intravenous immunoglobulin therapy, plasmapheresis.

MYELOFIBROSIS

Extramedullary hematopoiesis may cause extradural spinal cord compression, cerebral compression by calvarial-based intracranial mass, or orbital lesions with exophthalmos.

DISORDERS OF COAGULATION

Hematologic disorders or coagulopathies cause stroke in 4% to 17% of young patients and 1% of all patients with ischemic stroke. Most prothrombotic disorders associated with venous thrombosis at unusual sites.

ANTITHROMBIN (AT) DEFICIENCY

AT required for anticoagulant action of heparin. Deficiency inherited or acquired. Prevalence 1:2,000 to 1:5,000. Autosomal dominant. Cerebral thrombosis more commonly venous than arterial. Anticoagulation therapy ineffective.

PROTEIN S DEFICIENCY

Protein S cofactor for anticoagulant activity of activated protein C. Deficiency acquired or congenital (autosomal dominant). Thrombosis venous or arterial. Free level measurement sensitive, specific; test in absence of anticoagulation. Anticoagulation therapy used in patients with protein S deficiency and stroke.

PROTEIN C DEFICIENCY

Protein C, once activated, inhibits coagulation by inactivating factors Va, VIIIa. Deficiency inherited or acquired. Autosomal dominant. Deficiency in 6% to 8% of patients with stroke before age 40. Risk (often in association with second risk factor) for cerebral venous thrombosis, venous infarction. Anticoagulation with heparin or warfarin only for clinical thrombosis.

FACTOR V LEIDEN MUTATION

Most common known genetic risk factor for thrombosis. Factor Va resistance to degradation by activated protein C, predisposing to venous thrombosis (including brain).

AUTOANTIBODIES

Antiphospholipid antibodies (including lupus anticoagulant, anticardiolipin antibodies): most common acquired defect with thrombosis. Associated with ischemic stroke, often recurrent, particularly in young adults. Cerebral venous sinus thrombosis, dementia, chorea also seen.

PAROXYSMAL NOCTURNAL HEMOGLOBINURIA

Patients prone to hepatic vein and sagittal sinus thrombosis.

HEMOPHILIA

Intracranial hemorrhage in 3%, with 34% mortality.

CEREBROVASCULAR COMPLICATIONS OF CANCER

Found in 15% of patients with systemic malignancy at autopsy.
Nonbacterial thrombotic endocarditis ("marantic endocarditis"): most common cause of cerebral infarction in patients with systemic malignancy. Tumors usually lymphomas, mucin-producing adenocarcinomas. Role of anticoagulation controversial. Tumor emboli rarely cause cerebral infarction.

Coagulation disorders: due to tumor, chemotherapy, or radiotherapy, leading to spontaneous intraparenchymal or subarachnoid hemorrhage.

Hemorrhage into tumor: metastases of some tumors (melanoma, lung carcinoma, choriocarcinoma, hypernephroma), glioma.

Disseminated intravascular coagulation: acute (intracranial hemorrhage) or chronic (diffuse encephalopathy).

Superior sagittal sinus thrombosis: spontaneous or direct spread of tumor to dura.

Radiation-induced vasculopathy of carotid artery: may develop years after local radiation therapy.

OTHER DISORDERS

IDIOPATHIC HYPEREOSINOPHILIC SYNDROME

CNS affected in 15% of cases as encephalopathy, TIA, embolic infarction, or peripheral neuropathy.

LANGERHANS CELL HISTIOCYTOSIS (HISTIOCYTOSIS X)

Onset most commonly between one and four years of age, up to age 60. Bone, skin, liver, spleen, lymph nodes, bone marrow, lungs, orbits, oral cavity and teeth, ears, CNS may be involved.

CNS symptoms due to: dura compression by skull lesions; hypothalamic-pituitary involvement (diabetes insipidus); cranial nerve compression; intracerebral mass lesion.

Treatment: surgery, radiation therapy, chemotherapy, steroids.

NEUROLYMPHOMATOSIS

Lymphomatous infiltration of peripheral nerves. Mostly non-Hodgkin lymphoma with progressive sensorimotor peripheral neuropathy. Cranial neuropathy, bowel or bladder incontinence, gait ataxia, mental change also found. CSF: elevated protein, lymphocytic CSF pleocytosis in majority; abnormal cytology in 33%.

CHÉDIAK-HIGASHI SYNDROME

Partial oculocutaneous albinism, immunologic defects, bleeding diathesis, progressive neurologic dysfunction. Autosomal-recessive inheritance. Neurologic syndromes include spinocerebellar disorder, light-induced nystagmus, peripheral neuropathy.

CHAPTER 148 ■ HEPATIC DISEASE

Hepatic coma: acute hepatic necrosis; fulminant; delirium, convulsions, coma, decerebrate rigidity. Often fatal. Serum ammonia high.

Hepatic encephalopathy: usually with chronic liver disease. Failure of liver to detoxify blood from gastrointestinal system. Episodic ataxia, tremor, dysarthria, sensorial clouding, asterixis. May have progressive syndrome of dementia, ataxia, dysarthria, tremor, choreoathetosis (acquired chronic hepatocerebral degeneration). Convulsions rare in hepatic encephalopathy (vs. uremic encephalopathy).

Laboratory data: high serum ammonia, CSF glutamine content high.

Pathophysiology: increased sensitivity to inhibitory neurotransmitters such as gamma amino butyric acid (GABA) may underlie encephalopathy. Ammonia likely not responsible.

Differential diagnosis: acute ethanol intoxication, delirium tremens, Wernicke encephalopathy, Korsakoff syndrome, drug intoxication, other metabolic disorders (uremia, hyponatremia), consequences of head injury (e.g., subdural hematoma), Wilson disease.

Treatment: antibiotics (especially neomycin or metronidazole) decrease ammonia-producing intestinal organisms. Lactulose also beneficial.

Prognosis: recovery expected in mild cases. Cerebral edema in about 75%.

NEUROLOGIC COMPLICATIONS OF LIVER TRANSPLANTATION

Arise in 8% to 47% of liver transplant recipients. Range from mild encephalopathy to akinetic mutism or coma. Psychiatric syndromes: from mild anxiety or depression to hallucinatory psychosis. Other syndromes: seizures, myoclonus, tremor, cortical blindness, brachial plexopathy, peripheral neuropathy. Full recovery expected.

Graft-versus-host reactions: polyneuropathy, myasthenia gravis, polymyositis.

COMPLICATIONS OF IMMUNOSUPPRESSIVE THERAPY

Reversible posterior leukoencephalopathy (cyclosporine, tacrolimus): headache, visual disturbance, encephalopathy, seizures. Blood pressure usually elevated. MRI: occipital, parietal white matter changes. Complete resolution usually follows treatment of hypertension, reduction of dosage of immunosuppressive medication.

Other: central pontine myelinolysis (cyclosporine); seizures (cyclosporine, OKT3); aseptic meningitis (OKT3); opportunistic infections; demyelinating peripheral neuropathy (tacrolimus).

CHAPTER 149 ■ CEREBRAL COMPLICATIONS OF CARDIAC SURGERY

Neurologic complications (frequency about 1%): unresponsiveness after surgery, signs of cerebral infarction on awakening, stroke after surgery, dementia without focal signs. Transient encephalopathy after 3% to 12% of operations. Severe cognitive disability in 2% of patients 6 months after surgery.

Pathogenesis possibilities: atheromatous embolism, perioperative hypotension, air embolism. Important factors: oxygenator, cardiopulmonary bypass circuit, body temperature, arterial blood gases; arterial line filters.

Other risk factors for cerebral complications: infective endocarditis, prior cardiac operations, impaired left ventricular function, low cardiac output, sepsis, toxemia, impaired hemostasis.

INTERVENTIONAL CARDIAC PROCEDURES

Stroke or TIA after cardiac catheterization (0.1% to 1% of procedures), coronary angioplasty (0.2%), valvuloplasty (11% for aortic valve), coronary artery bypass graft (CABG; 1% to 5%). History of stroke increases likelihood of second stroke with CABG. Persistent postoperative coma in 1% of CABG patients.

CARDIAC TRANSPLANTATION

Perioperative period: stroke (up to 9%), reversible encephalopathy (10%), seizures, vascular headache.

Later: neurologic complications of immunosuppressive regimen (opportunistic infections, drug toxicity; see Chapter 148). Increased incidence of primary CNS lymphoma.

CAROTID STENOSIS AND CABG

Presence of carotid stenosis predicts worse outcome after cardiac surgery. Carotid endarterectomy prior to heart surgery, proposed to reduce stroke risk, does not offer proven benefit.

CHAPTER 150 ■ BONE DISEASE

OSTEITIS DEFORMANS (PAGET DISEASE)

Chronic disease of adult skeleton; bowing and irregular flattening of bones.

Any or all skeletal bones may be affected; tibia, skull, pelvis most frequent sites. Except for skeletal deformities and pain, disability only when skull or spine affected.

Pathology: imbalance between formation and resorption of bone.

Diagnosed at autopsy in 3% of patients older than 40. Onset age 30 to 70.

Symptoms and signs: result from (a) arteriosclerosis (a common accompaniment of Paget disease); (b) pressure on CNS or nerve roots by bony overgrowth. Most common symptoms: deafness (pressure on auditory nerves), unilateral facial palsy, monocular visual loss, spinal cord compression.

Laboratory data: normal serum calcium, increased serum alkaline phosphatase. Skull radiograph: areas of increased bone density with loss of normal architecture, mingled with areas of decreased bone density ("cotton wool" appearance).

Course: decades.

Treatment: calcitonin inhibits osteolytic process. Alternative: etidronate, pamidronate.

FIBROUS DYSPLASIA

Small areas of bony destruction or massive sclerotic overgrowth. Entire skull may be involved ("leontiasis ossea"), with exophthalmos, optic atrophy, cranial nerve palsies. Other symptoms: headache, convulsions, exophthalmos, optic atrophy, deafness. Onset: early adult years.

ACHONDROPLASIA

Most frequent skeletal dysplasia causing dwarfism. Neurologic symptoms: seizures, ataxia, paraplegia result from hydrocephalus, brainstem or spinal cord compression.

Treatment: shunting procedures for hydrocephalus; laminectomy for cord compression.

ANKYLOSING SPONDYLITIS

Inflammatory disorder of ligamentous insertions into bones. Spine becomes rigid. Cauda equina syndrome may appear late: symmetric pain, weakness, wasting, sensory loss in lumbosacral myotomes, with involvement of bladder and bowel.

ATLANTOAXIAL DISLOCATION

Subluxation of C1 on C2. Causes: trauma, congenital malformation; rheumatoid arthritis, Down syndrome. Risk of cervical myelopathy or medullary compression, sudden death. Surgical stabilization for symptomatic cases. Best treatment for asymptomatic cases uncertain.

CHAPTER 151 ■ RENAL DISEASE

Uremia: symptomatic renal failure.

UREMIC ENCEPHALOPATHY

Signs: dysarthria, unsteady gait, asterixis, tremor, multifocal myoclonus, obtundation. Day-to-day fluctuation.

Also: tetany, restless legs syndrome, meningismus (often with high CSF protein, pleocytosis). Seizures late manifestation. Renal failure alters drug clearance, protein-binding; follow free levels of anticonvulsant drugs.

Encephalopathy clears with hemodialysis.

UREMIC NEUROPATHY

Most common neurologic complication of chronic renal failure. Distal, symmetric, mixed sensorimotor neuropathy affects legs more than arms. Primarily axonal, secondary demyelination. Much more common in men than in women. Mononeuropathy may occur.

Variable rate of progression; may become stable or improve with hemodialysis; improves or disappears after renal transplantation.

DIALYSIS DYSEQUILIBRIUM SYNDROME

Headache, nausea, muscle cramps during or after hemodialysis. More rarely, obtundation, convulsions, or delirium. Syndrome self-limited, subsides in hours.

DIALYSIS DEMENTIA

Progressive, usually fatal encephalopathy in patients chronically dialyzed for >3 years.

Typical first symptoms: stammering, hesitant speech, speech arrest. EEG: bursts of high-voltage slowing in frontal leads. Progression: dysarthric, aphasic speech, dementia, delusions, myoclonic jerks, convulsions, asterixis.

Incidence greatly reduced, but not abolished, after removal of aluminum from dialysis water.

NEUROLOGIC COMPLICATIONS OF RENAL TRANSPLANTATION

Cerebral infarction (most common neurologic complication), primary CNS lymphoma, fungal brain abscess.
Complications of immunosuppressive therapy: see Chapter 148.

CHAPTER 152 ■ RESPIRATORY SUPPORT FOR NEUROLOGIC DISEASES

Most common neurologic indication for ICU: respiratory monitoring and support. Factors predisposing to pulmonary complications and respiratory failure: depressed consciousness; impaired airway due to depressed cough and gag reflexes; immobilization or paralysis; oropharyngeal and respiratory muscle weakness.

TABLE 152.1
PULMONARY FUNCTION TESTS IN NEUROMUSCULAR
RESPIRATORY FAILURE

	Normal	Criteria for intubation and weaning	Criteria for extubation
Vital capacity	40–70 mL/kg	15 mL/kg	25 mL/kg
Negative inspiratory pressure	>80 cm H_2O	20 cm H_2O	40 cm H_2O
Positive expiratory pressure	>140 cm H_2O	40 cm H_2O	50 cm H_2O

Adapted from Mayer SA. *Neurology* 1997;48[Suppl 5]:
S70–S75.

Respiratory failure: impaired gas exchange (Pao_2 <60 mm Hg or $Paco_2$ >50 mm Hg).

Premonitory signs: restlessness, insomnia, confusion, tachycardia, tachypnea, diaphoresis, asterixis, headache.

Causes of hypoxemia: low inspired oxygen concentration, alveolar hypoventilation, ventilation-perfusion mismatch, intracardiac right-to-left shunting, impaired diffusion.

Causes of hypercapnia: increased CO_2 production or inhalation, alveolar hypoventilation, ventilation-perfusion mismatching with "dead-space" ventilation.

Pulmonary function tests assess respiratory function in patients with neuromuscular respiratory failure (Table 152.1).

NEUROLOGIC DISEASES WITH PRIMARY RESPIRATORY DYSFUNCTION

BRAINSTEM DISEASE

Abnormal respiratory patterns from brainstem damage (see Chapter 4), often lead to endotracheal intubation.

Diagnosis of brain death includes formal **apnea testing:** pre-oxygenate patient with 100% oxygen, return Pco_2 to 40 mm Hg, turn off ventilator, allow Pco_2 to rise above 55 mm Hg.

Absence of chest wall or diaphragm movement by visual inspection confirms central apnea (if no neuromuscular impairment).

Other indications for endotracheal intubation in brainstem damage: altered consciousness, paralysis of pharyngeal and laryngeal muscles.

SPINAL CORD DISEASE

Lesion at C3 abolishes both diaphragmatic and intercostal muscle activity, leaving only accessory muscles. Result: hypercapnic respiratory failure.

Lesion at C5 to C6: transient decrease in vital capacity, with recovery months later.
High thoracic lesions: compromise intercostal and abdominal muscles.
Strychnine poisoning, tetanus: block spinal inhibitory interneurons; severe muscle spasms lead to apnea, respiratory failure.

MOTOR NEURON DISEASES

Respiratory complications: respiratory failure most common cause of death; usually late but may be first symptom of ALS; oropharyngeal weakness risk for aspiration pneumonia.

PERIPHERAL NEUROPATHIES

Respiratory failure typical of GBS, critical illness neuropathy (see Chapter 106).

DISORDERS OF NEUROMUSCULAR TRANSMISSION

Respiratory failure, aspiration pneumonitis complicate MG, botulism, neuromuscular blocking drugs. Severe dysarthria, dysphagia increase risk (see Chapters 121, 123).

MUSCLE DISEASE

Widespread skeletal muscle weakness: muscular dystrophies, myotonic disorders, inflammatory myopathies, periodic paralyses, metabolic myopathies (especially acid maltase deficiency), endocrine disorders (particularly thyroid disease), infectious myopathies, mitochondrial myopathies, toxic myopathies, myoglobinuria, electrolyte disorders (particularly hypophosphatemia, hypokalemia).

MANAGEMENT OF RESPIRATORY FAILURE IN NEUROLOGIC DISEASES

EXAMINATION

Signs of respiratory muscle fatigue: rapid, shallow breathing, impaired tidal volumes. Difficulty counting to 25 in single breath indicates severely curtailed ventilatory reserve.

Signs of severe oropharyngeal weakness: wet, gurgled voice; pooled oropharyngeal secretions; stridor; inability to sip 3 ounces of water without coughing.

MECHANICAL VENTILATION

Criteria for intubation and weaning listed in Tables 152.1, 152.2, and 152.3.

Volume-cycled positive pressure ventilation most common. Synchronous intermittent mandatory ventilation often adequate; ensures predetermined number of breaths per minute, adjusting timing of mechanical breaths without interfering with spontaneous breaths. Positive end-expiratory pressure maintained to prevent atelectasis.

TABLE 152.2

CRITERIA FOR INTUBATION AND MECHANICAL VENTILATION

Respiratory rate >35/min
Vital capacity <15 mL/kg
Peak inspiratory pressure <25 cm H_2O
Pao_2 <70 mm Hg with maximum oxygen by face mask
$Paco_2$ >50 mm Hg associated with acidosis (pH <7.35)
Severe oropharyngeal paresis with inability to protect the airway

These physiologic criteria are intended to serve only as guidelines; treatment decisions must be individualized. As a general rule, intubation in neurologic patients with impending respiratory failure should be performed *before* significant blood gas abnormalities develop.

TABLE 152.3

CRITERIA FOR WEANING FROM MECHANICAL
VENTILATION

Neurologic condition stable or improving
Vital capacity >15 mL/kg
Negative inspiratory pressure >20 mm Hg
PaO_2 >80 mm Hg with 40% oxygen
Patient free of fever, infection, fluid overload, anemia, gastric
distention, or other medical complications

Tracheostomy indicated if mechanical ventilation required
for >2 weeks; avoid pressure necrosis of tracheal mucosa by
pressure from balloon cuff of endotracheal tube.

Non-invasive continuous or bi-level positive-pressure ventilation (NPPV): helpful for transient, mild respiratory muscle
weakness.

CHAPTER 153 ■
PARANEOPLASTIC SYNDROMES

Definition: disorders caused by indirect damage from systemic
cancer to central or peripheral nervous system; not due to
metastasis.

Epidemiology: rare. Any cancer may be associated with paraneoplastic syndrome; most syndromes associated with specific cancer or particular group of cancer. Symptoms often
appear before cancer is manifest.

Pathogenesis: presumably autoimmune; antibodies against tumor cross-react with neural components. Tumor-secreted
hormones sometimes responsible.

CLINICAL SYNDROMES

Paraneoplastic cerebellar degeneration: ataxia of gait and
limbs, dysarthria, nystagmus, oscillopsia. Antibodies:

anti-Yo (ovarian cancer), anti-Hu (small-cell lung cancer [SCLC]), anti-Tr or anti-GluR1 (Hodgkin disease), anti-Ri (breast cancer). Pathology: Purkinje cell loss.

Sensory neuronopathy: painful paresthesias, CSF pleocytosis, loss of sensory evoked potentials; normal motor function. Anti-Hu antibody (SCLC).

Limbic encephalitis: personality and mood changes, delirium, dementia; CSF pleocytosis; enhancing signal sometimes present on MRI. Anti-Ma2 (testicular cancer), anti-Hu antibody (SCLC).

Brainstem encephalitis: cranial nerve, basal ganglia dysfunction; spreads to diffuse brain disease.

Opsoclonus-myoclonus: constant irregular rapid motion of eyes in random direction, myoclonus; mostly children with neuroblastoma.

Myelitis: spinal cord symptoms evolve in days to weeks. CSF: pleocytosis, high protein content, normal sugar, oligoclonal bands sometimes.

Motor neuron diseases: association with malignant tumor uncertain except for lymphoproliferative diseases.

Sensorimotor peripheral neuropathy: anti–myelin-associated glycoprotein (MAG) neuropathy; paraproteinemic polyneuropathy, paraneoplastic polyneuropathy. Cranial

---

TABLE 153.1

SELECTED ANTIBODIES ASSOCIATED WITH PARANEOPLASTIC SYNDROMES

Antibody	Syndrome	Associated tumors
Anti-amphiphysin	LEMS, sensory neuropathy, limbic encephalitis	Lung, breast, ovarian
Anti-Hu (ANNA-1)	Encephalomyelitis, sensory neuropathy	SCLC
Anti-Ri	Opsoclonus-myoclonus	Breast, SCLC
Anti-Ta	Limbic and brainstem encephalitis	Testicular
Anti-Tr	Subacute cerebellar disorder	Hodgkin disease
Anti-VGCC	LEMS	
Anti-Yo	Cerebellar disorder, brainstem encephalitis	Ovary, uterus, breast

ANNA-1, antineuronal nuclear antibody type 1; LEMS, Lambert-Eaton myasthenic syndrome; SCLC, small-cell lung carcinoma; VGCC, voltage-gated calcium channel of muscle.

symptoms usually absent. Slow course. May respond to immunotherapy (see Chapter 105).

Neuromuscular disorders: MG with thymoma (see Chapter 120). Other paraneoplastic conditions: Lambert-Eaton myasthenic syndrome (LEMS), neuromyotonia, stiff-person syndrome.

Myopathies: 20% patients with dermatomyositis after age 40 have associated tumor.

LABORATORY DATA

Demonstration of characteristic antibody accelerates diagnosis of paraneoplastic syndromes (Table 153.1).

TREATMENT

Sensorimotor polyneuropathy, LEMS often respond to IVIG or immunosuppressive drug therapy. Corticosteroid therapy often effective for opsoclonus-myoclonus syndrome in children.

CHAPTER 154 ■ NUTRITIONAL DISORDERS: MALABSORPTION, MALNUTRITION, VITAMIN DEFICIENCIES

VITAMIN B$_{12}$ (COBALAMIN) DEFICIENCY

Most common form: pernicious anemia; anemia, neurologic symptoms, atrophy of epithelial covering of tongue. Other causes: tropical sprue, gastric resection, ileal resection, jejunal diverticula.

PHYSIOLOGY

Animal products, sole dietary source for humans. Gastric acid needed for peptic digestion to release the vitamin from proteins. Intrinsic factor needed for absorption of B_{12}.

PATHOGENESIS

About 80% of adult-onset pernicious anemia attributed to lack of gastric intrinsic factor secondary to atrophic gastritis. Presumed autoimmune disorder.

PATHOLOGY

Symmetric loss of myelin sheaths, most prominent in posterior and lateral columns (***combined system disease***). Thoracic cord affected first; also sensorimotor neuropathy.

CLINICAL FEATURES

Neurologic symptoms or signs in 40% of patients with B_{12} deficiency. Age usually >60. Combined features of both myelopathy and peripheral neuropathy.

Symptoms: burning, painful or numb, tingling in hands and feet (most common symptom), sensory ataxia, memory loss, visual loss (optic neuropathy), orthostatic hypotension, anosmia, impaired taste, sphincter symptoms, impotence.

Sensory signs: glove-stocking sensory loss (especially vibratory and position sense), Romberg sign. Upper motor neuron signs: increased tone, impaired alternating movements, hyperactive tendon jerks, Babinski and Hoffmann signs. Cerebral signs: mild-to-severe dementia.

LABORATORY DATA

Blood levels of vitamin B_{12} <200 pg/mL. Serum methylmalonic acid, homocysteine increased in 99%. Severe anemia in only 20% of patients with neurologic findings.

MRI: increased T2-weighted signal and contrast enhancement of posterior and lateral columns of spinal cord. EMG: axonal or demyelinating sensorimotor neuropathy.

TREATMENT

B_{12} intramuscularly daily for first week, then weekly injections for first month, then monthly injections for life. About 50% left with some abnormality on examination; residual disability depends on duration of symptoms.

MALNUTRITION

Selected conditions ascribed to inadequate or inappropriate nutrition listed in Tables 154.1 and 154.2, with site of major neurologic involvement.

MALABSORPTION

Common syndromes: variable combinations of myopathy, sensorimotor peripheral neuropathy, degeneration of corticospinal

TABLE 154.1

NEUROLOGIC SYNDROMES ATTRIBUTED TO NUTRITIONAL DEFICIENCY

Site of major syndrome	Name
Encephalon	Hypocalcemia (lack of vitamin D), tetany, seizures
	Mental retardation (protein-calorie deprivation)
	Cretinism (lack of iodine)
	Wernicke-Korsakoff syndrome (thiamine)
Corpus callosum	Marchiafava-Bignami disease
Optic nerve	Nutritional deficiency optic neuropathy ("tobacco-alcohol amblyopia")
Brainstem	Central pontine myelinolysis
Cerebellum	Alcoholic cerebellar degeneration
	Vitamin E deficiency in bowel disease
Spinal cord	Combined system disease (B_{12} deficiency)
	Tropical spastic paraparesis (some forms?)
Peripheral nerves	Beriberi (thiamine), pellagra (nicotinic acid)
	Hypophosphatemia (?)
	Tetany (vitamin D deficiency)
Muscle	Myopathy of osteomalacia

TABLE 154.2
NEUROLOGIC SYNDROMES ATTRIBUTED TO DIETARY EXCESS

Syndrome	Condition	Agent
Increased intracranial pressure	Self-medication	Vitamin A
Encephalopathy	Phenylketonuria	Phenylalanine
	Water intoxication	Water
	Hepatic encephalopathy	Protein (and NH_3)
	Ketotic or nonketotic coma in diabetes	Glucose
Stroke	Hyperlipidemia	Lipid
Peripheral neuropathy	Self-medication	Pyridoxine
Mixed neuropathy/ myopathy	Insomnia, anxiety	Tryptophan
Myopathy	Anorexia nervosa, bulimia	Emetine, ipecac
Myoglobinuria	Constipation	Licorice

tracts and posterior columns, cerebellar abnormality. Less common: optic neuritis, atypical pigmentary degeneration of retina, dementia.

Common etiology: lack of vitamin E due to fat malabsorption, cholestatic liver disease, abetalipoproteinemia, autosomal-recessive absence of tocopherol transfer protein.

Celiac disease: malabsorption, abnormal small-bowel mucosa, intolerance to gluten; multiple autoantibodies often found (e.g., anti-gliadin). Neurologic complications from osteomalacic myopathy, B_{12} deficiency, hypokalemia, hypocalcemia. Gait ataxia may be prominent.

Crohn disease, ulcerative colitis increases risk of thromboembolism, myopathy; peripheral neuropathy with Crohn disease only.

Other malabsorption syndromes with neurologic complications: hypokalemia due to chronic diarrhea, acute hypophosphatemia, D-lactic acidosis, Whipple disease (see Chapter 35).

CHAPTER 155 ■ VASCULITIS SYNDROMES

Autoimmune diseases attributed to fibrinoid degeneration of blood vessels; manifest by arthritis, rash, visceral disease.

POLYARTERITIS NODOSA

Widespread panarteritis, mainly affecting medium-sized arteries. Onset ages 20 to 50 in >50%. CNS involved in 25%. Systemic manifestations: fever, malaise, tachycardia, sweating, fleeting edema, weakness, pains in joints, muscles, or abdomen.

Neurologic manifestations: mononeuritis multiplex; diffuse sensorimotor peripheral neuropathy. Poor prognosis; 5-year survival 50%.

Treatment: corticosteroids, immunosuppressive drugs.

TEMPORAL ARTERITIS (GIANT-CELL ARTERITIS)

Inflammation of temporal artery with multinucleated giant cells in media. Onset after age 50, primarily in white people.

Manifestations: headache, unilateral visual loss (14% to 33% of patients), jaw claudication, scalp tenderness in temporal region, malaise, fever, anorexia, weight loss, myalgia. ESR almost always >50 mm/h.

Treatment urgent to prevent visual loss. Early steroid therapy effective, unless visual loss already severe.

POLYMYALGIA RHEUMATICA

Shares with temporal arteritis: age onset; clinical syndrome, high ESR, pathology (giant-cell arteritis), course, response to steroid therapy. Headache, visual loss less frequent than in temporal arteritis. Excellent long-term outlook.

CHURG-STRAUSS SYNDROME AND WEGENER GRANULOMATOSIS

Both are types of ANCA-positive granulomatous giant-cell arteritis. Granulomas, necrosis more prominent than in other forms of arteritis above. (ANCA: anti-neuronal cytoplasmic autoantibody).

Churg-Strauss syndrome: eosinophilia, asthma. Sensorimotor neuropathy in 70%, sometimes visual loss.

Wegener granulomatosis: respiratory system, kidneys. About 90% ANCA positive. Sensorimotor peripheral neuropathy.

GRANULOMATOUS ANGIITIS OF THE BRAIN

Manifestations restricted to brain or spinal cord (granulomatous angiitis of spinal cord). Major syndrome: progressive encephalopathy (obtundation, cognitive loss); clinical strokes in 15%. Sometimes with herpes zoster, sarcoidosis, Hodgkin disease, AIDS.

Pathology: granulomatous change includes multinucleated giant cells.

Laboratory data: CSF pleocytosis (up to 500 mononuclear cells/high-power field), protein >100 mg/dL in 75%. Cerebral angiogram not diagnostic; "beading" of arteries in 10%. Cannot prove diagnosis without brain biopsy or autopsy; specimen includes brain parenchyma and meninges.

Usually fatal within a few years. Immunosuppressive drug therapy slows progression in some.

SYSTEMIC LUPUS ERYTHEMATOSUS

Widespread inflammatory change in connective tissue of skin and systemic organs. Immune complexes in small vessels. Onset age 20 to 40; 95% women.

Systemic manifestations: fever; erythematous rash; recurrent polyarthritis, pleuritis, pericarditis; anemia, leukopenia, thrombocytopenia, renal disease.

Neurologic manifestations: (a) cerebral lupus (encephalopathy, seizures, psychosis, dementia, chorea, cranial neuropathy; (b) transverse myelopathy; (c) sensorimotor peripheral neuropathy; (d) polymyositis.

Laboratory data: antinuclear antibodies (ANA), especially anti-double-stranded DNA. CSF glucose sometimes low.

Treatment and prognosis: intravenous methylprednisolone for 3 days, followed by low-dose oral therapy. Also cytotoxic drugs, anti-malarials. Steroids for peripheral neuropathy, myelitis, polymyositis. Ten-year survival 80% to 95%.

SYSTEMIC SCLEROSIS (SCLERODERMA)

Widespread scleroderma (hardening of skin) plus at least two of: sclerodactyly (skin changes on fingers); digital finger pad depressions from ischemic lesions; pulmonary fibrosis.

Polymyositis in 15%. Also migraine, trigeminal sensory neuropathy, transverse myelitis, sensorimotor axonal neuropathy, seizures, hemiparesis.

Treatment: D-penicillamine. Five-year survival 65%.

NEUROLOGIC SYNDROMES ASSOCIATED WITH OTHER COLLAGEN-VASCULAR DISEASES

Rheumatoid arthritis: aggressive polyneuropathy; atlantoaxial dislocation with cord compression.

Sjögren syndrome: peripheral neuropathy (primarily sensory or sensorimotor), trigeminal sensory neuropathy, polymyositis, venous sinus thrombosis, myelopathy, syndrome of motor neuron disease, aseptic meningitis.

Idiopathic hypereosinophilic syndrome: peripheral neuropathy.

CHAPTER 156 ■ HYPERTROPHIC PACHYMENINGITIS

Local or diffuse thickening of intracranial or spinal dura mater; often with adhesion to underlying leptomeninges. Attributed to infections (syphilis, tuberculosis, fungi); autoimmune or vasculitic diseases (Wegener granulomatosis, sarcoidosis, rheumatoid arthritis, Behçet disease, Sjögren syndrome, giant cell arteritis); malignancy (dural carcinomatosis, skull metastases, histiocytosis, lymphoma). Idiopathic hypertrophic pachymeningitis (IHP) considered autoimmune.

Clinical features: chronic headache, cranial neuropathies (compression of optic nerve may lead to blindness); cerebellar ataxia, hemiparesis, altered mentation, seizures, cervical myelopathy. Increased intracranial pressure, cerebral infarction due to dural venous sinus compression. Hypopituitarism, diabetes insipidus may occur.

Investigations: elevated ESR; CSF: lymphocytic pleocytosis, high protein. MRI: linear or nodular gadolinium enhancement, especially of falx, tentorium, cavernous sinus.

Treatment and course: headache, neurologic dysfunction usually improve with high-dose oral corticosteroids. MRI enhancement usually persists. Other therapies: pulse intravenous corticosteroid regimen; treatment with methotrexate, azathioprine, or cyclophosphamide. Surgical excision of thickened dura necessary in some patients. Progressive disorder.

CHAPTER 157 ■ NEUROLOGIC DISEASE DURING PREGNANCY

EPILEPSY

Women with preexisting epilepsy: seizure frequency increases during pregnancy in 35%, unchanged in 55%, reduced in 10%. Antiepileptic drug (AED) blood concentrations may change: non-protein-bound drug concentrations followed for highly protein-bound AEDs, including carbamazepine, phenytoin valproate.

Older AEDs (benzodiazepines, phenytoin, carbamazepine, phenobarbital, valproate) teratogenic. Major malformations 4% to 6%, compared to 2% to 4% in general population. Information about newer drugs not yet sufficient. Monitor lamotrigine levels (increase during pregnancy). Contact prospective registry for women who become pregnant while taking AEDs.

For all women of childbearing age who take AEDs, prescribe folic acid supplementation to reduce risk of neural tube defects. Vitamin K supplements recommended for last month of gestation to help prevent fetal hemorrhage.

Recommended AED regimen in pregnancy: monotherapy at lowest effective dose. Drug of choice: the one most likely to be effective and tolerated. If family history of neural tube defects, avoid carbamazepine and valproate.

Prenatal diagnostic testing: maternal serum alpha-fetoprotein and ultrasound at 14 to 18 weeks. Combination identifies neural tube defects in 95%.

Pregnant women with new-onset seizures: consider usual causes, also eclampsia. Magnetic resonance (MR) for imaging. Treatment guided by seizure type, etiology.

PREECLAMPSIA AND ECLAMPSIA

Mostly young primigravida women.

Preeclampsia: hypertension, proteinuria, edema. Associated with hepatic and coagulation abnormalities, hypoalbuminemia, increased urate levels, hemoconcentration.

Eclampsia: seizures, cerebral bleeding, death. Incidence in developed countries 1:2,000. Manifestations: confusion, seizures, cortical blindness, visual field defects, headaches, blurred vision. Main cause of death: pulmonary edema.

Differential diagnosis: subarachnoid hemorrhage, cerebral venous thrombosis.

Laboratory data: CT: hypodense regions in areas of cerebral edema. CSF usually normal in preeclampsia. In eclampsia, CSF protein moderately elevated; pressure may be increased.

Treatment: delivery of fetus, if appropriate. Magnesium sulfate may be best agent for treatment and prevention of eclamptic seizures.

CEREBRAL INFARCTION

Pregnancy a risk factor for stroke, especially postpartum. Risk increases with pregnancy-related hypertension, cesarean delivery.

Common etiologies: arterial occlusion (50% to 80%; mostly in second, third trimesters), cerebral venous thrombosis (mostly postpartum).

Treatment directed to specific cause. Heparin (including low-molecular-weight heparin) does not cross placenta. Warfarin crosses placenta and is teratogenic. Aspirin teratogenic, may cause bleeding in neonate; low-dose aspirin safe in second, third trimesters.

CEREBRAL HEMORRHAGE

Risk of cerebral hemorrhage increases in pregnancy. Occurs in 1 to 5 pregnancies per 10,000; fatal in 30% to 40%.

Subarachnoid hemorrhage: 50% of all intracranial bleeding in pregnancy. High mortality. Causes: cerebral aneurysm, arteriovenous malformation, eclampsia, cocaine abuse, coagulopathies, ectopic endometriosis, moyamoya disease, choriocarcinoma.

MULTIPLE SCLEROSIS

Rate of relapse declines in pregnancy; increases in first 3 months postpartum.

Interferon (IFN)-β1b, IFN-β1a, glatiramer acetate (copolymer 1) withheld during pregnancy. Short course of corticosteroid therapy for relapses.

MIGRAINE

Between 60% and 80% of migraine headaches improve with pregnancy. Medications limited during pregnancy. Acetaminophen, nonsteroidal antiinflammatory drugs (NSAIDs), codeine, other narcotics when necessary. Metoclopramide, prochlorperazine generally safe and effective for nausea, vomiting. Ergotamine, dihydroergotamine avoided. Triptan drugs: information still inadequate to assess teratogenicity.

NEOPLASMS

Tumor growth sometimes exacerbated by pregnancy, especially meningiomas. Choriocarcinoma the only systemic tumor specifically associated with pregnancy. Brain metastases in 3% to 20% at time of diagnosis of choriocarcinoma.

NEUROPATHIES

Risk for peripheral neuropathy increased during pregnancy and puerperium. Common types: carpal tunnel syndrome, facial nerve palsy, meralgia paresthetica, CIDP.

MYASTHENIA GRAVIS

During pregnancy and puerperium, symptoms are worse in one third of patients, unchanged in one third, improved in one third.

MOVEMENT DISORDERS

Most common: restless legs syndrome (see Chapter 145), chorea gravidarum, tardive syndromes (antiemetics such as metoclopramide, prochlorperazine).

CHAPTER 158 ■ HASHIMOTO ENCEPHALOPATHY

Hashimoto *thyroiditis*: goiter and thyroid dysfunction attributed to and defined by antithyroid (antimicrosomal or antithyroglobulin) antibodies.

Hashimoto *encephalopathy*: encephalopathy (clouding of consciousness); high titer of antithyroid antibodies. Thyroid function may be normal.

Clinical features: highly variable cerebral symptoms ("encephalopathy"). Discrete stroke-like episodes; progressive decline with dementia, psychiatric symptoms, obtundation. Also tremor, seizures, myoclonus.

Investigations: elevated serum antithyroglobulin or antithyroid peroxidase levels. TSH, T4 may be low, normal, or elevated.

ESR, C-reactive protein usually normal. CSF: increased protein in 76%. EEG: abnormal in >90% of patients (diffuse slowing most common). MRI: variable abnormalities.

Differential diagnosis: viral encephalitis, toxic-metabolic encephalopathy, Creutzfeldt-Jakob disease.

Treatment: >90% of patients respond well to corticosteroid therapy.

Section XXIII
Psychiatry

CHAPTER 159 ■ MOOD DISORDERS

MAJOR DEPRESSIVE DISORDER (MDD)

EPIDEMIOLOGY

18.8 million people affected in U.S. in 1998. Affects 1 in 33 children, 1 in 8 adolescents. Lifetime prevalence in US 12% in women, 5% in men. Death from suicide far more common in men. Incidence of postpartum depression up to 10%.

DIAGNOSIS

Profound sustained alteration in mood (depression or irritability) for at least 2 weeks, accompanied by 5 of the following: diminished interest or pleasure in almost all activities; weight loss without diet (5% or more of body weight); change in sleep pattern (insomnia or hypersomnia); psychomotor agitation or retardation; fatigue or loss of energy; continuous feelings of worthlessness or excessive or inappropriate guilt; diminished capacity for concentration or indecisiveness; recurrent thoughts of death, recurrent suicidal ideas, attempts, or plans.

DIFFERENTIAL DIAGNOSIS

Depressive episode precipitated by underlying medical condition, without underlying MDD: may be indistinguishable.

Depressive episode in bipolar disorder (bipolar depression): earlier onset, greater risk of suicide, positive family history, more frequent episodes of illness, prior manic episodes.

Milder forms of depression (fewer than required criteria for MDD): dysthymic disorders, adjustment disorders with depression, depressive personality disorders, seasonal affective disorders, chronic depression, masked depression, atypical depression.

PATHOPHYSIOLOGY

Unknown. Serotonin, norepinephrine implicated.

TREATMENT

Most effective initial treatment: combined pharmacotherapy, psychotherapy. Overall response rate near 80%. No proven superiority in effectiveness for any antidepressants (Table 159.1). Selective serotonin inhibitors (SSRIs) more tolerable than tricyclic antidepressants (TCAs). Individual response to given drug unpredictable, though family history of beneficial drug-response or previous response to medication may guide selection. Dose sensitivity varies up to 30-fold. Full benefit may take several weeks.

Relapse rate up to 20% of patients in 6 months, >30% in 1 year. Recurrence risk increases by 16% with each episode. With continued use of mood stabilizer, risk of antidepressant-induced mania is about 10%.

Treatment-refractory subjects: hospital admission; electro-convulsive therapy.

Suicide: risk factors include male gender, older age, living alone, access to firearm. Hospital admission, independent of patient's wishes, is standard of practice if suicide is considered imminent risk.

TABLE 159.1
ANTIDEPRESSANT MEDICATIONS

Tricyclic forms (dose range, mg)	SSRI derivatives (dose range, mg)	Miscellaneous (dose range, mg)
Amitriptyline (100–250)	Fluoxetine (10–60)	Venlafaxine (75–375)
Imipramine (150–300)	Sertraline (50–200)	Mirtazapine (15–45)
Nortriptyline (75–150)	Paroxetine (10–50)	Trazodone (200–500)
Doxepin (100–300)	Citalopram (10–40)	Bupropion (150–400)
Clomipramine (100–350)	Escitalopram (10–20)	
Desipramine (150–300)	Fluvoxamine (100–300)	

BIPOLAR DISORDER (BPD)

Type I: manic or psychotic manic episodes in addition to major depressive disorder. Type II: hypomanic episodes with one or more major depressive episodes.

Manic episode: expansive or irritable mood lasting at least one week, accompanied by at least 3 of the following: inflated self-esteem or grandiosity; decreased need for sleep (3 hours or less in 24 hours); increased talkativeness or pressure to continue talking; flight of ideas or racing thoughts; distractibility; psychomotor agitation or marked increase in multiple activities; excessive involvement in pleasurable activities with high risk for painful consequences (e.g., buying sprees, sexual indiscretion).

Hypomania: distinct period of expansive or irritable mood lasting throughout at least 4 days, accompanied by at least three of the following: inflated self esteem, decreased need for sleep, increased talkativeness, flight of ideas or racing thoughts, distractibility, psychomotor agitation, excessive involvement in pleasurable activities that may have painful consequences. Additional details of definition found in the Diagnostic and Statistical Manual IV (DSM-IV).

DIFFERENTIAL DIAGNOSIS

Seasonal affective disorder: mood disorder related to seasonal variation in light; depression occurs during fall or winter for at least 2 consecutive years with remission in spring or summer. Treatment: bright ambient light.

TREATMENT

Manic episode: lithium. Valproate or carbamazepine added if fast action required. Antipsychotics if psychosis present. Hospitalization usually necessary.

Prophylaxis: lithium, valproate, lamotrigine, carbamazepine. Combinations often used, along with psychosocial support.

Lithium responsible for 7-fold reduction in suicide rate. Contraindicated in patients with renal disease. Adverse effects include renal dysfunction, hypothyroidism, hyperparathyroidism, weight gain, tremor.

Suicide: rate higher than in any other psychiatric illness; 15-fold the rate in general population; responsible for death of 10–15% of patients.

MOOD DISORDERS DUE TO NEUROLOGIC CONDITIONS

25–40% of patients with neurologic conditions develop marked depressive syndrome at some point in course of illness. Treatment similar to MDD unrelated to neurologic conditions.

CHAPTER 160 ■ ANXIETY DISORDERS

Overall prevalence 7% to 9%. F:M, 2 to 3:1.

PANIC DISORDER

Recurrent, unexpected panic attacks (Table 160.1), accompanied by persistent concerns about repeated attacks or significant behavior change due to fear of repeated attacks. Onset often in young adulthood. Comorbid substance use (self-medication) common.

Treatment: cognitive behavioral therapy in combination with pharmacotherapy most helpful. Medications: include imipramine hydrochloride, benzodiazepines, selective serotonin reuptake inhibitors (SSRIs).

TABLE 160.1
CLINICAL MANIFESTATIONS OF PANIC ATTACK

Panic attack: defined by abrupt development (peaking within 10 minutes) of at least 4 of the following symptoms:

Palpitations, pounding heart, awareness of markedly accelerated heart rate
Sweating
Trembling or shaking
Sensations of shortness of breath, smothering
Choking feelings
Chest pain or discomfort
Nausea or abdominal distress
Feeling unsteady or faint, lightheaded
De-realization (feelings of unreality) or depersonalization (being detached from oneself)
Fear of dying
Fear of losing control or going crazy
Paresthesias (numbness or tingling)
Chills or hot flashes

SPECIFIC PHOBIAS AND SOCIAL PHOBIA

Phobia: specific marked, persistent fear of clearly discernible object or situation, with immediate excessive anxiety response on exposure. Duration at least six months. Examples: animals, insects; natural environment (storms, water, heights); situations (flying, driving, enclosed places). May be precipitated by life events, e.g., trauma.

Treatment: desensitization by gradual exposure. Hypnosis helpful for some. Pharmacotherapy not effective.

SOCIAL PHOBIA

Defined >20 years ago as distinct entity, but frequently overlaps depression, substance abuse, panic disorder generalized anxiety. Often early onset. Treatment: Cognitive behavioral therapy; SSRIs beneficial in about 60%; beta blockers, longer-acting benzodiazepines also used.

POST-TRAUMATIC STRESS DISORDER (PTSD)

Persistent re-experiencing of past traumatic event (threatened death or serious harm to self or others, accompanied by sense of fear, horror, or helplessness) in form of recurrent thoughts, dreams, flashbacks causing psychological or physiologic distress. Also: avoidance of stimuli associated with the trauma; persistent symptoms of increased arousal (hypervigilance, poor sleep, outbursts of irritability/anger). Symptom duration >4 weeks.

Treatment: Psychotherapy (may include cognitive behavioral, cognitive restructuring, supportive counseling) plus antidepressant medication (tricyclics, monoamine oxidase inhibitors, SSRIs). Benzodiazepines not effective.

OBSESSIVE COMPULSIVE DISORDER (OCD)

Obsessions: recurrent, intrusive thoughts, impulses, or images causing marked anxiety or distress.

Compulsions: repetitive behaviors (hand washing, checking) or mental acts (counting, repeating words silently), performed in response to an obsession or according to rigid rules, to reduce distress.

Person perceives obsessions or compulsions as excessive, interfering with normal routines, occupation, or social activities.

Obsessive compulsive disorder (OCD): chronic disorder. Onset usually in adolescence or early adult years. Men and women affected equally.

Treatment: cognitive-behavioral therapy alone or in combination with pharmacotherapy (SSRIs, clomipramine). Current guidelines recommend pharmacotherapy for at least 1 to 2 years.

GENERALIZED ANXIETY DISORDER

Apprehension, excessive worry that occur more days than not for at least 6 months and involve several events or activities.

Associated symptoms: restlessness, easy fatigability, difficulty concentrating, irritability, muscle tension, sleep disturbance. Often chronic; 40% of patients report symptoms for >5 years. Lifetime prevalence 5% in USA in one study.

Differential diagnosis: exclude substance abuse by history or blood/urine toxicology screen. Medical conditions: thyroid disease, other endocrinopathies, occult neoplasm.

Treatment: relaxation and behavioral anxiety treatments, hypnotherapy, psychoanalytic therapy have been described. Pharmacotherapy: benzodiazepines, venlafaxine. No specific guidelines exist for duration of treatment.

CHAPTER 161 ■ SCHIZOPHRENIA

Abnormalities in perception of reality, form, and content of thoughts and speech, emotional deficits, leading to disturbed sense of self, social dysfunction, apathy, peculiar behavior. Symptom onset usually in late adolescence, early adulthood. Prevalence about 1% of all people worldwide.

Psychosis: failure to distinguish between reality and thoughts (hallucinations, delusions). A feature of schizophrenia; also present in many medical diseases (Table 161.1), other psychiatric conditions (e.g., bipolar disorder, depression, dementia, substance use, acute and chronic post-traumatic stress disorders).

TABLE 161.1

DIFFERENTIAL DIAGNOSIS OF PSYCHOSIS: MEDICAL AND NEUROLOGIC DISORDERS

Epilepsy	Especially temporal lobe epilepsy
Neoplasm	Especially frontal, temporal lobe tumors
Cerebrovascular disease	
Traumatic brain injury	
Infectious	AIDS (progressive multifocal leukoencephalopathy, AIDS dementia, CNS lymphoma, toxoplasmosis, cryptococcal meningitis); herpes encephalitis; neurosyphilis
Inflammatory	Systemic lupus erythematosus, neurosarcoidosis
Metabolic	Acute intermittent porphyria, vitamin B_{12} deficiency, homocystinuria, pellagra, Wilson disease
Degenerative	Creutzfeldt-Jakob disease, frontotemporal dementia, Huntington disease, metachromatic leukodystrophy
Drug-related	Alcohol (delirium tremens, hallucinosis, Wernicke-Korsakoff syndrome), CNS depressants (barbiturate withdrawal), hallucinogens (LSD, phencyclidine [PCP]), stimulants (amphetamines, cocaine), corticosteroids
Other toxins	Carbon monoxide poisoning, heavy metal poisoning

CLINICAL FEATURES

Positive symptoms: hallucinations and delusions, disorganized thinking or behavior.

Negative symptoms: flat affect, alogia (impoverished thinking manifested by diminished speech output or content), apathy, avolition (lack of energy and drive), social withdrawal. Less responsive to treatment, confer worse prognosis than positive symptoms.

DSM-IV diagnostic criteria: presence of 2 or more of: (a) delusions, hallucinations; (b) disorganized speech; (c) grossly disorganized or catatonic behavior; (d) negative symptoms, for one month; accompanying social or occupational dysfunction.

COURSE AND ASSOCIATED FEATURES

Typical onset in late adolescence, early adult years with prodrome (attenuated psychotic symptoms, change in behavior, or global decline in function) for 6 to 12 months before first psychotic episode. Then becomes chronic with deterioration. Short prodrome (i.e., abrupt onset of psychosis), good premorbid function associated with better prognosis. Women have later onset and milder symptoms than men.

Alcohol and other substance abuse common. About 80% smoke tobacco. Patients with schizophrenia have increased medical morbidity and earlier death from cardiovascular disease, diabetes and other medical conditions (independent of cigarette smoking, medication effects). Suicide: 10% of patient deaths.

TREATMENT

ANTIPSYCHOTIC MEDICATION

First-Generation Antipsychotics

Dopamine (D_2) receptor antagonists. Include haloperidol, perphenazine, fluphenazine, and chlorpromazine (first antipsychotic agent, introduced 50 years ago). Common side effects: intense psychomotor restlessness (akathisia), parkinsonism, tardive dyskinesia (potentially irreversible), anticholinergic symptoms, prolongation of QT interval, neuroleptic malignant syndrome (Chapter 117). Galactorrhea, amenorrhea, gynecomastia, impotence can result from hyperprolactinemia (D_2 antagonism). All antipsychotic medications lower seizure threshold.

Newer Antipsychotics

Clozapine: lower affinity for D_2, higher affinity for serotonin 5-HT_{2A} receptor. Not associated with tardive dyskinesia below doses of 300 mg per day. Fatal agranulocytosis in 1% to 2%; monitor with weekly neutrophil counts. Other side effects: anticholinergic, antihistaminergic symptoms, hypersalivation, weight gain, diabetes.

Other second-generation antipsychotics: include risperidone, olanzapine, quetiapine, ziprasidone, and aripiprazole. Side effects include: weight gain (olanzapine, risperidone), somnolence (olanzapine, quetiapine, ziprasidone), diabetes (olanzapine), postural hypotension (quetiapine). Quetiapine has low rates of extrapyramidal symptoms.

OTHER PHARMACOTHERAPIES

Coexisting anxiety and mood disorders common; adjunctive anxiolytics, mood stabilizers, antidepressants may be used.

NONPHARMACOLOGIC THERAPIES

Negative symptoms (e.g., affect blunting, alogia, avolition), social dysfunction and cognitive impairment suboptimally treated by current drugs; predict unfavorable outcome. Other management strategies (e.g., cognitive behavioral therapy, social skills training) being studied.

CHAPTER 162 ■ SOMATOFORM DISORDERS

Somatoform disorders: conversion disorder, somatization disorder, pain disorder, hypochondriasis, body dysmorphic disorder.

Somatizing disorders: besides somatoform disorders, also include malingering, factitious disorders, psychological factors affecting a medical condition (Table 162.1).

Physical symptoms in somatoform disorders: (a) suggest general medical condition but not explained by any general medical disorder, substance effect, or other psychiatric

TABLE 162.1
SOMATIZING DISORDERS: DEFINING CHARACTERISTICS

	Conscious intentionality	Primary gain	Secondary gain	Coexisting psychopathology	Prognosis
Somatoform Disorders	Absent	Repress unacceptable wishes, feelings or conflicts	Any pragmatic benefits, if present, are secondary	Highly variable: May include affective, anxiety, dissociative, psychotic, developmental or personality disorders	Highly variable: depends on chronicity, coexisting psychopathology, patient resilience, support network, treatment
Factitious Disorders	Present	Assume the sick role	Generally no significant pragmatic benefits; if present, are secondary	Often includes dependent, histrionic, borderline or antisocial personality features	Often poor, especially if chronic
Malingering	Present	Pragmatic benefit: financial, legal, drugs	Circumvent authority	Often includes antisocial personality disorder	Symptoms are relinquished only when the goal is either obtained or seen as clearly unobtainable
Psychological Factors Affecting a Medical Condition	Variable	None	Any pragmatic benefits, if present, are secondary	Highly variable	Highly variable, depending on medical condition, chronicity, patient resilience, support network, treatment

657

disorder; (b) cause clinically meaningful distress or functional impairment; (c) not intentionally produced (vs. factitious disorders, malingering). Psychological factors judged to play major role in symptom onset.

Conversion disorder: symptoms affecting voluntary motor or sensory function, suggesting a neurologic or other general medical condition. Antecedent psychological stressors usually difficult to identify without extensive psychiatric evaluation.

Somatization disorder: multiple, recurring somatic complaints that result in medical treatment or functional impairment. Begins before age 30, persists for years. DSM-IV criteria: a) pain related to at least 4 different sites or functions; b) at least 2 gastrointestinal symptoms other than pain; c) at least 1 sexual or reproductive symptom other than pain; and d) at least 1 symptom, other than pain, suggesting neurologic disorder. Coexisting depressive, anxiety and personality disorders frequent.

Pain disorder: pain is primary problem.

Hypochondriasis: preoccupation with fear of having serious disease based on misinterpreting one or more bodily signs or symptoms. Partial insight into disproportionate concern often present.

Body dysmorphic disorder: preoccupation with imagined defect in appearance.

CLINICAL EVALUATION

Clues to diagnosis: incongruities in history (e.g., tremor of sudden onset); inconsistencies in exam findings (e.g., accurately reaching for hand to shake in spite of subjective blindness). Absence of clear psychological factors on initial evaluation does not rule out diagnosis.

Thorough assessment for any condition, other than somatoform disorder, that could explain clinical presentation.

Informing patient of diagnosis: 1) validate clinical manifestations as physical findings with psychological basis; 2) emphasize potential reversibility of symptoms; 3) clarify nature of referral to psychiatrist as enlisting help in management (not "dumping" the patient).

TREATMENT

Team approach recommended: neurologist (monitors nature, progression of physical manifestations); psychiatrist (identifies, treats psychological conflict and related disorders); physical and occupational therapists (devise exercises to help reestablish voluntary control over affected systems). Combination of treatments often required, specific for individual patient.

Psychotherapy: identify conflict underlying physical symptoms; techniques may include hypnosis.

Behavior modification: strategies to alter environmental factors contributing to expression of psychological conflict through physical symptoms.

Physical therapy: helpful in cases of limb weakness, fixed postures, gait abnormality.

Pharmacotherapy: often indicated for coexisting psychiatric condition (e.g., depression, anxiety, psychosis).

Other: family therapy; speech therapy; direct environmental intervention (to deal with contributory stressors or secondary gain influences.

Some patients with chronic symptoms or severe functional impairment benefit from hospital inpatient admission to: 1) facilitate acceptance of diagnosis, 2) initiate intensive clinical treatment trial.

Section XXIV
Environmental Neurology

CHAPTER 163 ■ ALCOHOLISM

Ethanol-related deaths >100,000 each year; 5% of all deaths in United States. Problem drinkers: 7% of all adults, 19% of adolescents in United States addicted to ethanol or have problems when they drink.

ETHANOL INTOXICATION

Signs of cerebral disinhibition (euphoria, jocularity, sociability) precede signs of global cerebral depression (lethargy, stupor, coma).

Alcoholic blackout: amnesia for period of intoxication, sometimes hours, although consciousness at times seemingly undisturbed.

Acute ethanol poisoning can be fatal due to respiratory depression. In stuporous alcoholic patients, consider also subdural hematoma, meningitis, hypoglycemia. Serum osmolarity may be increased (measured > calculated).

Treatment: respiratory support; correct hypovolemia, acid-base or electrolyte imbalance, hypoglycemia (give both glucose and thiamine); return temperature to normal. Avoid sedatives.

Takes 6 hours to clear mildly intoxicating alcohol level (blood ethanol concentration [BEC] of 100 mg/dL); BEC of 400 mg/dL takes 20 hours to return to zero in nonhabitual drinker. Hemodialysis or peritoneal dialysis for: BEC >600 mg/dL; severe acidosis; concurrent ingestion of methanol, ethylene glycol, or other dialyzable drugs; also for severely intoxicated children. Magnesium sulfate may further depress sensorium in intoxicated patient.

ETHANOL-DRUG INTERACTIONS

Combination of ethanol with other drugs, often in suicide attempts, causes 2,500 deaths annually. Alcohol particularly dangerous with: barbiturates (lowered lethal dose of either drug), morphine (increased potency when repeatedly used together), propoxyphene (death reported).

ETHANOL DEPENDENCE AND WITHDRAWAL

Dependence: confirmed by signs of withdrawal during abstinence.

EARLY WITHDRAWAL (HOURS TO DAYS)

Onset 0 to 48 hours. Duration to 2 weeks; usually few days.

Tremulousness: increasing severity with insomnia, easy startle, agitation, facial and conjunctival flushing, sweating, anorexia, nausea, retching, weakness, tachypnea, tachycardia, hypertension.

Perceptual disturbances: in about 25%; nightmares, illusions, hallucinations (visual, auditory, tactile, olfactory, or combination). May progress to persistent auditory hallucinosis.

Seizures: (a) ethanol can precipitate seizures in any person with epilepsy. (b) "Alcohol-related" seizures (otherwise nonepileptic person) early in withdrawal; during active drinking or after >1 week of abstinence. Focal features in 25%. Electroencephalogram abnormal in <10%.

Phenytoin does not prevent seizures during withdrawal. Status epilepticus treated as in other situations. Long-term anticonvulsants superfluous for ethanol withdrawal seizures or abstainers; drinkers do not take them.

LATE WITHDRAWAL (DELIRIUM TREMENS)

Onset 48 to 72 hours after last drink. Duration up to few days. Mortality up to 15%.

Agitated confusion typical, typically alternating with periods of lucidity. Inattention, tremulousness, fever, tachycardia, profuse sweating. Patient picks at bed clothes, stares wildly about, shouts at or fends off hallucinated people or objects. Seizures rare; suspect other diagnosis if present.

Treatment: sedatives (benzodiazepines) for prevention in any heavy drinker undergoing sudden abstinence (admission to hospital for other reason); also for treatment of active syndrome. Sometimes need ICU.

WERNICKE-KORSAKOFF SYNDROME

Two clinically distinct syndromes. Same pathology. Both caused by thiamine deficiency.

Wernicke syndrome: (a) global confusion, appearing over days or weeks; disordered perception common. (b) Eye movement abnormalities (nystagmus, lateral rectus palsy, conjugate gaze palsy, ophthalmoplegia). (c) Truncal ataxia present in >80%.

Korsakoff syndrome: mental syndrome dominated by amnesia; emerges as Wernicke syndrome responds to treatment. Amnesia both anterograde (inability to retain new information) and retrograde (randomly lost recall for events months or years ago). Other signs: decreased spontaneous speech or activity, confabulation, impaired insight, anosognosia for mental symptoms.

Treatment: thiamine replacement (with glucose). Untreated syndrome fatal; mortality 10% of treated patients.

OTHER ALCOHOL-RELATED NEUROLOGIC SYNDROMES

Alcoholic cerebellar degeneration: ataxia dominant in trunk and legs. Nystagmus, dysarthria rare. Symptoms eventually stable.

Alcoholic polyneuropathy: onset with paresthesias, burning or lancinating pains. Sensorimotor, demyelinating and axonal. Etiology probably nutritional. Becomes stable or improves with abstinence and adequate diet.

Peripheral nerve pressure palsies: radial, peroneal most common. Recovery in days or weeks.

Alcoholic amblyopia: visual impairment progresses days to weeks; central or centrocecal scotoma, temporal disc pallor. Demyelination of optic nerves, chiasm, tracts. Nutritional etiology. Improves (often incompletely) with nutritional replacement.

Pellagra: nicotinic acid deficiency in alcohol users. Skin, gastrointestinal, neurologic symptoms. Altered mentation progresses for hours, days to amnesia, delusions, hallucinations, delirium.

Alcoholic liver disease: nearly all cirrhosis deaths in people older than 45 caused by ethanol. Syndromes include hepatic encephalopathy, "acquired chronic hepatocerebral degeneration" (see Chapter 148).

Hypoglycemia: due to impaired gluconeogenesis, depletion of glycogen stores (starvation). Altered behavior, seizures, coma, focal neurologic signs. Residual symptoms common.

Alcoholic ketoacidosis: β-hydroxybutyric acid, lactic acid accumulate with heavy drinking. Typically chronic alcoholic young women. Vomiting, dehydration, confusion, obtundation, Kussmaul respiration ensues. Large anion gap. Treatment: glucose-thiamine; correct dehydration or hypotension; replace electrolytes. Insulin usually not needed.

Infection in alcoholics: alteration of white blood cell (WBC) function contributes to predisposition to infection. Alcoholic intoxication a risk factor for HIV infection.

Trauma in alcoholics: thrombocytopenia, abnormalities of clotting factors (direct effect of ethanol or consequence of cirrhosis) increase likelihood of intracranial hematoma after head injury.

Alcohol and cancer: ethanol in moderate amounts increases risk of carcinoma of mouth, esophagus, pharynx, larynx, liver, breast.

Alcohol and stroke: low-to-moderate amounts of ethanol decrease risk of ischemic stroke; higher amounts increase it. Risk for hemorrhagic stroke increased at any dose.

Alcoholic myopathy: (a) subclinical (elevated serum CK levels, EMG changes); (b) chronic; (c) acute myoglobinuria. Likely due to ethanol toxicity.

Alcoholic dementia: progressive mental decline in alcoholics without other cause.

Central pontine myelinolysis, Marchiafava-Bignami disease:
see Chapters 135 and 136.
Fetal alcohol syndrome: see Chapter 168.

TREATMENT OF CHRONIC ALCOHOLISM

Daily disulfiram induces unpleasant reaction when alcohol
taken. Helps only patients with strong desire to abstain. Reaction may be dangerous.

CHAPTER 164 ■ DRUG DEPENDENCE

Psychic dependence (addiction): craving, drug-seeking behavior. Physical dependence: withdrawal symptoms and signs with
abstinence. May occur separately or together. Addiction: psychic dependence. Selected classes of recreational drugs listed in
Table 164.1.

TABLE 164.1

SELECTED CLASSES OF RECREATIONAL DRUGS AND THEIR EFFECTS

Drug class	Examples	Intoxication	Overdose	Treatment	Withdrawal
Opioids	Heroin	Drowsy euphoria, analgesia, cough suppression, miosis. Often nausea, vomiting, sweating, pruritus, hypothermia, postural hypotension, constipation, decreased libido. "Rush" from parenteral route	Coma, respiratory depression, pinpoint (but reactive) pupils	Respiratory support, naloxone, close observation	Irritability, lacrimation, rhinorrhea, sweating, yawning, mydriasis, myalgia, muscle spasms, piloerection, nausea, vomiting, abdominal cramps, fever, hot flashes, tachycardia, hypertension, orgasm. Often fatal in newborn

Stimulants	Cocaine, amphetamine, methamphetamine, methylphenidate, ephedrine, phenylpropanolamine	Alert, euphoria, increased motor activity and physical endurance. "Rush" when taken parenterally or smoked ("crack," "ice")	Headache, chest pain, tachycardia, hypertension, flushing, sweating, fever, excitement delirium, cardiac arrhythmia, seizures, stroke, myoglobinuria, shock, coma, death	Sedation, correct acidosis, anticonvulsants, cooling, antihypertensives respiratory and blood pressure support, cardiac monitoring	Fatigue, depression, increased hunger and sleep
Sedatives	Barbiturates, benzodiazepines, glutethimide, ethchlorvynol, methaqualone, zolpidem, gamma-hydroxybutyric acid (GHB)	Similar to ethanol intoxication	Similar to ethanol intoxication	Supportive, flumazenil (benzodiazepine antagonist)	Tremor, seizures, delirium tremens

(continued)

TABLE 164.1
SELECTED CLASSES OF RECREATIONAL DRUGS AND THEIR EFFECTS (*Continued*)

Drug class	Examples	Intoxication	Overdose	Treatment	Withdrawal
Cannabinoids	Marijuana, hashish	Relaxed, dreamy euphoria, jocularity, disinhibition, depersonalization, subjective slowing of time, conjunctival injection, tachycardia, postural hypotension	Auditory or visual hallucinations, confusion, psychosis		Craving
Hallucinogens	Psilocybin, psilocin, mescaline, lysergic acid diethylamide (LSD), 3,4-methylenedioxy methamphetamine (MDMA, "ecstasy")	Perceptual distortions or hallucinations (usually visual, elaborately formed), depersonalization, altered mood, dizziness, tremor, paresthesias. Acute panic, delayed "flashbacks" sometimes seen	Hypertension, obtundation, seizures	Calm environment, reassurance, sedation	None

					Craving
Inhalants	Nitrous oxide, trichloroethylene, toluene (from aerosols, spot removers, glues, lighter fluid, fire-extinguishing agents, bottled fuel gas, marker pens, paints, gasoline)	Similar to ethanol intoxication	Hallucinations, seizures, coma, death	Respiratory and cardiac monitoring	
Phencyclidine ("angel dust")		Euphoria or dysphoria, feeling of numbness	Agitation, nystagmus, tachycardia, hypertension, fever, sweating, ataxia, paranoid or catatonic psychosis, hallucinations, myoclonus, myoglobinuria, seizures, coma, respiratory depression, death	Calm environment, sedation, gastric suctioning, activated charcoal, forced diuresis, cooling, antihypertensives, anticonvulsants, monitoring of cardiorespiratory and renal function. Avoid neuroleptics	None

(*continued*)

671

TABLE 164.1

SELECTED CLASSES OF RECREATIONAL DRUGS AND THEIR EFFECTS (*Continued*)

Drug class	Examples	Intoxication	Overdose	Treatment	Withdrawal
Anticholinergics	Plant *Datura stramonium*, antiparkinsonian drugs, amitriptyline	Decreased sweating, tachycardia, dry mouth, dilated unreactive pupils, delirium with hallucinations	Myoclonus, seizures, coma, and death	Intravenous physostigmine, gastric lavage, cooling, bladder catheterization, respiratory and cardiovascular monitoring, anticonvulsants. Neuroleptics contraindicated	None

CHAPTER 165 ■ IATROGENIC DISEASE

Selected adverse neurologic reactions due to drugs or diagnostic procedures listed in Table 165.1.

TABLE 165.1

ADVERSE NEUROLOGIC REACTIONS DUE TO DRUGS OR PROCEDURES FOR DIAGNOSIS OR THERAPY

Adverse reaction	Drug or procedure
Aseptic meningitis	Trimethoprim, sulfadiazine, ibuprofen, intravenous immunoglobulin azathioprine, sulindac, tolmetin, naproxen, OKT3
Basal ganglia syndromes (parkinsonism, tardive dyskinesia, other dyskinesias)	Butyrophenones, levodopa, phenothiazines, reserpine, tetrabenazine
Brain tumor	Immunosuppression (CNS lymphoma) Radiotherapy (meningioma)
Central pontine myelinolysis	Rapid correction of hyponatremia
Encephalopathy	Anticonvulsant drugs, cimetidine, corticosteroids, hemodialysis, insulin (hypoglycemia), lithium, methotrexate, metrizamide, monoamine oxidase inhibitors, overhydration (water intoxication), penicillin, pentazocine, propoxyphene, radiotherapy, vincristine
Leukoencephalopathy	Methotrexate, radiation, vaccines
Neuroleptic malignant syndrome	Neuroleptic drugs
Meningoencephalitis (viral, yeast, toxoplasmosis)	Immunosuppression
Malignant hyperthermia	Succinylcholine, halothane, others

(continued)

TABLE 165.1

ADVERSE NEUROLOGIC REACTIONS DUE TO DRUGS OR PROCEDURES FOR DIAGNOSIS OR THERAPY (*Continued*)

Adverse reaction	Drug or procedure
Myopathies and myoglobinuria	Anticonvulsants (with osteomalacia), bacterial toxins with tampon use (toxic shock syndrome), chloroquine, corticosteroids, emetine, epsilon caproic acid, hypophosphatemia, ipecac, kaliuretic diuretics (furosemide, thiazides), licorice (glycyrrhiza), lovastatin, penicillamine, zidovudine
Muscle fibrosis	Meperidine, pentazocine
Myotonia	Diazacholesterol
Myelopathy	Intrathecal injections, delayed arachnoiditis after myelography, radiotherapy, spinal anesthesia, spinal angiography, vaccination
Neuromuscular disorders	
MG	Antiepileptic drugs, penicillamine
Other neuromuscular blockade	Aminoglycoside antibiotics, succinylcholine
Optic neuropathy	Chloroquine, ethambutol, isoniazid, penicillamine, vincristine
Peripheral neuropathy	Anticoagulants (nerve compression by hematoma), barbiturates (in acute porphyria), disopyramide, disulfiram, ethambutol, hypophosphatemia, isoniazid, metronidazole, nitrofurantoin, nitrous oxide, perihexilene, phenytoin, procarbazine, vincristine, vitamin B_6 excess
Pseudotumor cerebri	Corticosteroids, nalidixic acid, tetracycline, vitamin A
Stroke	Amphetamines, anticoagulants, cerebral angiography and intraarterial interventional therapies, chiropractic manipulation of neck, induced hypotension for surgery, induced cardiac arrest, insulin-induced hypoglycemia, massage of carotid sinus, open heart surgery and cardiopulmonary bypass, oral contraceptives, overcorrection of hypertension, radiotherapy of neck or cranium

CHAPTER 166 ■ COMPLICATIONS OF CANCER CHEMOTHERAPY

Tables 166.1, 166.2 list neurologic complications of cancer treatments.

TABLE 166.1

NEUROTOXICITY OF ANTINEOPLASTIC DRUGS

Neurologic disorder	Drug
Peripheral neuropathy	Carboplatin, cisplatin, cytarabine, docetaxel, etoposide, fludarabine, oxaliplatin, paclitaxel, procarbazine, suramin, vinblastine, vincristine, vinorelbine
Cranial neuropathy	Carmustine, cisplatin, 5-fluorouracil, ifosfamide, vinblastine, vincristine
Autonomic neuropathy	Cisplatin, paclitaxel, procarbazine, vinblastine, vincristine, vinorelbine
Encephalopathy	Asparaginase, busulfan, carmustine, cisplatin, cytarabine, 5-fluorouracil, fludarabine, ifosfamide, methotrexate, procarbazine
Cerebellar syndrome	Cytarabine, 5-fluorouracil, procarbazine
Acute myelopathy	Cytarabine, methotrexate, thiotepa

TABLE 166.2

NEUROLOGIC COMPLICATIONS OF MISCELLANEOUS CANCER TREATMENTS

Treatment category	Drug	Neurologic disorder	Special features
Immunosuppressant drugs	Cyclosporine	Tremor, paresthesias, seizures, lethargy, ataxia, quadriparesis	Frequency 8% to 47%
		Cerebral blindness (usually reversible)	Occurs with serum level > 500 mg/dL. CT: posterior cerebral white matter lesions
	OKT3	Altered mental function, seizures, lethargy, aseptic meningitis, visual loss, transient sensorineural hearing loss	
	FK-506 (tacrolimus)	Acute tremor, headache, paresthesias Leukoencephalopathy	Frequency 5% to 10% Similar to cyclosporine leukoencephalopathy
Biologic response modifiers	Cytokines	Vertigo, memory loss, confusion, emotional instability, somnolence, depression, seizures, hemiparesis	Corticosteroid treatment may help
Bone marrow transplantation		Cerebral hemorrhage (4%), metabolic encephalopathy (3%), CNS infections (2%) Polymyositis, MG, sensorimotor neuropathy, aseptic meningitis, leukoencephalopathy	Associated with chronic graft-versus-host disease

CHAPTER 167 ■ OCCUPATIONAL AND ENVIRONMENTAL NEUROTOXICOLOGY

Table 167.1 lists selected neurotoxic syndromes.

ADDITIONAL CONSIDERATIONS

Exposure may be acute high dose or chronic low dose.

Short or long latency may separate exposure and symptoms.

Preexisting or coincidental disease may complicate diagnosis.

Symptoms may be numerous, nonspecific.

Susceptibility varies in populations, and between humans and experimental animals.

Damage may be reversible or irreversible.

A cascade of effects may have secondary and systemic complications as well as psychological problems.

Secondary gain, issues may complicate diagnosis.

Neurologic signs may be absent or subtle within recognized syndromes.

Laboratory data may be nonspecific despite symptoms and signs of neurologic disorder.

Exclude other possible causes.

TABLE 167.1

NEUROTOXIC SYNDROMES

Agent	Occupational or other exposure	Syndrome	
		Acute	Chronic
Metals			
Arsenic	Pesticides, pigments, paint, electroplating, seafood, smelter, semiconductors	Encephalopathy	Neuropathy
Lead	Solder, lead shot, illicit whiskey, insecticides, auto body shop, storage battery manufacture, smelter, paint, water pipes, gasoline sniffing	Encephalopathy	Encephalopathy, neuropathy, motor neuron disease–like syndrome
Manganese	Iron industry, welding, mining smelter, fireworks, fertilizer, dry cell batteries	Encephalopathy	Parkinsonism
Mercury	Thermometers, other gauges; dental office (amalgams); felt hat manufacture; electroplating; photography	Headache, tremor	Neuropathy, encephalopathy with dementia, tremor
Tin	Canning industry, solder, electronics, plastics, fungicides	Delirium	Encephalomyelopathy
Solvents			
Carbon disulfide	Rayon manufacture, preservatives, textiles, rubber cement, varnish, electroplating	Encephalopathy	Neuropathy, parkinsonism

Agent	Source	Acute	Chronic
Trichlorethylene	Paints, degreasers, spot removers, decaffeination, dry cleaning, rubber solvents	Narcosis	Encephalopathy, trigeminal neuropathy
Hexacarbons[a]	Paints, paint removers, varnish, degreasers, rapid-drying ink, glues, cleaning agents, glues for making shoes in poorly ventilated cottage industry; glue sniffing, MNBK in plastics	Narcosis	Neuropathy, encephalopathy, ataxia
Insecticides			
Organophosphates, carbamates	Manufacture, application	Cholinergic syndrome	Ataxia, neuropathy, myelopathy
Carbon monoxide	Accidental or deliberate exposure in motor vehicles, faulty gasoline-fueled heaters	Anoxic encephalopathy	
Methyl alcohol	Contaminated illicit whiskey	Retinal blindness	
Recreation abuse			
Nitrous oxide	Dental offices	Encephalopathy	B_{12}-deficient myelopathy
Seafood			
Ciguatera		Sensory neuropathy with temperature inversion	
Shellfish		Acute neuropathy	

[a]Hexacarbons: *n*-hexane, methyl *n*-butyl ketone (MNBK).

CHAPTER 168 ■ HIV, FETAL ALCOHOL AND DRUG EFFECTS, AND THE BATTERED CHILD

PEDIATRIC AIDS AND HIV INFECTION

Incidence of neurologic abnormalities in HIV-infected cohorts has dropped from around 30% to <2% with antiretroviral drugs. Progressive neurologic dysfunction first evidence of progression to AIDS in 10% of infected children.

HIV ENCEPHALOPATHY IN CHILDREN

Progressive or static. Progressive encephalopathy: loss of developmental milestones, progressive pyramidal tract dysfunction, acquired microcephaly or impaired brain growth. Fulminant, progressive, or stepwise. Static encephalopathy less well defined. Imaging may reveal atrophy, foci of demyelination.

FOCAL MANIFESTATIONS

Rare in HIV encephalopathy. Focal signs, seizures raise possibility of neoplasm, strokes, opportunistic infection.

Primary CNS lymphoma: most common cause of focal cerebral signs in HIV-infected children (3% to 4% of cases). Seizures in 33% of patients. Differentiation from toxoplasmic brain abscess may require brain biopsy.
Stroke: risk increased with HIV infection (1.3% per year in HIV-infected children). About 50% of strokes hemorrhagic. Nonhemorrhagic stroke, subarachnoid hemorrhage attributed to arteriopathy of large vessels or meninges. Vasculopathy presumed infectious (HIV, varicella zoster virus [VZV]); check VZV PCR in CSF; treat with appropriate antiviral medications. Steroids not indicated, may worsen vasculopathy.
Opportunistic CNS infection: rare in HIV-infected children.

TABLE 168.1

TYPICAL FEATURES OF FETAL ALCOHOL SYNDROME

Pre- and postnatal growth retardation (weight, length, and/or
  head size <10th percentile)
Cerebral involvement (neurologic or cognitive impairment,
  developmental delay)
Dysmorphic features
  Microcephaly (head circumference <5th percentile)
  Microphthalmia, short palpebral fissures, or both
  Poorly developed philtrum
  Thin upper lip
  Flattening of the maxillary area

FETAL ALCOHOL SYNDROME

Affects children of chronic alcoholic women; also occurs with
binge drinking (≥5 drinks per occasion). Fetal susceptibility to
alcohol greatest during first trimester of pregnancy. 2 to 4 per
1,000 live births. Clinical features: see Table 168.1.

Postnatal alcohol exposure: alcohol transferred through breast
  milk impairs motor development but not mental development at age 1 year.
Withdrawal syndrome: rare. Restlessness, agitation, tremulousness, opisthotonus, seizures shortly after birth. Resolves
  in a few days.

FETAL COCAINE EFFECTS

Cocaine use during pregnancy linked to intrauterine growth
retardation, impaired fetal brain growth.
  Neonatal period: irritability, excitability, poor feeding,
sleep disturbances, movement abnormalities. Increased risk
of stroke, porencephaly, intraventricular hemorrhage. Focal
seizures occur with stroke.
  Sequelae in childhood include irritability, impulsivity, aggressive behavior.
  Cocaine exposure in childhood: seizures chief manifestation of symptomatic intoxication.

THE BATTERED CHILD

Suspect nonaccidental head trauma when severity of injury (e.g., skull fracture) is not consistent with history given or child's age and development.

Shaken baby syndrome: usually seen in infants <1 year, shaken to stop crying. Clinical features: depressed mental status, seizures, retinal hemorrhages, signs of raised ICP. External signs of trauma usually absent. Brain imaging: bilateral subdural hematomas or subarachnoid hemorrhage. Skeletal survey may reveal fractures in other sites (ribs, long bones); help confirm nonaccidental injury. Neurologic sequelae include hydrocephalus, blindness, developmental delay, mental retardation, microcephaly, spastic quadriparesis.

CHAPTER 169 ■ FALLS IN THE ELDERLY

More than a third of people age 65 or older fall each year. 5% to 10% of falls in elderly result in injury. Fatality rate increases with age. Likelihood of admission to nursing home increases with number of falls.

Risk factors for falls: residence in long-term care facility; taking more than one drug; antidepressant drugs (for residents of nursing homes); Parkinson disease; previous stroke; arthritis; dementia.

Propensity to falls generated by cumulative handicaps: poor vision, poor balance, unsteady gait, stooped posture, impaired proprioception. Likelihood of falling also increased by disequilibrium of unknown cause: subjectively impaired balance; impaired gait on examination; no cause discerned by medical, neurologic, vestibular examination.

Cerebral white matter disease (MRI) associated with gait and balance dysfunction.

Prevention: (1) multidisciplinary health, environmental screening to correct falling risk factors; (2) muscle strengthening, balance training at home; (3) home hazard assessment in people with history of falls; (4) withdrawal of psychotropic medications; (5) cardiac pacing for fallers with cardioinhibitory carotid sinus sensitivity; (6) Tai Chi over 15 weeks as group exercise.

Section XXV
Rehabilitation

CHAPTER 170 ■ NEUROLOGIC REHABILITATION

Approaches: (a) bypass neurologic impediment by teaching adaptive techniques using preserved neurologic function (e.g., practice using normal hand for person with paretic arm); (b) facilitate return of neurologic function (e.g., tasks to improve strength of paretic arm). Functional outcome improved by treatment in comprehensive rehabilitation program.

OCCUPATIONAL THERAPY

Goal: promote maximum independence in activities of daily living by improving arm function, cognitive skills. Examples: prevent permanent disability from complications of temporary neurologic impairment (splinting to prevent wrist-flexor contractures from radial nerve palsy); teach new techniques for self-care; prescribe adaptive equipment to compensate for impairment.

PHYSICAL THERAPY

Goal: maximize function and mobility. Examples: strengthening exercises, gait and balance training, spasticity reduction through stretching or medication, surgical release of shortened tendons, bracing, assistive devices (cane, walker), use of wheelchair.

DYSPHAGIA THERAPY

Goal: evaluate and treat dysphagia, dysarthria. Performed by speech therapist.

Dysphagia evaluation indicated for: esophageal obstruction, aspiration pneumonia, malnutrition; coughing, choking, or nasal regurgitation while eating; dysarthria; diseases associated with dysphagia (motor neuron disease, MG).

Treatment: teach techniques that improve swallowing, reduce aspiration (chin tucking before swallowing).

LANGUAGE AND COGNITIVE THERAPIES

Speech therapist characterizes and treats specific language-based cognitive dysfunction. Neuropsychologist defines cognitive problems and monitors improvement.

Examples: speech therapy for aphasia; introduce adaptive techniques (writing, visual imagery, picture board, computer-assisted communication).

INCONTINENCE THERAPY

Performed by rehabilitation nurse.

Bladder hyperreflexia: bladder contracts at low urine volumes; failure of voluntary inhibition of bladder contraction, sphincter relaxation fails. Treatment: scheduled voiding at 2-hour intervals.

Bladder dyssynergia: bladder contraction, sphincter relaxation are dissociated; bladder contracts against closed sphincter. Treatment: bladder antispasmodic drugs, intermittent catheterization.

Bladder flaccidity: bladder emptying incomplete and at low pressures; incontinence between voluntary voidings. Treatment: cholinergic agents, intermittent catheterization.

Constipation: bowel obstruction may result from immobility. Prevention combines high-fiber diet, stool softeners, laxatives, enemas timed to stimulate evacuation on regular schedule.

Section XXVI
Ethical and Legal Guidelines

CHAPTER 171 ■ END-OF-LIFE ISSUES IN NEUROLOGY

Informed consent: patient may accept or refuse treatment or diagnostic test after learning about anticipated benefits, risks, and alternative options. Patient autonomy requires accurate information about prognosis.

Advance directives: legal documents (living wills) that specify individual's preferences for end-of-life treatment under specific circumstances. Surrogate decision maker (health care proxy) appointed for possibility that individual may not be competent to make decisions at some future time.

Refusal of life-sustaining treatment: included in doctrine of informed consent (refusal, a decision not to provide consent). When patient loses capacity to make decisions, right to consent or refuse treatment transferred to legally authorized surrogate decision maker. Not necessary to consult lawyer before withdrawing life-sustaining therapy.

Double effect: morally and ethically acceptable action may have foreseeable but unintended and undesirable outcomes; morality of the action depends on morality of intended outcome, not the unintended one. In practice, this principle makes it possible to administer sufficient analgesic and sedative medication to keep patient comfortable even though the treatment will not prolong life.

Palliative care: "comfort care"; treatment intended to relieve pain and suffering rather than to cure the disease, restore patient to health, or prolong life. Oral or parenteral morphine in amounts sufficient to control pain and maintain comfort.

Physician-assisted suicide: Giving prescription for possibly lethal drug; legal in only one state in United States (Oregon).

Terminal sedation: right to forgo treatment includes refusal of food and water. Pain or other discomfort ameliorated by standard palliative measures, may include sedation to unconsciousness; patient then dies as a result of underlying disease, dehydration, or both.

Euthanasia: administration of lethal drug by physician in compliance with patient's request. Illegal in the United States; permitted in the Netherlands.

Note: A "t" after a page number indicates a table.